Physical Examination
AND HISTORY TAKING

BATES'
Pocket Guide to
Physical
Examination
AND HISTORY TAKING

SIXTH EDITION

Lynn S. Bickley, MD
Associate Dean for Curriculum and Professor of Internal Medicine
School of Medicine
Texas Tech University Health Sciences Center
Lubbock, Texas

Peter G. Szilagyi, MD, MPH
Professor of Pediatrics
Chief, Division of General Pediatrics
University of Rochester School of Medicine and Dentistry
Rochester, New York

Wolters Kluwer | Lippincott Williams & Wilkins
Health
Philadelphia · Baltimore · New York · London
Buenos Aires · Hong Kong · Sydney · Tokyo

Acquisitions Editor: Peter Darcy
Development Editor: Renee Gagliardi
Senior Production Editor: Sandra Cherrey Scheinin
Director of Nursing Production: Helen Ewan
Senior Managing Editor/Production: Erika Kors
Design Coordinator: Joan Wendt
Art Director, Illustration: Brett MacNaughton
Manufacturing Coordinator: Karin Duffield
Indexer: Gaye Tarallo
Compositor: Circle Graphics

Care has been taken to confirm the accuracy of the information
presented and to describe generally accepted practices. However, the
authors, editors, and publisher are not responsible for errors or omis-
sions or for any consequences from application of the information in
this book and make no warranty, expressed or implied, with respect
to the currency, completeness, or accuracy of the contents of the
publication. Application of this information in a particular situation
remains the professional responsibility of the practitioner; the clinical treatments described and recommended may not be considered
absolute and universal recommendations.

The authors, editors, and publisher have exerted every effort to
ensure that drug selection and dosage set forth in this text are in
accordance with the current recommendations and practice at the
time of publication. However, in view of ongoing research, changes
in government regulations, and the constant flow of information
relating to drug therapy and drug reactions, the reader is urged to
check the package insert for each drug for any change in indications
and dosage and for added warnings and precautions. This is particularly important when the recommended agent is a new or infre-
quently employed drug.

Some drugs and medical devices presented in this publication
have Food and Drug Administration (FDA) clearance for limited use
in restricted research settings. It is the responsibility of the health
care provider to ascertain the FDA status of each drug or device
planned for use in his or her clinical practice.

*To Robert A. Hoekelman, master pediatrician,
whose legacy of blending science with humanism for
faculty, students, and patients lives on in this book,
which he helped pioneer.*

CONTENTS

CHAPTER 1   **Overview: Physical Examination and History Taking 1**

CHAPTER 2   **Clinical Reasoning, Assessment, and Recording Your Findings 17**

CHAPTER 3   **Interviewing and the Health History 37**

CHAPTER 4   **Beginning the Physical Examination: General Survey, Vital Signs, and Pain 55**

CHAPTER 5   **Behavior and Mental Status 75**

CHAPTER 6   **The Skin, Hair, and Nails 93**

CHAPTER 7   **The Head and Neck 111**

CHAPTER 8   **The Thorax and Lungs 141**

CHAPTER 9   **The Cardiovascular System 163**

CHAPTER 10   **The Breasts and Axillae 181**

CHAPTER 11   **The Abdomen 193**

CHAPTER 12   **The Peripheral Vascular System 215**

CHAPTER 13   **Male Genitalia and Hernias 229**

CHAPTER 14   **Female Genitalia 241**

CHAPTER 15   **The Anus, Rectum, and Prostate 259**

CHAPTER 16   **The Musculoskeletal System 271**

CHAPTER 17   **The Nervous System 311**

CHAPTER 18   **Assessing Children: Infancy Through Adolescence 349**

CHAPTER 19   **The Pregnant Woman 389**

CHAPTER 20   **The Older Adult 403**

Index 427

INTRODUCTION

The *Pocket Guide to Physical Examination and History Taking*, 6/E is a concise, portable text that:

- Describes how to interview the patient and take the health history
- Provides an illustrated review of the physical examination
- Reminds students of common, typical findings
- Describes special techniques of assessment that students may need in specific instances
- Provides succinct aids to interpretation of selected findings

There are several ways to use the *Pocket Guide*:

To review and remember the content of a health history.

To review and rehearse the techniques of examination. This can be done while learning a single section and again while combining the approaches to several body systems or regions into an integrated examination (see Chap. 1).

To review common variations of normal and selected abnormalities. Observations are keener and more precise when the examiner knows what to look, listen, and feel for.

To look up special techniques as the need arises. Maneuvers such as doing an Allen test are included in the relevant sections of the examination and highlighted by a shaded blue-green bar.

To look up additional information about possible findings, including abnormalities and standards of normal.

The *Pocket Guide* is not intended to serve as a primary text for learning the skills of taking a history or performing a physical examination. Its detail is insufficient for these purposes. It is intended instead as an aid for student review and recall and as a convenient, brief, and portable reference.

Overview: Physical Examination and History Taking

This chapter provides a road map to clinical proficiency in two critical areas: the health history and the physical examination.

For adults, the comprehensive history includes *Identifying Data and Source of the History, Chief Complaint(s), Present Illness, Past History, Family History, Personal and Social History,* and *Review of Systems.* New patients in the office or hospital merit a *comprehensive health history;* however, in many situations a more flexible *focused,* or *problem-oriented, interview* is appropriate. The components of the comprehensive health history structure the patient's story and the format of your written record, but the order shown on pp. 3–7 should not dictate the sequence of the interview. The interview is more fluid and should follow the patient's leads and cues, as described in Chapter 3.

● The History and Physical Examination: Comprehensive or Focused?

Comprehensive Assessment	Focused Assessment
• Is appropriate for new patients in the office or hospital	• Is appropriate for established patients, especially during routine or urgent care visits
• Provides fundamental and personalized knowledge about the patient	
• Strengthens the clinician-patient relationship	• Addresses focused concerns or symptoms
• Helps identify or rule out physical causes related to patient concerns	• Assesses the specific body systems relevant to the patient's concerns
• Develops proficiency in the essential skills of physical examination	

Be sure to distinguish *subjective* from *objective* data.

Subjective Data	Objective Data
What the patient tells you	What you detect during the examination
The history, from Chief Complaint through Review of Systems	All physical examination findings

---

COMPONENTS OF THE ADULT HEALTH HISTORY

Identifying Data

- *Identifying data*—such as age, gender, occupation, marital status
- *Source of the history*—usually the patient, but can be a family member or friend, letter of referral, or the medical record
- If appropriate, establish *source of referral*, because a written report may be needed

Reliability

- Varies according to the patient's memory, trust, and mood

Chief Complaint(s)

- The one or more symptoms or concerns causing the patient to seek care

Present Illness

- Amplifies the *Chief Complaint*, describes how each symptom developed, gives the seven features of every symptom (see p. 3)
- Includes patient's thoughts and feelings about the illness
- Includes pertinent positives and negatives based on relevant portions of the *Review of Systems* (see pp. 5–7)
- May include *medications, allergies*, habits of *smoking and alcohol*, which are frequently pertinent to the present illness

Past History

- Lists childhood illnesses
- Lists adult illnesses with dates for at least four categories: medical; surgical; obstetric/gynecologic; and psychiatric

(continued)

COMPONENTS OF THE ADULT HEALTH HISTORY (CONTINUED)

- Includes *Health Maintenance* practices such as immunizations, screening tests, lifestyle issues, and home safety

Family History

- Outlines or diagrams age and health, or age and cause of death, of siblings, parents, and grandparents.
- Documents presence or absence of specific illnesses in family, such as hypertension, coronary artery disease, etc.

Personal and Social History

- Described educational level, family of origin, current household, personal interests, and lifestyle

Review of Systems

- Documents presence or absence of common symptoms related to each major body system

THE COMPREHENSIVE ADULT HEALTH HISTORY

As you elicit the adult health history, be sure to include the following: date and time of history; identifying data, which include age, gender, marital status, and occupation; and reliability, which reflects the quality of information the patient provides.

CHIEF COMPLAINT(S)

Quote the patient's own words. "My stomach hurts and I feel awful"; or "I have come for my regular check-up."

PRESENT ILLNESS

This section is a complete, clear, and chronologic account of the problems prompting the patient to seek care. It should include the problem's onset, the setting in which it has developed, its manifestations, and any treatments.

Every principal symptom should be well characterized, with descriptions of the seven features listed below and *pertinent positives* and *negatives* from relevant areas of the Review of Systems.

- Location
- Quality
- Quantity or severity
- Timing, including onset, duration, and frequency
- Setting in which they occur
- Aggravating and relieving factors
- Associated manifestations

In addition, list **medications,** including name, dose, route, and frequency of use; **allergies,** including *specific reactions* to each medication; **tobacco** use; and **alcohol** and **drug** use.

 PAST HISTORY

List **childhood illnesses,** then list **adult illnesses** in each of four areas:

- *Medical* (e.g., diabetes, hypertension, hepatitis, asthma, HIV), with dates of onset; also information about hospitalizations with dates; number and gender of sexual partners; risky sexual practices
- *Surgical* (dates, indications, and types of operations)
- *Obstetric/gynecologic* (obstetric history, menstrual history, birth control, and sexual function)
- *Psychiatric* (illness and time frame, diagnoses, hospitalizations, and treatments)

Also discuss **health maintenance,** including *immunizations,* such as tetanus, pertussis, diphtheria, polio, measles, rubella, mumps, influenza, varicella, hepatitis B, *Haemophilus influenzae* type b, and pneumococcal vaccine; and *screening tests,* such as tuberculin tests, Pap smears, mammograms, stools for occult blood, and cholesterol tests, together with the results and the dates they were last performed.

FAMILY HISTORY

Outline or diagram the age and health, or age and cause of death, of each immediate relative, including grandparents, parents, siblings, children, and grandchildren. Record the following conditions as either *present or absent* in the family: hypertension, coronary artery disease, elevated cholesterol levels, stroke, diabetes, thyroid or renal disease, cancer (specify type), arthritis, tuberculosis, asthma or lung disease, headache, seizure disorder, mental illness, suicide, alcohol or drug addiction, and allergies, as well as symptoms that the patient reports.

 PERSONAL AND SOCIAL HISTORY

Include occupation and the last year of schooling; home situation and significant others; sources of stress, both recent and long-term; important life experiences, such as military service; leisure activities; religious affiliation and spiritual beliefs; and activities of daily living (ADLs). Also include lifestyle habits such as *exercise* and *diet, safety measures,* and *alternative health care* practices.

 REVIEW OF SYSTEMS

These questions go from "head to toe." Start with a fairly general question. This allows you to shift to more specific questions about systems that may be of concern. For example, "How are your ears and hearing?" "How about your lungs and breathing?" "Any trouble with your heart?" "How is your digestion?" The *Review of Systems* questions may uncover problems that the patient overlooked. *Remember to move major health events to the Present Illness or Past History in your write-up.*

Some clinicians do the *Review of Systems* during the physical examination. If the patient has only a few symptoms, this combination can be efficient. If he or she has multiple symptoms, the flow of both the history and the examination can be disrupted.

General.   Usual weight, recent weight change, any clothes that fit more tightly or loosely than before; weakness, fatigue, fever.

Skin.   Rashes, lumps, sores, itching, dryness, color change, changes in hair or nails, changes in size or color of moles.

Head, Eyes, Ears, Nose, Throat (HEENT). *Head:* Headache, head injury, dizziness, lightheadedness. *Eyes:* Vision, glasses or contact lenses, last examination, pain, redness, excessive tearing, double or blurred vision, spots, specks, flashing lights, glaucoma, cataracts. *Ears:* Hearing, tinnitus, vertigo, earache, infection, discharge. If hearing is decreased, use or nonuse of hearing aid. *Nose and sinuses:* Frequent colds, nasal stuffiness, discharge or itching, hay fever, nosebleeds, sinus trouble. *Throat (or mouth and pharynx):* Condition of teeth and gums; bleeding gums; dentures, if any, and how they fit; last dental examination; sore tongue; dry mouth; frequent sore throats; hoarseness.

Neck.   Lumps, "swollen glands," goiter, pain, stiffness.

Breasts.   Lumps, pain or discomfort, nipple discharge, self-examination practices.

Respiratory.   Cough, sputum (color, quantity), hemoptysis, dyspnea, wheezing, pleurisy, last chest x-ray. You may wish to include asthma, bronchitis, emphysema, pneumonia, and tuberculosis.

Cardiovascular.   Heart trouble, hypertension, rheumatic fever, heart murmurs, chest pain or discomfort, palpitations, dyspnea, orthopnea, paroxysmal nocturnal dyspnea, edema, past electrocardiographic or other heart test results.

Gastrointestinal.   Trouble swallowing, heartburn, appetite, nausea, bowel movements, color and size of stools, change in bowel habits, rectal bleeding or black or tarry stools, hemorrhoids, constipation, diarrhea. Abdominal pain, food intolerance, excessive belching or passing of gas. Jaundice, liver or gallbladder trouble, hepatitis.

Urinary.   Frequency of urination, polyuria, nocturia, urgency, burning or pain on urination, hematuria, urinary infections, kidney stones, incontinence; in males, reduced caliber or force of urinary stream, hesitancy, dribbling.

Genital.   *Male:* Hernias, discharge from or sores on penis, testicular pain or masses, history of sexually transmitted diseases (STDs) and treatments, testicular self-examination practices. Sexual habits, interest, function, satisfaction, birth control methods, condom use, problems. Exposure to HIV infection. *Female:* Age at menarche; regularity, frequency, and duration of periods; amount of bleeding, bleeding between periods or after intercourse, last menstrual period; dysmenorrhea, premenstrual tension; age at menopause, menopausal symptoms, postmenopausal bleeding. In patients born before 1971, exposure to diethylstilbestrol (DES) from maternal use during pregnancy. Vaginal discharge, itching, sores, lumps, STDs and treatments. Number of pregnancies, number and type of deliveries, number of abortions (spontaneous and induced); complications of pregnancy; birth control methods. Sexual preference, interest, function, satisfaction, problems (including dyspareunia). Exposure to HIV infection.

Peripheral Vascular.   Intermittent claudication; leg cramps; varicose veins; past clots in veins; swelling in calves, legs, or feet; color change in fingertips or toes during cold weather; swelling with redness or tenderness.

Musculoskeletal.   Muscle or joint pain, stiffness, arthritis, gout, backache. If present, describe location of affected joints or muscles, any swelling, redness, pain, tenderness, stiffness, weakness, or limitation of motion or activity; include timing of symptoms (e.g., morning or evening), duration, and any history of trauma. Neck or low back pain. Joint pain with systemic features such as fever, chills, rash, anorexia, weight loss, or weakness.

Psychiatric.   Nervousness; tension; mood, including depression, memory change, suicide attempts, if relevant.

Neurologic.   Changes in mood, attention, or speech; changes in orientation, memory, insight, or judgment; headache, dizziness, vertigo; fainting, blackouts, seizures, weakness, paralysis, numbness or loss of sensation, tingling or "pins and needles," tremors or other involuntary movements; seizures.

Hematologic.   Anemia, easy bruising or bleeding, past transfusions, transfusion reactions.

Endocrine.   Thyroid trouble, heat or cold intolerance, excessive sweating, excessive thirst or hunger, polyuria, change in glove or shoe size.

THE PHYSICAL EXAMINATION: APPROACH AND OVERVIEW

Conduct a *comprehensive physical examination* on most new patients or patients being admitted to the hospital. For more *problem-oriented*, or *focused*, *assessments*, the presenting complaints will dictate which segments you elect to perform.

- *The key to a thorough and accurate physical examination is a systematic sequence of examination*. With effort and practice, you will acquire your own routine sequence. This book recommends examining from the patient's *right side*.

- Apply the techniques of inspection, palpation, auscultation, and percussion to each body region, but be sensitive to the whole patient.

- *Minimize the number of times you ask the patient to change position* from supine to sitting, or standing to lying supine.

- For an overview of the physical examination, study the sequence that follows. *Note that clinicians vary in where they place different segments, especially for the musculoskeletal and nervous systems.*

BEGINNING THE EXAMINATION: SETTING THE STAGE

Take the following steps to prepare for the physical examination.

Preparing for the Physical Examination

- Reflect on your approach to the patient.
- Adjust the lighting and the environment.
- Make the patient comfortable.
- Determine the scope of the examination.
- Choose the sequence of the examination.
- Observe the correct examining position (the patient's right side) and handedness.

Think through your approach, your professional demeanor, and how to make the patient comfortable and relaxed. *Wash your hands in the patient's presence before beginning.*

THE PHYSICAL EXAMINATION: SUMMARY OF SUGGESTED SEQUENCE

- General survey
- Vital signs
- Skin: upper torso, anterior and posterior
- Head and neck, including thyroid and lymph nodes
- *Optional:* Nervous system (mental status, cranial nerves, upper extremity motor strength, bulk, tone; cerebellar function)
- Thorax and lungs
- Breasts
- Musculoskeletal as indicated: upper extremities
- Cardiovascular, including JVP, carotid upstrokes and bruits, PMI, etc.
- Cardiovascular, for S_3 and murmur of mitral stenosis
- Nervous system: lower extremity motor strength, bulk, tone: sensation; reflexes; Babinskis

- Musculoskeletal, as indicated
- *Optional:* Skin, anterior and posterior
- *Optional:* Nervous system, including gait
- *Optional:* Musculoskeletal, comprehensive
- *Women:* Pelvic and rectal examination
- *Men:* Prostate and rectal examination
- Cardiovascular, for murmur of aortic insufficiency
- *Optional:* Thorax and lungs — anterior
- Breasts and axillae
- Abdomen
- Peripheral vascular; *Optional:* Skin—lower torso and extremities

---

Key to the Symbols for the Patient's Position

Sitting	Lying supine, with hips flexed, abducted, and externally rotated, and knees flexed (lithotomy position)
Lying supine, with head of bed raised 30 degrees	
Same, turned partly to left side	Lying on the left side (left lateral decubitus)
Standing	Sitting, leaning forward
	Lying supine

Each symbol pertains until a new one appears. Two symbols separated by a slash indicate either or both positions.

Reflect on Your Approach to the Patient.   Identify yourself as a student. Try to appear calm, organized, and competent, even if you feel differently. If you forget to do part of the examination, this is not uncommon, especially at first! Simply examine that area out of sequence, but smoothly.

Adjust Lighting and the Environment.   Adjust the bed to a convenient height (be sure to lower it when finished!). Ask the patient to move toward you if this makes it easier to do your physical examination.

Good lighting and a quiet environment are important. *Tangential lighting* is optimal for structures such as the jugular venous pulse, the thyroid gland, and the apical impulse of the heart. It throws contours, elevations, and depressions, whether moving or stationary, into sharper relief.

Make the Patient Comfortable.   Show concern for privacy and modesty.

- Close nearby doors and draw curtains before beginning.

- Acquire the art of *draping the patient* with the gown or draw sheet as you learn each examination segment in future chapters. *The goal is to visualize one body area at a time.*

- As you proceed, keep the patient informed, as when checking for the femoral pulse. Also try to gauge how much the patient wants to know.

- Make sure your instructions to the patient at each step are courteous and clear.

- Watch the patient's facial expression and even ask "Is it okay?" as you move through the examination.

When you have finished, tell the patient your general impressions and what to expect next. Lower the bed to avoid risk of falls and raise the bedrails if needed. As you leave, clean your equipment, dispose of waste materials, and wash your hands.

Determine the Scope of the Examination.   *Comprehensive or Focused?* Choose whether to do a *comprehensive* or *focused examination.*

Choose the Sequence of the Examination.   The sequence of the examination should

- maximize the patient's comfort
- avoid unnecessary changes in position, and
- enhance the clinician's efficiency.

In general, move from head to toe. An important goal as a student is to develop your own sequence with these principles in mind. See Chapter 1 for a suggested examination sequence.

Observe the Correct Examining Position and Handedness.
Note that it is more reliable to estimate jugular venous pressure from the right, the palpating hand rests more comfortably on the apical impulse, the right kidney is more frequently palpable than the left, and examining tables are frequently positioned to accommodate a right-handed approach. To examine the *supine patient,* you can examine the head, neck, and anterior chest. Then roll the patient onto each side to listen to the lungs, examine the back, and inspect the skin. Roll the patient back and finish the rest of the examination with the patient again supine.

 ## THE COMPREHENSIVE ADULT PHYSICAL EXAMINATION

General Survey.   Continue this survey throughout the patient visit. Observe general state of health, height, build, and sexual development. Note posture, motor activity, and gait; dress, grooming, and personal hygiene; and any odors of the body or breath. Watch facial expressions and note manner, affect, and reactions to persons and things in the environment. Listen to the patient's manner of speaking and note the state of awareness or level of consciousness.

Vital Signs.   Ask the patient **to sit** on the edge of the bed or examining table, unless this position is contraindicated. Stand in front of the patient, moving to either side as needed. Measure the blood pressure. Count pulse and respiratory rate. If indicated, measure body temperature.

Skin. Observe the face. Identify any lesions, noting their location, distribution, arrangement, type, and color. Inspect and palpate the hair and nails. Study the patient's hands. Continue to assess the skin as you examine the other body regions.

HEENT. Darken the room to promote pupillary dilation and visibility of the fundi. ***Head:*** Examine the hair, scalp, skull, and face. ***Eyes:*** Check visual acuity and screen the visual fields. Note position and alignment of the eyes. Observe the eyelids. Inspect the sclera and conjunctiva of each eye. With oblique lighting, inspect each cornea, iris, and lens. Compare the pupils, and test their reactions to light. Assess extraocular movements. With an ophthalmoscope, inspect the ocular fundi. ***Ears:*** Inspect the auricles, canals, and drums. Check auditory acuity. If acuity is diminished, check lateralization (Weber test) and compare air and bone conduction (Rinne test). ***Nose and sinuses:*** Examine the external nose; using a light and nasal speculum, inspect nasal mucosa, septum, and turbinates. Palpate for tenderness of the frontal and maxillary sinuses. ***Throat (or mouth and pharynx):*** Inspect the lips, oral mucosa, gums, teeth, tongue, palate, tonsils, and pharynx. *(You may wish to assess the Cranial Nerves at this point in the examination.)*

Neck. Move behind the sitting patient to feel the thyroid gland and to examine the back, posterior thorax, and lungs. Inspect and palpate the cervical lymph nodes. Note any masses or unusual pulsations in the neck. Feel for any deviation of the trachea. Observe sound and effort of the patient's breathing. Inspect and palpate the thyroid gland.

Back. Inspect and palpate the spine and muscles.

Posterior Thorax and Lungs. Inspect and palpate the spine and muscles of the *upper* back. Inspect, palpate, and percuss the chest. Identify the level of diaphragmatic dullness on each side. Listen to the breath sounds; identify any adventitious (or added) sounds, and, if indicated, listen to the transmitted voice sound (see p. 148).

Breasts, Axillae, and Epitrochlear Nodes. The patient is **still sitting**. Move to the front again. ***Female:*** Inspect the breasts with patient's arms relaxed, then elevated, and then with her hands pressed on her hips. ***Male and Female:*** Inspect the axillae and feel for the axillary nodes; feel for the epitrochlear nodes.

A Note on the Musculoskeletal System: By now, you have made preliminary observations of the musculoskeletal system, including the hands, the upper back, and, in women, the shoulders' range of motion (ROM). Use these observations to decide whether a full musculoskeletal examination is warranted: *with the patient still sitting,* examine the hands, arms, shoulders, neck, and temporomandibular joints. Inspect and palpate the joints and check their ROM. *(You may choose to examine upper-extremity muscle bulk, tone, strength, and reflexes at this time, or you may decide to wait.)*

Palpate the breasts, while continuing your inspection.

○—— **Anterior Thorax and Lungs.** **The patient position is supine.** Ask the patient to lie down. Stand at the *right side* of the patient's bed. Inspect, palpate, and percuss the chest. Listen to the breath sounds, any adventitious sounds, and, if indicated, transmitted voice sounds.

○—— **Cardiovascular System.** **Elevate head of bed to about 30°,** adjusting as necessary to see the jugular venous pulsations. Observe the jugular venous pulsations, and measure the jugular venous pressure in relation to the sternal angle. Inspect and palpate the carotid pulsations. Listen for carotid bruits.

○+ /○—— Ask the patient to roll partly onto the left side while you listen at the apex. Then have the patient roll back to supine while you listen to the rest of the heart. Ask the patient to sit, lean forward, and exhale while you listen for the murmur of aortic regurgitation. Inspect and palpate the precordium. Note the location, diameter, amplitude, and duration of the apical impulse. Listen at the apex and the lower sternal border with the bell of a stethoscope. Listen at each auscultatory area with the diaphragm. Listen for S_1 and S_2 and for physiologic splitting of S_2. Listen for any abnormal heart sounds or murmurs.

○— /| **Peripheral Vascular System.** **With the patient supine,** palpate the femoral pulses and, if indicated, popliteal pulses. Palpate the inguinal lymph nodes. Inspect for edema, discoloration, or ulcers in the lower extremities. Palpate for pitting edema. **With the patient standing,** inspect for varicose veins.

○— **Abdomen.**   Lower the head of the bed to the flat position. **The patient should be supine.** Inspect, auscultate, and percuss. Palpate lightly, then deeply. Assess the liver and spleen by percussion and then palpation. Try to feel the kidneys; palpate the aorta and its pulsations. If you suspect kidney infection, percuss posteriorly over the costovertebral angles.

○— /⌐ **Lower Extremities.**   Examine the legs, assessing the three systems (see next page) while the patient is still supine. Each of these systems can be further assessed when the patient stands.

⌐/○— **Nervous System.**   **The patient is sitting or supine.** The examination of the nervous system can also be divided into the upper-extremity examination (when the patient is still sitting) and the lower-extremity examination (when the patient is supine) after examination of the peripheral nervous system.

- **Mental Status:** If indicated and not done during the interview, assess orientation, mood, thought process, thought content, abnormal perceptions, insight and judgment, memory and attention, information and vocabulary, calculating abilities, abstract thinking, and constructional ability.

- **Cranial Nerves:** If not already examined, check sense of smell, funduscopic examination, strength of the temporal and masseter muscles, corneal reflexes, facial movements, gag reflex, strength of the trapezia and sternomastoid muscles, and protrusion of tongue.

- **Motor System:** Muscle bulk, tone, and strength of major muscle groups. *Cerebellar function:* rapid alternating movements (RAMs), point-to-point movements such as finger to nose (F → N) and heel to shin (H → S); gait. Observe patient's gait and ability to walk heel to toe, on toes, and on heels; to hop in place; and to do shallow knee bends. Do a Romberg test; check for pronator drift.

- **Sensory System:** Pain, temperature, light touch, vibrations, and discrimination. Compare right and left sides and distal with proximal areas on the limbs.

- **Reflexes:** Include biceps, triceps, brachioradialis, patellar, Achilles deep tendon reflexes; also plantar reflexes or Babinski reflex (see p. 328-331)

Additional Examinations.   The *rectal* and *genital* examinations are often performed at the end of the physical examination. Patient positioning is as indicated.

Male Genitalia and Hernias.   Examine the penis and scrotal contents. Check for hernias.

Rectal Examination in Men.   The patient is **lying on his left side** for the rectal examination. Inspect the sacrococcygeal and perianal areas. Palpate the anal canal, rectum, and prostate. (If the patient cannot stand, examine the genitalia before doing the rectal examination.)

Genital and Rectal Examination in Women.   The patient is **supine in the lithotomy position.** Sit during the examination with the speculum, then stand during bimanual examination of uterus, adnexa, and rectum. Examine the external genitalia, vagina, and cervix. Obtain a Pap smear. Palpate the uterus and adnexa. Do a bimanual and rectal examination.

 ## STANDARD AND UNIVERSAL PRECAUTIONS

The Centers for Disease Control and Prevention (CDC) have issued several guidelines to protect patients and examiners from the spread of infectious disease. All clinicians examining patients are well advised to study and observe these precautions at the CDC Web-sites. Advisories for standard and methicillin-resistant *Staphylococcus aureus* (MRSA) precautions and for universal precautions are briefly summarized below.

- *Standard and MRSA precautions:* Standard precautions are based on the principle that all blood, body fluids, secretions, excretions except sweat, nonintact skin, and mucous membranes may contain transmissible infectious agents. These practices apply to all patients in any setting. They include: hand hygiene; when to use gloves, gowns, and mouth, nose, and eye protection; respiratory hygiene and cough etiquette; patient isolation criteria; precautions relating to equipment, toys and solid surfaces, and handling of laundry; and safe needle injection practices.

Be sure to wash your hands before and after examining the patient. This will show your concern for the patient's welfare and display your awareness of a critical component of patient safety. Antimicrobial fast-drying soaps are often within easy reach. *Change your white coat frequently* since cuffs can become damp and smudged.

- *Universal precautions:* Universal precautions are a set of precautions designed to prevent transmission of HIV, hepatitis B virus (HBV), and other bloodborne pathogens when providing first aid or health care. The following fluids are considered potentially infectious: all blood and other body fluids containing visible blood, semen, and vaginal secretions; and cerebrospinal, synovial, pleural, peritoneal, pericardial, and amniotic fluids. Protective barriers include gloves, gowns, aprons, masks, and protective eyewear. All healthcare workers should *observe the important precautions for safe injections and prevention of injury from needlesticks, scalpels, and other sharp instruments and devices.* Report to your health service immediately if such injury occurs.

Clinical Reasoning, Assessment, and Recording Your Findings

2

ASSESSMENT AND PLAN: THE PROCESS OF CLINICAL REASONING

Because assessment takes place in the clinician's mind, the process of clinical reasoning often seems inaccessible to beginning students. As an active learner, ask your teachers and clinicians to elaborate on the fine points of their clinical reasoning and decision making.

As you gain experience, your thinking will begin at the outset of the patient encounter, not at the end. Listed below are principles underlying the process of clinical reasoning and certain explicit steps to help guide your thinking.

IDENTIFYING PROBLEMS AND MAKING DIAGNOSES: STEPS IN CLINICAL REASONING

- **Identify abnormal findings.** Make a list of the patient's *symptoms,* the *signs* you observed during physical examination, and any available results of laboratory reports.
- **Localize these findings anatomically.** The symptom of a scratchy throat and the sign of an erythematous inflamed pharynx, for example, clearly localize the problem to the pharynx. Some symptoms and signs, such as fatigue or fever, cannot be localized but are useful in the next steps.
- **Interpret the findings in terms of the probable process.** There are a number of *pathologic* processes, including congenital, inflammatory or infectious, immunologic, neoplastic, metabolic, nutritional, degenerative,

(continued)

IDENTIFYING PROBLEMS AND MAKING DIAGNOSES: STEPS IN CLINICAL REASONING (CONTINUED)

vascular, traumatic, and toxic. Other problems are *pathophysiologic,* reflecting derangements of biologic functions, such as congestive heart failure. Still other problems are *psychopathologic,* such as headache as an expression of a somatization disorder.

- **Make hypotheses about the nature of the patient's problems.** Draw on your knowledge, experience, and reading about patterns of abnormalities and diseases. By consulting the clinical literature, you will embark on the lifelong goal of *evidence-based decision making.* The following steps should help:
  1. Select the most specific and critical findings to support your hypothesis.
  2. Match your findings against all the conditions you know that can produce them.
  3. Eliminate the diagnostic possibilities that fail to explain the findings.
  4. Weigh the competing possibilities and select the most likely diagnosis.
  5. Give special attention to potentially life-threatening and treatable conditions. One rule of thumb is *always to include "the worst case scenario"* in your list of differential diagnoses and make sure you have ruled out that possibility based on your findings and patient assessment.
- **Test your hypotheses.** You may need further history, additional maneuvers on physical examination, or laboratory studies or x-rays to confirm or to rule out your tentative diagnosis or to clarify which of a few possible diagnoses is most likely.
- **Establish a working diagnosis.** Make this at the highest level of explicitness and certainty that the data allow. You may be limited to a symptom, such as "tension headache, cause unknown." At other times, you can define a problem explicitly in terms of its structure, process, and cause, such as "bacterial meningitis, pneumococcal." Routinely listing *Health Maintenance* helps you track several important health concerns more effectively: immunizations, screening measures (e.g., mammograms, prostate examinations),

(continued)

IDENTIFYING PROBLEMS AND MAKING DIAGNOSES: STEPS IN CLINICAL REASONING (CONTINUED)

instructions regarding nutrition and breast or testicular self-examinations, recommendations about exercise or use of seat belts, and responses to important life events.

● **Develop a plan agreeable to the patient.** Identify and record a *Plan* for each patient problem, ranging from tests to confirm or further evaluate a diagnosis; to consultations for subspecialty evaluation; to additions, deletions, or changes in medication; or to arranging a family meeting.

THE CASE OF MRS. N

Now study the case of Mrs. N. Scrutinize the findings recorded, apply your clinical reasoning, and analyze the assessment and plan.

Health History

8/30/08 11:00 AM
Mrs. N is a pleasant, 54-year-old widowed saleswoman residing in Amarillo, Texas.
Referral. None
Source and Reliability. Self-referred; seems reliable.

Chief Complaint: "My head aches."

Present Illness: For about 3 months, Mrs. N has had increasing problems with frontal headaches. These are usually bifrontal, throbbing, and mild to moderately severe. She has missed work on several occasions because of associated nausea and vomiting. Headaches now average once a week, usually are related to stress, and last 4 to 6 hours. They are relieved by sleep and putting a damp towel over the forehead. There is little relief from aspirin. No associated visual changes, motor-sensory deficits, or paresthesias.

(continued)

"Sick headaches" with nausea and vomiting began at age 15, recurred throughout her mid-20s, then decreased to one every 2 or 3 months and almost disappeared.

The patient reports increased pressure at work from a new and demanding boss; she is also worried about her daughter (see *Personal and Social History*). She thinks her headaches may be like those in the past but wants to be sure, because her mother died following a stroke. She is concerned that they interfere with her work and make her irritable with her family. She eats three meals a day and drinks three cups of coffee per day; cola at night.

> *Medications.* Aspirin, 1 to 2 tablets every 4 to 6 hours as needed. "Water pill" in the past for ankle swelling, none recently.
>
> **Allergies.* Ampicillin causes rash.
>
> *Tobacco.* About 1 pack of cigarettes per day since age 18 (36 pack-years).
>
> *Alcohol/drugs.* Wine on rare occasions. No illicit drugs.

Past History

Childhood Illnesses. Measles, chickenpox. No scarlet fever or rheumatic fever.

Adult Illnesses. **Medical:** Pyelonephritis, 1998, with fever and right flank pain; treated with ampicillin; developed generalized rash with itching several days later. Reports kidney x-rays were normal; no recurrence of infection. **Surgical:** Tonsillectomy, age 6; appendectomy, age 13. Sutures for laceration, 2001, after stepping on glass. **Ob/Gyn:** 3-3-0-3, with normal vaginal deliveries. 3 living children. Menarche age 12. Last menses 6 months ago. Little interest in sex, and not sexually active. No concerns about HIV infection. **Psychiatric:** None.

Health Maintenance. **Immunizations:** Oral polio vaccine, year uncertain; tetanus shots × 2, 1991, followed with booster 1 year later; flu vaccine, 2000, no reaction. **Screening tests:** Last Pap smear, 2004, normal. No mammograms to date.

(continued)

---

*You may wish to add an asterisk or underline important points.

Family History

Train accident | 43
Stroke, varicose veins, headaches | 67

High blood pressure 67
58
54 Heart attack
Infancy

Migraine headaches 33
Headaches 31
27

/ Indicates patient

▨ Deceased male

◉ Deceased female

▢ Living male

◯ Living female

OR

Father died at age 43 in train accident. Mother died at age 67 from stroke; had varicose veins, headaches.

One brother, 61, with hypertension, otherwise well; second brother, 58, well except for mild arthritis; one sister, died in infancy of unknown cause.

Husband died at age 54 of heart attack.

Daughter, 33, with migraine headaches, otherwise well; son, 31, with headaches; son, 27, well.

No family history of diabetes, tuberculosis, heart or kidney disease, cancer, anemia, epilepsy, or mental illness.

Personal and Social History: Born and raised in Lake City, finished high school, married at age 19. Worked as sales clerk for 2 years, then moved with husband to Amarillo, had 3 children. Returned to work 15 years ago because of financial pressures. Children all married. Four years ago Mr. N died suddenly of a heart attack, leaving little savings. Mrs. N has moved to small apartment to be near daughter, Dorothy. Dorothy's husband, Arthur, has an alcohol problem. Mrs. N's apartment now a haven for Dorothy and her 2 children, Kevin, 6 years, and

(continued)

Linda, 3 years. Mrs. N feels responsible for helping them; feels tense and nervous but denies depression. She has friends but rarely discusses family problems: "I'd rather keep them to myself. I don't like gossip." No church or other organizational support. She is typically up at 7:00 A.M., works 9:00 to 5:30, eats dinner alone.

> *Exercise and diet.* Gets little exercise. Diet high in carbohydrates.
>
> *Safety measures.* Uses seat belt regularly. Uses sunblock. Medications kept in an unlocked medicine cabinet. Cleaning solutions in unlocked cabinet below sink. Mr. N's shotgun and box of shells in unlocked closet upstairs.

Review of Systems

General. *Has *gained* about 10 lbs in the past 4 years.

Skin. No rashes or other changes.

Head, Eyes, Ears, Nose, Throat (HEENT). See *Present Illness.* No history of head injury. *Eyes:* Reading glasses for 5 years, last checked 1 year ago. No symptoms. *Ears:* Hearing good. No tinnitus, vertigo, infections. *Nose, sinuses:* Occasional mild cold. No hay fever, sinus trouble. **Throat (or mouth and pharynx):* Some bleeding of gums recently. Last dental visit 2 years ago. Occasional canker sore.

Neck. No lumps, goiter, pain. No swollen glands.

Breasts. No lumps, pain, discharge. Does breast self-exam sporadically.

Respiratory. No cough, wheezing, shortness of breath. Last chest x-ray, 1986, St. Mary's Hospital; unremarkable.

Cardiovascular. No known heart disease or high blood pressure; last blood pressure taken in 2003. No dyspnea, orthopnea, chest pain, palpitations. Has never had an electrocardiogram (ECG).

Gastrointestinal. Appetite good; no nausea, vomiting, indigestion. Bowel movement about once daily, *though sometimes has hard stools for 2 to 3 days when especially tense; no diarrhea or bleeding. No pain, jaundice, gallbladder or liver problems.

(continued)

Urinary. No frequency, dysuria, hematuria, or recent flank pain; nocturia × 1, large volume. *Occasionally loses some urine when coughs hard.

Genital. No vaginal or pelvic infections. No dyspareunia.

Peripheral Vascular. Varicose veins appeared in both legs during first pregnancy. For 10 years, has had swollen ankles after prolonged standing; wears light elastic pantyhose; tried "water pill" 5 months ago, but it didn't help much; no history of phlebitis or leg pain.

Musculoskeletal. Mild, aching, low back pain, often after a long day's work; no radiation down the legs; used to do back exercises but not now. No other joint pain.

Psychiatric. No history of depression or treatment for psychiatric disorders. See also *Present Illness* and *Personal and Social History.*

Neurologic. No fainting, seizures, motor or sensory loss. Memory good.

Hematologic. Except for bleeding gums, no easy bleeding. No anemia.

Endocrine. No known thyroid trouble, temperature intolerance. Sweating average. No symptoms or history of diabetes.

Physical Examination

Mrs. N is a short, overweight, middle-aged woman, who is animated and responds quickly to questions. She is somewhat tense, with moist, cold hands. Her hair is fixed neatly and her clothes are immaculate. Her color is good, and she lies flat without discomfort.

Vital Signs. Ht (without shoes) 157 cm (5'2"). Wt (dressed) 65 kg (143 lb). BMI 26. BP 164/98 right arm, supine; 160/96 left arm, supine; 152/88 right arm, supine with wide cuff. Heart rate (HR) 88 and regular. Respiratory rate (RR) 18. Temperature (oral) 98.6°F.

Skin. Palms cold and moist, but color good. Scattered cherry angiomas over upper trunk. Nails without clubbing, cyanosis.

Head, Eyes, Ears, Nose, Throat (HEENT). *Head:* Hair of average texture. Scalp without lesions, normocephalic/atraumatic (NC/AT). *Eyes:* Vision 20/30 in each eye. Visual fields full by confrontation. Conjunctiva pink; sclera white. Pupils 4 mm

(continued)

constricting to 2 mm, round, regular, equally reactive to light. Extraocular movements intact. Disc margins sharp, without hemorrhages, exudates. No arteriolar narrowing or A-V nicking. *Ears:* Wax partially obscures right tympanic membrane (TM); left canal clear, TM with good cone of light. Acuity good to whispered voice. Weber midline. AC > BC. *Nose:* Mucosa pink, septum midline. No sinus tenderness. *Mouth:* Oral mucosa pink. Several interdental papillae red, slightly swollen. Dentition good. Tongue midline, with 3 × 4 mm shallow white ulcer on red base on undersurface near tip; tender but not indurated. Tonsils absent. Pharynx without exudates.

Neck. Neck supple. Trachea midline. Thyroid isthmus barely palpable, lobes not felt.

Lymph Nodes. Small (<1 cm), soft, nontender, and mobile tonsillar and posterior cervical nodes bilaterally. No axillary or epitrochlear nodes. Several small inguinal nodes bilaterally, soft and nontender.

Thorax and Lungs. Thorax symmetric with good excursion. Lungs resonant. Breath sounds vesicular with no added sounds. Diaphragms descend 4 cm bilaterally.

Cardiovascular. Jugular venous pressure 1 cm above the sternal angle, with head of examining table raised to 30°. Carotid upstrokes brisk, without bruits. Apical impulse discrete and tapping, barely palpable in the 5th left interspace, 8 cm lateral to the midsternal line. Good S_1, S_2; no S_3 or S_4. A II/VI medium-pitched midsystolic murmur at the 2nd right interspace; does not radiate to the neck. No diastolic murmurs.

Breasts. Pendulous, symmetric. No masses; nipples without discharge.

Abdomen. Protuberant. Well-healed scar, right lower quadrant. Bowel sounds active. No tenderness or masses. Liver span 7 cm in right midclavicular line; edge smooth, palpable 1 cm below right costal margin (RCM). Spleen and kidneys not felt. No costovertebral angle tenderness (CVAT).

Genitalia. External genitalia without lesions. Mild cystocele at introitus on straining. Vaginal mucosa pink. Cervix pink, parous, and without discharge. Uterus anterior, midline, smooth, not enlarged. Adnexa not palpated due to obesity and poor relaxation. No cervical or adnexal tenderness. Pap smear taken. Rectovaginal wall intact.

(continued)

Rectal. Rectal vault without masses. Stool brown, negative for occult blood.

Extremities. Warm and without edema. Calves supple, nontender.

Peripheral Vascular. Trace edema at both ankles. Moderate varicosities of saphenous veins in both lower extremities. No stasis pigmentation or ulcers. Pulses (2 + = brisk, or normal):

	Radial	Femoral	Popliteal	Dorsalis Pedis	Posterior Tibial
RT	2+	2+	2+	2+	2+
LT	2+	2+	2+	Absent	2+

Musculoskeletal. No joint deformities. Good range of motion in hands, wrists, elbows, shoulders, spine, hips, knees, ankles.

Neurologic. *Mental Status:* Tense but alert and cooperative. Thought coherent. Oriented to person, place, and time. *Cranial Nerves:* II–XII intact. *Motor:* Good muscle bulk and tone. Strength 5/5 throughout (see p. 321 for grading system). *Cerebellar:* Rapid alternating movements (RAMs), point-to-point movements intact. Gait stable, fluid. *Sensory:* Pinprick, light touch, position sense, vibration, and stereognosis intact. Romberg negative. *Reflexes:*

	Biceps	Triceps	Brachio-radialis	Patellar	Achilles	Plantar
RT	2+	2+	2+	2+	1+	↓
LT	2+	2+	2+	2+/2+	1+	↓

Laboratory Data

None Currently. See Plan.

ASSESSMENT AND PLAN

1. **Migraine headaches.** A 54-year-old woman with migraine headaches since childhood, with a throbbing vascular pattern and frequent nausea and vomiting. Headaches are associated with stress and relieved by sleep and cold compresses. There is no papilledema, and there are no motor or sensory deficits on the neurologic examination. The differential diagnosis includes tension headache, also associated with stress, but there is no relief with massage, and the pain is more throbbing than aching. There are no fever, stiff neck, or focal findings to suggest meningitis, and the lifelong recurrent pattern makes subarachnoid hemorrhage unlikely (usually described as "the worst headache of my life").

   Plan:
   - Discuss features of migraine vs. tension headaches.
   - Discuss biofeedback and stress management.
   - Advise patient to avoid caffeine, including coffee, colas, and other caffeinated beverages.
   - Start NSAIDs for headache, as needed.
   - If needed next visit, begin prophylactic medication, because patient is having more than three migraines per month.

2. **Elevated blood pressure.** Systolic hypertension with wide cuff is present. May be related to obesity, also to anxiety from first visit. No evidence of end-organ damage to retina or heart.

   Plan:
   - Discuss standards for assessing blood pressure.
   - Recheck blood pressure in 1 month, using wide cuff.
   - Check basic metabolic panel; review urinalysis.
   - Introduce weight reduction and/or exercise programs (see #4).
   - Reduce salt intake.

3. **Cystocele with occasional stress incontinence.** Cystocele on pelvic examination, probably related to bladder relaxation. Patient is perimenopausal. Incontinence reported with coughing, suggesting alteration in bladder neck

(continued)

ASSESSMENT AND PLAN (CONTINUED)

anatomy. No dysuria, fever, flank pain. Not taking any contributing medications. Usually involves small amounts of urine, no dribbling, so doubt urge or overflow incontinence.

Plan:

- Explain cause of stress incontinence.
- Review urinalysis.
- Recommend Kegel's exercises.
- Consider topical estrogen cream to vagina next visit if no improvement.

4. **Overweight.** Patient 5'2", weighs 143 lbs. BMI is ~26.

   Plan:

   - Explore diet history; ask patient to keep food intake diary.
   - Explore motivation to lose weight; set target for weight loss by next visit.
   - Schedule visit with dietitian.
   - Discuss exercise program, specifically, walking 30 minutes most days each week.

5. **Family stress.** Son-in-law with alcohol problem; daughter and grandchildren seeking refuge in patient's apartment, leading to tensions in these relationships. Patient also has financial constraints. Stress currently situational. No evidence of major depression at present.

   Plan:

   - Explore patient's views on strategies to cope with stress.
   - Explore sources of support, including Al-Anon for daughter and financial counseling for patient.
   - Continue to monitor for depression.

6. **Occasional musculoskeletal low back pain.** Usually with prolonged standing. No history of trauma or motor vehicle accident. Pain does not radiate; no tenderness or motor-sensory deficits on examination. Doubt disc or nerve root compression, trochanteric bursitis, sacroiliitis.

   Plan:

   - Review benefits of weight loss and exercises to strengthen low back muscles.

(continued)

ASSESSMENT AND PLAN (CONTINUED)

7. **Tobacco abuse.** 1 pack per day for 36 years.

   Plan:
   - Check peak flow or FEV_1/FVC on office spirometry.
   - Give strong warning to stop smoking.
   - Offer referral to tobacco cessation program.
   - Offer patch, current treatment to enhance abstinence.

8. **Varicose veins, lower extremities.** No complaints currently.

9. **History of right pyelonephritis, 1998.**

10. **Ampicillin allergy.** Developed rash but no other allergic reaction.

11. **Health maintenance.** Last Pap smear 2004; has never had a mammogram.

    Plan:
    - Teach patient breast self-examination; schedule mammogram.
    - Schedule Pap smear next visit.
    - Provide three stool guaiac cards; next visit discuss screening colonoscopy.
    - Suggest dental care for mild gingivitis.
    - Advise patient to move medications and caustic cleaning agents to locked cabinet—if possible, above shoulder height.

APPROACHING THE CHALLENGES OF CLINICAL DATA

As you can see from the case of Mrs. N, organizing the patient's clinical data poses several challenges. The following guidelines will help you address these challenges.

- **Clustering data into single vs. multiple problems.** The patient's *age* may help. Young people are more likely to have a single disease, while older people tend to have multiple diseases. The *timing* of symptoms is often useful. For example, an episode of pharyngitis 6 weeks ago probably is unrelated to fever, chills, pleuritic chest pain, and cough that prompt an office visit today.

If symptoms and signs are in a single system, one disease may explain them. Problems in different, apparently unrelated systems often require more than one explanation. Again, knowledge of disease patterns is necessary.

Some diseases involve *multisystem conditions.* To explain cough, hemoptysis, and weight loss in a 60-year-old plumber who has smoked cigarettes for 40 years, you probably even now would rank lung cancer high in your list of differential diagnoses.

- **Sifting through an extensive array of data.** Try to *tease out separate clusters of observations and analyze one cluster at a time.* You also can *ask a series of key questions* that may steer your thinking in one direction. For example, you may ask what produces and relieves the patient's chest pain. If the answer is exercise and rest, you can focus on the cardiovascular and musculoskeletal systems and set the gastrointestinal system aside.

- **Assessing the quality of the data.** To avoid errors in interpreting clinical information, acquire the habits of skilled clinicians, summarized in the following.

TIPS FOR ENSURING THE QUALITY OF YOUR PATIENT ASSESSMENT

- Ask open-ended questions and listen carefully and patiently to the patient's story.
- Craft a thorough and systematic sequence to history taking and physical examination.
- Keep an open mind toward the patient, the patient's story, and your physical findings.
- Always include "the worst-case scenario" in your list of possible explanations of the patient's problem, and make sure it can be eliminated safely.
- Analyze any mistakes in data collection or interpretation.
- Confer with colleagues and review the pertinent medical literature to clarify uncertainties.
- Apply principles of evidence-based data analysis to patient information and testing.

- **Improving your assessment of clinical data and laboratory tests.** Apply several key principles for selecting and using clinical data and tests: *reliability, validity, sensitivity, specificity,* and *predictive value.* Learn to apply these principles to your clinical findings and the tests you order.

- **Displaying clinical data.** To use these principles, it is important to display the data in the 2 × 2 format diagrammed on page 32. Always using this format will ensure the accuracy of your calculations of sensitivity, specificity, and predictive value.

Principles of Test Selection and Use

Reliability: The reproducibility of a measurement. It indicates how well repeated measurements of the same relatively stable phenomenon will give the same result, also known as **precision.** Reliability may be measured for one observer or more observers.

> *Example.* If on several occasions one clinician consistently percusses the same span of a patient's liver dullness, *intraobserver reliability* is good. If, on the other hand, several observers find quite different spans of liver dullness on the same patient, *interobserver reliability* is poor.

Validity: The closeness with which a measurement reflects the true value of an object. It indicates how closely a given observation agrees with "the true state of affairs," or the best possible measure of reality.

> *Example.* Blood pressure measurements by mercury-based sphygmomanometers are less valid than intra-arterial pressure tracings.

Sensitivity: Identifies the proportion of people who test positive in a group of people known to have the disease or condition, or the proportion of people who are *true positives* compared with the total number of people who actually have the disease. When the observation or test is negative in people who have the disease, the result is termed *false negative. Good observations or tests have a sensitivity of more than 90% and*

(continued)

PRINCIPLES OF TEST SELECTION AND USE (CONTINUED)

help "rule out" disease because false negatives are few. Such observations or tests are especially useful for screening.
    Example. The sensitivity of Homan's sign in the diagnosis of deep venous thrombosis (DVT) of the calf is 50%. In other words, compared with a group of patients with DVT confirmed by phlebogram, a much better test, only 50% will have a positive Homan's sign, so this sign, if absent, is not helpful, because 50% of patients may have DVT.

Specificity: Identifies the proportion of people who test negative in a group known to be *without* a given disease or condition, or the proportion of people who are *true negatives* compared with the total number of people without the disease. When the observation or test is positive in people without the disease, the result is termed *false positive. Good observations or tests have a specificity of more than 90% and help "rule in" disease, because the test is rarely positive when disease is absent, and false positives are few.*
    Example: The specificity of serum amylase in patients with possible acute pancreatitis is 70%. In other words, of 100 patients without pancreatitis, 70% will have a normal serum amylase; in 30%, the serum amylase will be falsely elevated.

Predictive value: Indicates how well a given symptom, sign, or test result—either positive or negative—predicts the presence or absence of disease. *Positive predictive value* is the probability of disease in a patient with a positive (abnormal) test, or the proportion of "true positives" out of the total population tested. *Negative predictive value* is the probability of not having the condition or disease when the test is negative (normal), or the proportion of "true negatives" out of the total population tested.
    Examples. In a group of women with palpable breast nodules in a cancer screening program, the proportion with confirmed breast cancer would constitute the *positive predictive value* of palpable breast nodules for diagnosing breast cancer. In a group of women without

(continued)

PRINCIPLES OF TEST SELECTION AND USE (CONTINUED)

palpable breast nodules in a cancer screening program, the proportion without confirmed breast cancer constitutes the *negative predictive value* of absence of breast nodules.

Sensitivity, specificity, and *predictive values* are illustrated in a 2 × 2 table, as shown below in an example of 200 people, half of whom have the disease in question. In this example, the disease prevalence of 50% is much higher than in most clinical situations. Because the positive predictive value increases with prevalence, its calculated value here is unusually high.

	Disease		
	Present	**Absent**	
+	95 true positive observations *a*	95 false positive observations *b*	105 total positive observations
Observation			
−	5 false negative observations *c*	*d* 90 true negative observations	95 total negative observations
	100 total persons with the disease	100 total persons without the disease	200 total persons

$$\text{Sensitivity} = \frac{a}{a+c} = \frac{95}{95+5} \times 100 = 95\%$$

$$\text{Specificity} = \frac{d}{b+d} = \frac{90}{90+10} \times 100 = 90\%$$

$$\text{Positive predictive value} = \frac{a}{a+b} = \frac{95}{95+10} \times 100 = 90.5\%$$

$$\text{Negative predictive value} = \frac{d}{c+d} = \frac{90}{90+5} \times 100 = 94.7\%$$

ORGANIZING THE PATIENT RECORD

A clear, well-organized clinical record is one of the most important adjuncts to your patient care. Think about the *order and readability* of the record and the *amount of detail* needed. Use the following checklist to make sure your record is clear, informative, and easy to follow.

CHECKLIST FOR YOUR PATIENT RECORD

Is the order clear?

Order is imperative. Make sure that future readers, including you, can find specific points of information easily. Keep the *subjective* items of the history, for example, in the history; do not let them stray into the physical examination. Did you . . .

- Make the headings clear?
- Accent your organization with indentations and spacing?
- Arrange the *Present Illness* in chronologic order, starting with the current episode, then filling in relevant background information?

Do the data included contribute directly to the assessment?

Spell out the supporting data—both positive and negative— for every problem or diagnosis that you identify.

Are pertinent negatives specifically described?

Often portions of the history or examination suggest a potential or actual abnormality.
> *Examples.* For the patient with notable bruises, record the "pertinent negatives," such as the absence of injury or violence, familial bleeding disorders, or medications or nutritional deficits that might lead to bruising.
> For the patient who is depressed but not suicidal, record both facts. In the patient with a transient mood swing, on the other hand, a comment on suicide is unnecessary.

(continued)

CHECKLIST FOR YOUR PATIENT RECORD (CONTINUED)

Are there overgeneralizations or omissions of important data?

Remember that data not recorded are data lost. No matter how vividly you can recall selected details today, you probably will not remember them in a few months. The phrase "neurologic exam negative," even in your own handwriting, may leave you wondering in a few months' time, "Did I really do the sensory exam?"

Is there too much detail?

Avoid burying important information in a mass of excessive detail, to be discovered by only the most persistent reader. *Omit most negative findings* unless they relate directly to the patient's complaints or to specific exclusions in your diagnostic assessment. *Do not list abnormalities that you did not observe. Instead, concentrate on a few major ones,* such as "no heart murmurs," and try to describe structures concisely and positively.

> *Examples.* "Cervix pink and smooth" indicates you saw no redness, ulcers, nodules, masses, cysts, or other suspicious lesions, but the description is shorter and much more readable.

You can omit certain body structures even though you examined them, such as normal eyebrows and eyelashes.

Are phrases and short words used appropriately? Is there unnecessary repetition of data?

Omit unnecessary words, such as those in parentheses in the examples below. This saves valuable time and space.

> *Examples.* "Cervix is pink (in color)." "Lungs are resonant (to percussion)." "Liver is tender (to palpation)." "Both (right and left) ears with cerumen." "II/VI systolic ejection murmur (audible)." "Thorax symmetric (bilaterally)."

Omit repetitive introductory phrases such as "The patient reports no . . . ," because readers assume the patient is the source of the history unless otherwise specified.

Use short words instead of longer, fancier ones when they mean the same thing, such as "felt" for "palpated" or "heard" for "auscultated."

(continued)

CHECKLIST FOR YOUR PATIENT RECORD (CONTINUED)

Describe what you observed, not what you did. "Optic discs seen" is less informative than "disc margins sharp," even if it marks your first glimpse as an examiner!

Is the written style succinct? Is there excessive use of abbreviations?

Records are scientific and legal documents, so they should be clear and understandable. Using words and brief phrases instead of whole sentences is common, but abbreviations and symbols should be used only if they are readily understood. Likewise, an overly elegant style is less appealing than a concise summary.

Be sure your record is legible; otherwise, all that you have recorded is worthless to your readers.

Are diagrams and precise measurements included where appropriate?

Diagrams add greatly to the clarity of the record.

Examples. Study the examples below:

(continued)

CHECKLIST FOR YOUR PATIENT RECORD (CONTINUED)

To ensure accurate evaluations and future comparisons, make measurements in centimeters, not in fruits, nuts, or vegetables. *Example.* "1 × 1 cm lymph node" vs. "a pea-sized lymph node. . ." Or "2 × 2 cm mass on the left lobe of the prostate" vs. "a walnut-sized prostate mass."

Is the tone of the write-up neutral and professional?

It is important to be objective. Hostile, moralizing, or disapproving comments have no place in the patient's record. Never use words, penmanship, or punctuation that are inflammatory or demeaning.

Example. Comments such as "Patient DRUNK and LATE TO CLINIC AGAIN!!" are unprofessional and set a bad example for other providers reading the chart. They also might prove difficult to defend in a legal setting.

Once you have completed your assessment and written record, you will find it helpful to generate a *Problem List* that summarizes the patient's problems for the front of the office or hospital chart. A sample *Problem List* for Mrs. N is provided next.

● Sample Problem List

Date Entered	Problem No.	Problem
8/30/08	1	Migraine headaches
	2	Elevated blood pressure
	3	Cystocele with occasional stress incontinence
	4	Overweight
	5	Family stress
	6	Low back pain
	7	Tobacco abuse
	8	Varicose veins
	9	History of right pyelonephritis
	10	Allergy to ampicillin
	11	Health maintenance

Interviewing and the Health History

The health history is a conversation with a purpose. Unlike social conversation, in which you express your own needs and interests with responsibility only for yourself, the primary goal of the clinician–patient interview is the well-being of the patient. The purpose of patient history taking is three-fold: to establish a trusting and supportive relationship, to gather information, and to offer information.

The interviewing process differs significantly from the format for the health history presented in Chapter 1. Both are fundamental to your work with patients but serve different purposes.

- The **health history format** is a structured framework for organizing patient information in written or verbal form for other health care providers.

- The **interview** that actually generates this information is more fluid. It requires knowledge of the information you need to obtain, the ability to elicit accurate and detailed information, and interpersonal skills that allow you to respond to the patient's feelings and elicit the **patient's story** in his or her **own words.**

For new patients in the office, hospital, or long-term care setting, you will do a *comprehensive health history,* described for adults in Chapter 1. For patients who seek care for a specific complaint, such as painful urination, a more limited interview, tailored to that specific problem— sometimes called a *focused* or *problem-oriented history,* may be indicated.

GETTING READY: THE APPROACH TO THE INTERVIEW

Interviewing patients to elicit their health history requires planning.

- **Take time for self-reflection.** As clinicians, we encounter a wide variety of people, each one unique. Because we bring our own values, assumptions, and biases to every encounter, we must look inward to clarify how our expectations and reactions may affect what we hear and how we behave. *Self-reflection brings a deepening personal awareness to our work with patients and is one of the most rewarding aspects of providing patient care.*

- **Review your clinical behavior and appearance.** Consciously or not, you send messages through your behavior. Posture, gestures, eye contact, and tone of voice all can express interest, attention, acceptance, and understanding. The skilled interviewer seems calm and unhurried, even when time is limited. Reactions that betray disapproval, embarrassment, impatience, or boredom block communication. Patients find cleanliness, neatness, conservative dress, and a nametag reassuring.

- **Review the chart.** Before seeing the patient, review the medical record, or chart. It often provides valuable information about past diagnoses and treatments; however, data may be incomplete or even disagree with what you learn from the patient, so be open to developing new approaches or ideas.

- **Adjust the environment.** Always consider the patient's privacy. Pull shut any bedside curtains. Suggest moving to an empty room rather than having a conversation that can be overheard.

- **Set goals for the interview.** Clarify your goals for the interview. A clinician must balance **provider-centered goals** with **patient-centered goals.** The clinician's task is to balance these multiple agendas.

- **Take notes.** Jot down short phrases, specific dates, or words rather than trying to put them into a final format. Maintain good eye contact, and whenever the patient is talking about sensitive or disturbing material, put down your pen.

LEARNING ABOUT THE PATIENT: THE SEQUENCE OF THE INTERVIEW

In general, an interview moves through several stages. *Throughout this sequence, you, as the clinician, must always stay attuned to the patient's feelings, help the patient express them, respond to their content, and validate their significance.* Whether the interview is comprehensive or focused, be attentive to the patient's feelings and affect.

- **Greet the patient and establish rapport.** *Greet the patient* by name and introduce yourself, giving your name. If possible, shake hands. If this is the first contact, explain your role, including your status as a student and how you will be involved in the patient's care. Using a title to address the patient (e.g., Mr. O'Neil, Ms. Wu) is always best. **Avoid first names** unless you have specific permission from the patient.

  Whenever visitors are present, *maintain confidentiality.* Let the **patient** decide if visitors or family members should remain in the room, and ask for the patient's permission before conducting the interview in front of them.

  Attend to the patient's comfort. Ask how he or she is feeling and if you are coming at a convenient time. Look for signs of discomfort, such as frequent changes of position or facial expressions that show pain or anxiety. Arranging the bed may make the patient more comfortable.

  Consider the best way to *arrange the room.* Choose a distance that facilitates conversation and good eye contact. Try to sit at eye level with the patient. Move any physical barriers between you and the patient, such as desks or bedside tables, out of the way.

  Give the patient your undivided attention. Try not to look down to take notes or read the chart, and spend enough time on small talk to put the patient at ease.

- **Establish an agenda.** It is important to identify both your own and the patient's issues at the beginning of the encounter. Often, you may need to focus the interview by asking the patient which problem is most pressing. For example, "Do you have some special concerns today? Which one are you most concerned about?" Some patients may not have a specific complaint or problem. *It is still important to start with the patient's story.*

- **Invite the patient's story.** As you probe the patient's concern, begin with **open-ended questions** that allow full freedom of response: "Tell me more about . . . ." Avoid questions that restrict the patient to a minimally informative "yes" or "no" answer. *Listen to the patient's answers without interrupting.*

  Train yourself to *follow the patient's leads.* Use verbal and nonverbal cues that prompt patients to recount their stories spontaneously. Use *continuers,* especially at the outset, such as nodding your head and using phrases such as "Uh huh," "Go on," and "I see."

- **Identify and respond to the patient's emotional cues.** Patients offer various clues to their concerns that may be direct or indirect, verbal or nonverbal; they may express them as ideas or emotions. Acknowledging and responding to these clues help build rapport, expand the clinician's understanding of the illness, and improve patient satisfaction. A taxonomy of the clues about the patient's perspective on illness is provided in the box below.

CLUES TO THE PATIENT'S PERSPECTIVE ON ILLNESS

- Direct statement(s) by the patient of explanations, emotions, expectations, and effects of the illness
- Expression of feelings about the illness
- Attempts to explain or understand symptoms
- Speech clues (e.g., repetition, prolonged reflective pauses)
- Sharing a personal story
- Behavior clues indicative of unidentified concerns, dissatisfaction, or unmet needs such as reluctance to accept recommendations, seeking a second opinion, or early appointment

(Source: Lang F, Floyd MR, Beine KL. Clues to patients' explanations and concerns about their illnesses: a call for active listening. Arch Fam Med 9(3):222–227, 2000.)

- **Expand and clarify the patient's story.** Each symptom has attributes that must be clarified, including context, associations, and chronology, especially for pain. It is critical to understand fully every symptom's essential characteristics. *Always elicit the seven features of every symptom.*

THE SEVEN ATTRIBUTES OF A SYMPTOM

1. **Location.** Where is it? Does it radiate?
2. **Quality.** What is it like?
3. **Quantity or severity.** How bad is it? (For pain, ask for a rating on a scale of 1–10.)
4. **Timing.** When did (does) it start? How long did (does) it last? How often did (does) it occur?
5. **Setting in which it occurs.** Include environmental factors, personal activities, emotional reactions, or other circumstances that may have contributed to the illness.
6. **Remitting or exacerbating factors.** Does anything make it better or worse?
7. **Associated manifestations.** Have you noticed anything else that accompanies it?

Use language that is understandable and appropriate to the patient. Technical language confuses patients and blocks communication. Whenever possible, *use the patient's words, making sure you clarify their meaning.*

Learn to facilitate the patient's story by using different types of questions and the techniques of skilled interviewing on pp. 43–45. Often you will need to *use directed questions* (see pp. 43–44) that ask for specific information the patient has not already offered. *In general, the patient interview moves back and forth from an open-ended question to a directed question and then on to another open-ended question.*

Establishing the sequence and time course of the patient's symptoms is important. You can encourage a chronologic account by asking such questions as "What then?" or "What happened next?"

- **Generate and test diagnostic hypotheses.** As you listen to the patient's concerns, you will begin to *generate* *hypotheses* about what disease process might be the cause. Identifying the various attributes of the patient's symptoms and pursuing specific details are fundamental to recognizing patterns of disease and differentiating one disease from another.

- **Create a shared understanding of the problem.** The *disease/illness model* helps you understand the difference between your perspective and the patient's perspective. In this model, *disease* is the explanation that the *clinician* brings to the symptoms. It is the way that the clinician organizes what he or she learns from the patient into a coherent picture that leads to a clinical diagnosis and treatment plan. *Illness* can be defined as how the *patient* experiences symptoms. *The health history interview needs to include both of these views of reality.*

  Learning how patients perceive illness means asking patient-centered questions in the four domains listed below, which follow the mnemonic "FIFE"—Feelings, Ideas, effect on Function, and Expectations. This is crucial to patient satisfaction, effective health care, and patient follow-through.

EXPLORING THE PATIENT'S PERSPECTIVE

- The patient's **F**eelings, including fears or concerns, about the problem
- The patient's **I**deas about the nature and the cause of the problem
- The effect of the problem on the patient's life and **F**unction
- The patient's **E**xpectations of the disease, of the clinician, or of health care, often based on prior personal or family experiences

---

- **Negotiate a plan.** Learning about the disease and conceptualizing the illness give you and the patient the basis for planning further evaluation (physical examination, laboratory tests, consultations, etc.).

- **Plan for follow-up and closing.** Make sure the patient fully understands the plans you have developed together.

You can say, "We need to stop now. Do you have any questions about what we've covered?" Review future evaluation, treatments, and follow-up. Give the patient a chance to ask any final questions.

BUILDING A THERAPEUTIC RELATIONSHIP: THE TECHNIQUES OF SKILLED INTERVIEWING

Skilled interviewing requires the use of specific learnable techniques. Practice these techniques and find ways to be observed or recorded so that you can receive feedback on your progress.

Active Listening.   This requires listening closely to what the patient is communicating, being aware of the patient's emotional state, and using verbal and nonverbal skills to encourage the speaker to continue and expand.

Guided Questioning.   Learn to adapt your questioning to the patient's verbal and nonverbal cues.

ADAPTIVE QUESTIONING: OPTIONS FOR CLARIFYING THE PATIENT'S STORY

- Moving from open-ended to focused questions
- Questioning to elicit a graded response
- Asking a series of questions, one at a time
- Offering multiple choices for answers
- Clarifying what the patient means
- Using continuers
- Echoing

Proceed from the general to the specific. Directed questions should not be leading questions that call for a "yes" or "no" answer: not "Did your stools look like tar?" but "Please describe your stools."

Ask questions that require *a graded response* rather than a single answer. "What physical activity do you do that makes you short of breath?" is better than "Do you get short of breath climbing stairs?" Be sure to *ask one question at a time*. Try "Do you have any of the following problems?" Be sure to pause and establish eye contact as you list each problem.

Sometimes patients seem unable to describe symptoms. *Offer multiple-choice answers.*

For patients using words that are ambiguous, *request clarification*, as in "Tell me exactly what you meant by 'the flu.' "

Posture, actions, or words encourage the patient to say more but do not specify the topic. Nod your head or remain silent. Lean forward, make eye contact, and use **continuers** like "Mm-hmm," "Go on," or "I'm listening."

Repetition and **echoing** of the patient's words encourage the patient to express both factual details and feelings.

Nonverbal Communication. Being sensitive to nonverbal messages allows you both to "read the patient" more effectively and to send messages of your own. Pay close attention to eye contact, facial expression, posture, head position and movement such as shaking or nodding, interpersonal distance, and placement of the arms or legs, such as crossed, neutral, or open. Physical contact (like placing your hand on the patient's arm) can convey empathy or help the patient gain control of feelings. You also can mirror the patient's *paralanguage,* or qualities of speech such as pacing, tone, and volume, to increase rapport. Be sensitive to cultural variations in uses and meanings of nonverbal behaviors.

Empathic Responses. Patients may express—with or without words—feelings they have not consciously acknowledged. *To empathize with your patient you must first identify his or her feelings.* Inquire about them rather than assuming how the patient feels.

Respond with understanding and acceptance. Responses may be as simple as "I understand," "That sounds upsetting," or "You seem sad." Empathy also may be nonverbal—for example, offering a tissue to a crying patient.

Validation.   An important way to make a patient feel accepted is to provide verbal support that legitimizes or validates the patient's emotional experience.

Reassurance.   Avoid premature or false reassurance. Such reassurance may block further disclosures, especially if the patient feels that exposing anxiety is a weakness. *The first step to effective reassurance is identifying and accepting the patient's feelings without offering reassurance at that moment.*

Partnering.   Express your desire to work with patients in an ongoing way. Reassure patients that regardless of what happens with their disease, as their provider you are committed to a continuing partnership. Even in your role as a student, such support can make a big difference.

Summarization.   Giving a capsule summary lets the patient know that you have been listening carefully. It also clarifies what you know and what you don't know. Summarization allows you to organize your clinical reasoning and to convey your thinking to the patient, which makes the relationship more collaborative.

Transitions.   Tell patients when you are changing directions during the interview. This gives patients a greater sense of control.

Empowering the Patient.   The clinician–patient relationship is inherently unequal. Patients have many reasons to feel vulnerable: pain, worry, feeling overwhelmed with the health care system, lack of familiarity with the clinical evaluation process. Differences of gender, ethnicity, race, or class may also create power differentials. Ultimately patients must be empowered to take care of themselves and feel confident about following through on your advice. Review the principles below.

PRINCIPLES FOR EMPOWERING THE PATIENT

- Inquire about the patient's perspective.
- Express interest in the person, not just the problem.
- Follow the patient's lead.
- Elicit emotional content.
- Share information with the patient (e.g., transitions).
- Make your clinical reasoning transparent to the patient.
- Reveal the limits of your knowledge.

ADAPTING YOUR INTERVIEW TO SPECIFIC SITUATIONS

Always remember the importance of listening to the patient and clarifying the patient's agenda.

Silent Patient. Silence has many meanings and purposes. Watch closely for nonverbal cues such as difficulty controlling emotions. You may need to shift your inquiry to symptoms of depression or begin an exploratory mental status examination. Silence may be the patient's response to how you are asking questions. Are you asking too many direct questions? Have you offended the patient?

Confusing Patient. Some patients have *multiple symptoms* or a somatization disorder. Focus on the meaning or function of the symptoms and guide the interview into a psychosocial assessment. At other times you may be baffled, frustrated, and confused. The history is vague and difficult to understand, and patients may describe symptoms in bizarre terms. Try to learn more about the unusual symptoms. Watch for delirium in acutely ill or intoxicated patients and for dementia in the elderly. When you suspect a psychiatric or neurologic disorder, shift to a mental status examination, focusing on level of consciousness, orientation, and memory.

Patient With Altered Capacity. Some patients cannot provide their own histories because of delirium, dementia, or other conditions. Others cannot relate certain parts of the history. In such cases, determine whether the patient has *decision-making capacity,* or the ability to understand information related to health, to make medical choices based on reason and a consistent set of values and to declare preferences about treatments. Many patients with psychiatric or cognitive deficits still retain the ability to make decisions.

For patients **with capacity,** obtain their consent before talking about their health with others. Maintain confidentiality and clarify what you can discuss with others. Your knowledge about the patient can be quite comprehensive, yet others may offer surprising and important information. Consider dividing the interview into two segments—one with the patient and the other with both the patient and a second informant. Also learn the tenets of the *Health Insurance Portability and*

Accountability Act (HIPAA) passed by Congress in 1996, which sets strict standards for disclosure for both institutions and providers when sharing patient information. These can be found at www.hhs.gov/ocr/hipaa/.

For patients **with impaired capacity,** find a *surrogate informant* or *decision-maker* to assist with the history. Check whether the patient has a *durable power of attorney for health care* or a *health care proxy.* If not, in many cases a spouse or family member can represent the patient's wishes.

Talkative Patient. With a garrulous, rambling patient, several techniques are helpful. For the first 5 or 10 minutes, listen closely. Does the patient seem obsessively detailed or unduly anxious? Is there a flight of ideas or disorganized thought process? Try to focus on what seems most important to the patient. "You've described many concerns. Let's focus on the hip pain first. Can you tell me what it feels like?"

Crying Patient. Usually crying is therapeutic, as is quiet acceptance of the patient's distress. Make a facilitating or supportive remark like "I'm glad that you got that out."

Angry or Disruptive Patient. Many patients have reasons to be angry: they are ill, they have suffered a loss, they lack accustomed control over their own lives, and they feel relatively powerless. They may direct this anger toward you. *Accept angry feelings from patients and allow them to express such emotions without getting angry in return.* Validate their feelings without agreeing with their reasons. "I understand that you felt very frustrated by the long wait and answering the same questions over and over." Some angry patients become hostile and disruptive. Before approaching them, alert security. It is important to stay calm, appear accepting, and avoid being challenging. Keep your posture relaxed and nonthreatening. Once you have established rapport, gently suggest moving to a different location.

Patient With a Language Barrier. The ideal interpreter is a neutral, objective person trained in both languages and cultures. Avoid using family members or friends as interpreters: confidentiality may be violated. As you begin working with the interpreter, *make questions clear, short, and simple.* Speak directly to the patient. Bilingual written questionnaires are valuable.

GUIDELINES FOR WORKING WITH AN INTERPRETER

- Choose a professional interpreter in preference to a hospital worker, volunteer, or family member. Use the interpreter as a resource for cultural information.
- Orient the interpreter to the components you plan to cover in the interview; include reminders to translate everything the patient says.
- Arrange the room so that you and the patient have eye contact and can read each other's nonverbal cues.
- Seat the interpreter next to you (or even behind you) and allow the interpreter and the patient to establish rapport.
- Address the patient directly. Reinforce your questions with nonverbal behaviors.
- Keep sentences short and simple. Focus on the most important concepts to communicate.
- Verify mutual understanding by asking the patient to report back what he or she has heard.
- Be patient. The interview will take more time yet provide less information.

Patient With Low Literacy. Assess ability to read. Some patients may try to hide their reading problems. Ask the patient to read whatever instructions you have written. Simply handing the patient written material upside-down to see if the patient turns it around may settle the question.

Patient With Impaired Hearing. Find out the patient's preferred method of communicating. Patients may use American Sign Language, a unique language with its own syntax, or various other communication forms combining signs and speech. Determine whether the patient identifies with the Deaf or Hearing culture. Handwritten questions and answers may be the best solution. When patients have *partial hearing impairment* or can *read lips,* face them directly, in good light. If the patient has a *unilateral hearing loss,* sit on the hearing side. If the patient has a *hearing aid,* make sure it is working. Eliminate background noise such as television.

Patient With Impaired Vision.   Shake hands to establish contact and explain who you are and why you are there. If the room is unfamiliar, orient the patient to the surroundings.

Patient With Limited Intelligence.   Patients of moderately limited intelligence usually can give adequate histories. Pay special attention to the patient's schooling and ability to function independently. How far has the patient gone in school? If he or she didn't finish, why not? Assess simple calculations, vocabulary, memory, and abstract thinking. For patients with severe mental retardation, obtain the history from the family or caregivers. Avoid "talking down" or using condescending behavior. The sexual history is equally important and often overlooked.

Patient With Personal Problems.   Patients may ask you for advice about personal problems outside the range of health. Letting the patient talk through the problem is usually more valuable and therapeutic than any answer you could give.

SENSITIVE TOPICS THAT CALL FOR SPECIFIC APPROACHES

The Sexual History.   You can introduce questions about sexual function and practices at multiple points in a patient's history. An orienting sentence or two is often helpful. "Now I'd like to ask you some questions about your sexual health and practices" or "I routinely ask all patients about their sexual function."

- "When was the last time you had intimate physical contact with someone?" "Did that contact include sexual intercourse?"

- "Do you have sex with men, women, or both?" The health implications of heterosexual, homosexual, or bisexual experiences are significant.

- "How many sexual partners have you had in the last 6 months?" "In the last 5 years?" "In your lifetime?"

- Because no explicit risk factors may be present, it is important to ask all patients "Do you have any concerns about HIV disease or AIDS?" Also ask about routine use of condoms.

Mental Health History.   Cultural constructs of mental illness vary widely, causing marked differences in acceptance and attitudes. Ask open-ended questions initially: "Have you ever had any problem with emotional or mental illnesses?" Then move to more specific questions: "Have you ever visited a counselor or psychotherapist?" "Have you taken medication for emotional issues?" "Have you or a family member ever been hospitalized for a mental health problem?"

Be sensitive to reports of mood changes or symptoms such as fatigue, tearfulness, appetite or weight changes, insomnia, and vague somatic complaints. Two opening screening questions are: "Over the past 2 weeks, have you felt down, depressed, or hopeless?" and "Over the past 2 weeks, have you felt little interest or pleasure in doing things?" Ask about thoughts of suicide: "Have you ever thought about hurting yourself or ending your life?" Evaluate severity.

Many patients with schizophrenia or other psychotic disorders can function in the community and tell you about their diagnoses, symptoms, hospitalizations, and medications. Investigate their symptoms and assess any effects on mood or daily activities.

The Alcohol and Drug History.   Clinicians should routinely ask about current and past use of alcohol or drugs, patterns of use, and family history. "What do you like to drink?" or "Tell me about your use of alcohol" are good opening questions that avoid the easy yes or no response. The most widely used screening questions are the CAGE questions. Two or more affirmative answers to the CAGE questions suggest alcoholism.

THE CAGE QUESTIONS

● Have you ever felt the need to **Cut down** on drinking?
● Have you ever felt **Annoyed** by criticism of drinking?
● Have you ever felt **Guilty** about drinking?
● Have you ever taken a drink first thing in the morning (**Eye-opener**) to steady your nerves or get rid of a hangover?

(Adapted from Mayfield D, McLeod G, Hall P. The CAGE questionnaire: validation of a new alcoholism screening instrument. Am J Psychiatry 131:1121–1123, 1974.)

Also ask about blackouts (loss of memory for events during drinking), seizures, accidents or injuries while drinking, job loss, marital conflict, or legal problems. Ask specifically about drinking while driving or operating machinery.

Questions about drugs are similar. "How much marijuana do you use? Cocaine? Heroin? Amphetamines?" (Ask about each one by name.) "How about prescription drugs such as sleeping pills?" "Diet pills?" "Painkillers?" Use the CAGE questions but relate them to drug use. With adolescents, it may be helpful to ask about substance use by friends or family members first. "A lot of young people are using drugs these days. How about at your school? Your friends?"

Family Violence.   Many authorities recommend routine screening of all female patients for domestic violence. Start with general "normalizing" questions: "Because abuse is common in many women's lives, I've begun to ask about it routinely." "Are there times in your relationships that you feel unsafe or afraid?" Consider physical abuse in the following settings:

- If injuries are unexplained, seem inconsistent with the patient's story, are concealed by the patient, or cause embarrassment

- If the patient has delayed getting treatment for trauma

- If there is a past history of repeated injuries or "accidents"

- If the patient or a person close to the patient has a history of alcohol or drug abuse

- If a partner tries to dominate the interview, will not leave the room, or seems unusually anxious or solicitous

Death and the Dying Patient.   Work through your own feelings with the help of reading and discussion. Kubler-Ross has described five stages in our response to loss or the anticipatory grief of impending death: denial and isolation, anger, bargaining, depression or sadness, and acceptance. These stages may occur sequentially or overlap in different combinations.

Dying patients rarely want to talk about their illnesses all the time, nor do they wish to confide in everyone they meet. Give them opportunities to talk and then listen receptively, but be supportive if they prefer to stay at a social level.

Understanding the patient's wishes about treatment at the end of life is an important clinician responsibility. Even if discussions of death and dying are difficult, you must learn to ask specific questions. Ask about Do Not Resuscitate (DNR) status. Find out about the patient's frame of reference. "What experiences have you had with the death of a close friend or relative?" "What do you know about cardiopulmonary resuscitation (CPR)?" Assure patients that relieving pain and taking care of their other spiritual and physical needs will be a priority.

Encourage any adult, but especially the elderly or chronically ill, to establish a *health care proxy,* an individual who can act for the patient in life-threatening situations.

Society and Ethics: Cultural Humility. As you provide care for an ever-expanding and diverse group of patients, it is important to understand how culture shapes not just the patient's beliefs, but your own. *Culture* is a system of shared ideas, rules, and meanings that influences how we view the world, experience it emotionally, and behave in relation to other people. This definition of culture is broader than the term *ethnicity.* The influence of culture is not limited to minority groups—it is relevant to everyone.

Clinicians are increasingly challenged to adopt *cultural humility,* a "process that requires humility as individuals continually engage in self-reflection and self-critique as lifelong learners and reflective practitioners." This process includes "the difficult work of examining cultural beliefs and cultural systems of both patients and providers to locate the points of cultural dissonance or synergy that contribute to patients' health outcomes." It calls for clinicians to "bring into check the power imbalances that exist in the dynamics of (clinician)-patient communication" and maintain mutually respectful and dynamic partnerships with patients and communities. The three-point framework below will help you.

- **Self-awareness.** As clinicians, we face the task of bringing our own values and biases to a conscious level. *Values* are the standards we use to measure our own and others' beliefs and behaviors. *Biases* are the attitudes or feelings that we attach to perceived differences, for example, the way an individual relates to time, which can be a culturally determined phenomenon. Are you always on time—a positive value in the dominant Western culture? Or do you tend to run a little late? How do you feel about people whose habits are opposite to yours? Think about the role of physical appearance. Do you consider yourself thin, midsize, or heavy? How do you feel about people who have different weights?

- **Enhanced Communication and Learning From the Patient.** Maintain an open, respectful, and inquiring attitude. "What did you hope to get from this visit?" If you have established rapport and trust, patients will be willing to teach you. Be ready to acknowledge your ignorance or bias. "I mistakenly made assumptions about you that are not right. I apologize. Would you be willing to tell me more about yourself and your future goals?"

  Learn about different cultures: do some reading; go to movies that are made in different countries; learn about different consumer health agendas.

- **Collaborative Partnerships.** Communication based on trust, respect, and a willingness to reexamine assumptions helps allow patients to express concerns that run counter to the dominant culture. You, the clinician, must be willing to listen to and validate these feelings, and not let your own feelings prevent you from exploring painful areas. You also must be willing to reexamine your beliefs.

Sexuality in the Clinician–Patient Relationship. The emotional and physical intimacy of the clinician–patient relationship may lead to sexual feelings. If you become aware of such feelings, accept them as a normal human response, and bring them to the conscious level so they will not affect your behavior. Denying these feelings makes it more likely that you will act inappropriately. *Any* sexual contact or romantic relationship with patients is *unethical;* keep your relationship with the patient within professional bounds and seek help if you need it.

Ethical Considerations. Fundamental maxims are as follows:

- *Nonmaleficence* or *primum non nocere,* commonly stated as "First, do no harm"

- *Beneficence,* or the dictum that the clinician needs to "do good" for the patient. As clinicians, our actions need to be motivated by what is in the patient's best interest.

- *Autonomy,* whereby patients have the right to determine what is in their own best interest

- *Confidentiality,* meaning that we are obligated not to tell others what we learn from our patients

The Tavistock Principles guide behavior in health care for both individuals and institutions.

THE TAVISTOCK PRINCIPLES

Rights: People have a right to health and health care.

Balance: Care of individual patients is central, but the health of populations is also our concern.

Comprehensiveness: In addition to treating illness, we have an obligation to ease suffering, minimize disability, prevent disease, and promote health.

Cooperation: Health care succeeds only if we cooperate with those we serve, each other, and those in other sectors.

Improvement: Improving health care is a serious and continuing responsibility.

Safety: Do no harm.

Openness: Being open, honest, and trustworthy is vital in health care.

Beginning the Physical Examination: General Survey, Vital Signs, and Pain

Common or Concerning Symptoms

- Changes in weight
- Fatigue and weakness
- Fever, chills, night sweats
- Pain

Changes in Weight.   Good opening questions include "How often do you check your weight?" and "How is it compared to a year ago?"

- *Weight gain* occurs when caloric intake exceeds caloric expenditure over time. It also may reflect abnormal accumulation of body fluids.

- *Weight loss* has many causes: decreased food intake, dysphagia, vomiting, and insufficient supplies of food; defective absorption of nutrients; increased metabolic requirements; and loss of nutrients through the urine, feces, or injured skin. Be alert for signs of malnutrition.

Fatigue and Weakness.   *Fatigue* is a nonspecific symptom with many causes. Use open-ended questions to explore the attributes of the patient's fatigue, and encourage the patient to fully describe what he or she is experiencing.

Weakness differs from fatigue. It denotes a demonstrable loss of muscle power and will be discussed later with other neurologic symptoms.

Fever, Chills, and Night Sweats. Ask about fever if the patient has an acute or chronic illness. Find out whether the patient has used a thermometer to measure the temperature. Distinguish between subjective *chilliness* and a *shaking chill*, with shivering throughout the body and chattering of teeth. *Night sweats* raise concerns about tuberculosis or malignancy.

Focus your questions on the timing of the illness and its associated symptoms. Become familiar with patterns of infectious diseases that may affect your patient. Inquire about travel, contact with sick people, or other unusual exposures. Be sure to inquire about medications, since they may cause fever. In contrast, recent ingestion of aspirin, acetaminophen, corticosteroids, and nonsteroidal anti-inflammatory drugs may mask it.

Pain. Approximately 70 million Americans report persisting or intermittent pain, often underassessed. Adopt the comprehensive approach found on pp. 67–69.

HEALTH PROMOTION AND COUNSELING

Important Topics for Health Promotion and Counseling

- Optimal weight, nutrition, and diet
- Exercise

Optimal Weight, Nutrition, and Diet. Less than half of U.S. adults maintain a healthy weight (BMI ≥ 19 but ≤ 25). Obesity has increased in every segment of the population. More than 50% of people with type 2 diabetes and roughly 20% of those with hypertension or elevated cholesterol levels are overweight or obese. Increasing obesity in children has been linked to rising rates of childhood diabetes.

Diet recommendations hinge on assessment of the patient's motivation and readiness to lose weight and individual risk factors. The *Clinical Guidelines on the Identification, Evaluation, and Treatment of Overweight and Obesity in Adults* recommend the following general guidelines:

- A 10% weight reduction over 6 months, or a decrease of 300 to 500 kcal/day, for people with BMIs between 27 and 35

- A weight loss goal of ½ to 1 pound per week, because more rapid weight loss does not lead to better results at 1 year

Exercise. Thirty minutes of moderate activity (defined as walking 2 miles in 30 minutes, or its equivalent, on most days of the week) is recommended. Patients can increase exercise by such simple measures as parking further away from their place of work or using stairs instead of elevators.

TECHNIQUES OF EXAMINATION

EXAMINATION TECHNIQUES	POSSIBLE FINDINGS
GENERAL SURVEY	
Apparent State of Health	Acutely or chronically ill, frail, robust, vigorous
Level of Consciousness. Is the patient awake, alert, and interactive?	If not, promptly assess level of consciousness (see p. 333).
Signs of Distress	
• Cardiac or respiratory distress	Clutching the chest, pallor, diaphoresis; labored breathing, wheezing, cough
• Pain	Wincing, sweating, protecting painful area
• Anxiety or depression	Anxious face, fidgety movements, cold and moist palms; inexpressive or flat affect, poor eye contact, psychomotor slowing
Skin Color and Obvious Lesions. See Chapter 6, *The Skin, Hair, and Nails,* for details.	Pallor, cyanosis, jaundice, rashes, bruises

EXAMINATION TECHNIQUES	POSSIBLE FINDINGS

Dress, Grooming, and Personal Hygiene

- Is the patient wearing any unusual jewelry? Where? Is there any body piercing?

- Note patient's hair, fingernails, and use of cosmetics.

Facial Expression. Watch for eye contact. Is it natural? Sustained and unblinking? Averted quickly? Absent? | Stare of hyperthyroidism; flat or sad affect of depression. Decreased eye contact may be cultural or may suggest anxiety, fear, or sadness.

Odors of Body and Breath. Odors can be important diagnostic clues. | Breath odor of alcohol, acetone, uremia, or liver failure. Fruity odor of diabetes. (Never assume that alcohol on a patient's breath explains changes in mental status or neurologic findings.)

Posture, Gait, and Motor Activity | Preference to sit up in left-sided heart failure and to lean forward with arms braced in chronic obstructive pulmonary disease (COPD)

HEIGHT AND WEIGHT

Height. Measure the patient's height in stocking feet. Note the build—muscular or unconditioned, tall or short. Observe the body proportions.

EXAMINATION TECHNIQUES | POSSIBLE FINDINGS

Weight. Is the patient emaciated? Plump? If obese, is there central or dispersed distribution of fat? Weigh the patient with shoes off.

Calculate the *Body Mass Index* (BMI), which incorporates estimated but more accurate measurements of body fat than weight alone.

More than 50% of U.S. adults are overweight (BMI > 25); nearly 25% are obese (BMI > 30). These excesses are proven risk factors for diabetes, heart disease, stroke, hypertension, osteoarthritis, sleep apnea syndrome, and some forms of cancer.

● Methods to Calculate Body Mass Index (BMI)

Unit of Measure	Method of Calculation
Weight *in pounds,* height *in inches*	1. Body Mass Index Chart (see p. 60)
	2. $\dfrac{\left(\dfrac{\text{Weight (lbs)} \times 700^{*}}{\text{Height (inches)}}\right)}{\text{Height (inches)}}$
Weight *in kilograms,* height *in meters squared*	3. $\dfrac{\text{Weight (kg)}}{\text{Height (m}^2)}$
Either	4. BMI Calculator at Web site www. nhlbisupport.com/bmi/bmicalc.htm

*Several organizations use 704.5, but the variation in BMI is negligible.
Conversion formulas: 2.2 lbs = 1 kg; 1.0 inch = 2.54 cm; 100 cm = 1 meter
(Source: National Institutes of Health and National Heart, Lung and Blood Institute. Body Mass Index Calculator. Available at: www.nhlbisupport. com/bmi/bmicalc.htm. Accessed December 12, 2007.)

- If the BMI falls *above* 25, engage the patient in a 24-hour dietary recall and compare the intake of food groups and number of servings per day with

EXAMINATION TECHNIQUES   POSSIBLE FINDINGS

current recommendations.
Or choose a screening
tool and provide appro-
priate counseling or
referral.

● If the BMI falls *below* 17,
  be concerned about
  possible anorexia nervosa,
  bulimia, or other medical

● **Body Mass Index Chart**

	19	20	21	22	23	24	25	26	27	28	29	30	31	32	33	34	35
Height (inches)							Body Weight (pounds)	Overweight						Obese			
58	91	96	100	105	110	115	119	124	129	134	138	143	148	153	158	162	167
59	94	99	104	109	114	119	124	128	133	138	143	148	153	158	163	168	173
60	97	102	107	112	118	123	128	133	138	143	148	153	158	163	168	174	179
61	100	105	111	116	122	127	132	137	143	148	153	158	164	169	174	180	185
62	104	109	115	120	126	131	136	142	147	153	158	164	169	175	180	185	191
63	107	113	118	124	130	135	141	145	152	158	163	169	174	180	185	191	197
64	110	116	122	128	134	140	145	151	157	163	169	174	180	185	192	197	204
65	114	120	126	132	138	144	150	156	162	168	174	180	186	192	198	204	210
66	118	124	130	136	142	148	155	161	167	173	179	186	192	198	204	210	216
67	121	127	134	140	146	153	159	166	172	178	185	191	198	204	211	217	223
68	125	131	138	144	151	158	164	171	177	184	190	197	203	210	216	223	230
69	128	135	142	149	155	162	169	176	182	189	196	203	209	216	223	230	236
70	132	139	146	153	160	167	174	181	188	189	196	203	209	216	223	230	236
71	136	143	150	157	165	172	179	186	193	200	208	215	222	229	236	243	250
72	140	147	154	162	169	177	184	191	199	206	213	221	228	235	242	250	258
73	144	151	159	166	174	182	189	197	204	212	219	227	235	242	250	257	265
74	148	155	163	171	179	186	194	202	210	218	225	233	241	249	256	264	272
75	152	160	168	176	184	192	200	208	216	224	232	240	248	256	264	272	279
76	156	164	172	180	189	197	205	213	221	230	238	246	254	263	271	279	287

(Source: National Institutes of Health and National Heart, Lung
and Blood Institute. Clinical Guidelines on the Identification,
Evaluation, and Treatment of Overweight and Obesity in Adults,
June 1998.)

EXAMINATION TECHNIQUES   POSSIBLE FINDINGS

conditions (see Table 4-1, p. 70).

If the BMI is ≤35, measure the *waist circumference* just above the hip bones. The patient may have excess body fat if the waist measures ≥40 inches for men.

THE VITAL SIGNS: BLOOD PRESSURE, HEART RATE, RESPIRATORY RATE, AND TEMPERATURE

Blood Pressure.   To measure blood pressure accurately, choose a cuff of appropriate size and ensure careful technique.

SELECTING THE CORRECT BLOOD PRESSURE CUFF

- Width of the inflatable bladder of the cuff should be about 40% of upper-arm circumference (about 12–14 cm in the average adult).
- Length of inflatable bladder should be about 80% of upper-arm circumference (almost long enough to encircle the arm)

STEPS TO ENSURE ACCURATE BLOOD PRESSURE RECORDINGS

- Ideally, ask the patient to avoid smoking or drinking caffeinated beverages for 30 minutes before the blood pressure is taken and to rest for at least 5 minutes.
- Check to make sure the examining room is quiet and comfortably warm.
- Make sure the arm selected is *free of clothing*. There should be no arteriovenous fistulas for dialysis, scarring

(continued)

EXAMINATION TECHNIQUES

STEPS TO ENSURE ACCURATE BLOOD PRESSURE RECORDINGS (CONTINUED)

from prior brachial artery cutdowns, or signs of lymphedema (seen after axillary node dissection or radiation therapy).
- Palpate the brachial artery to confirm that it has a viable pulse.
- Position the arm so that the brachial artery, at the antecubital crease, is *at heart level*—roughly level with the 4th interspace at its junction with the sternum.
- If the patient is seated, rest the arm on a table a little above the patient's waist; if standing, try to support the patient's arm at the midchest level.

MEASURING BLOOD PRESSURE

- Center the inflatable bladder over the brachial artery. The lower border of the cuff should be about 2.5 cm above the antecubital crease. Secure the cuff snugly. Position the patient's arm so that it is slightly flexed at the elbow.
- To determine how high to raise the cuff pressure, first estimate the systolic pressure by palpation. As you feel the radial artery with the fingers of one hand, rapidly inflate the cuff until the radial pulse disappears. Read this pressure on the manometer and add 30 mm Hg to it. Use of this sum as the target for subsequent inflations prevents discomfort from unnecessarily high cuff pressures. It also avoids the occasional error caused by an auscultatory gap—a silent interval between the systolic and diastolic pressures.
- Deflate the cuff promptly.
- Now place the bell of a stethoscope lightly over the brachial artery, taking care to make an air seal with its full rim. Because the sounds to be heard *(Korotkoff sounds)* are relatively low in pitch, they are heard better with the **bell.**

(continued)

EXAMINATION TECHNIQUES

MEASURING BLOOD PRESSURE (CONTINUED)

- Inflate the cuff rapidly again to the level just determined, and then deflate it slowly, at a rate of about 2 to 3 mm Hg per second. Note the level at which you hear the sounds of at least two consecutive beats. This is the **systolic pressure.**
- Continue to lower the pressure slowly. The disappearance point, usually only a few mm Hg below the muffling point, is the best estimate of **diastolic pressure.**
- Read both the systolic and diastolic levels to the nearest 2 mm Hg. Wait 2 or more minutes and repeat. Average your readings. If the first two readings differ by more than 5 mm Hg, take additional readings.
- Take blood pressure in both arms at least once.
- In patients taking antihypertensive medications or with a history of fainting, postural dizziness, or possible depletion of blood volume, take the blood pressure in two positions— supine and standing (unless contraindicated). A fall in systolic pressure of 20 mm Hg or more, especially when accompanied by symptoms, indicates orthostatic (postural) hypotension.

In 2003, the Joint National Committee on Detection, Evaluation, and Treatment of High Blood Pressure (JNC) categorized four levels of systolic blood pressure (SBP) and diastolic blood pressure (DBP).

● JNC VII Blood Pressure Classification—Adults Older Than 18 Years		
Category	Systolic (mm Hg)	Diastolic (mm Hg)
Normal	<120	<80
Prehypertension	120–139	80–89
Hypertension		
Stage 1	140–159	90–99
Stage 2	≥160	≥100

Note that the blood pressure goal for patients with hypertension, diabetes, or renal disease is <130/80.

EXAMINATION TECHNIQUES | POSSIBLE FINDINGS

When the systolic and diastolic levels fall in different categories, use the higher category. For example, 170/92 mm Hg is Stage 2 hypertension; 135/100 mm Hg is Stage 1 hypertension. In *isolated systolic hypertension*, systolic blood pressure is ≥140 mm Hg, and diastolic blood pressure is <90 mm Hg.

Heart Rate. The radial pulse is used commonly to assess heart rate. With the pads of your index and middle fingers, compress the radial artery until you detect a maximal pulsation. If the rhythm is regular, count the rate for 15 seconds and multiply by 4. If the rate is unusually fast or slow, count it for 60 seconds. When the rhythm is irregular, evaluate the rate by auscultation at the cardiac apex (the apical pulse).

Heart Rhythm. Feel the radial pulse. Check the rhythm again by listening with your stethoscope at the cardiac apex. Is the rhythm regular or irregular? If irregular, try to identify a pattern: (1) Do early beats appear in a basically regular rhythm? (2) Does the irregularity vary consistently with respiration? (3) Is the rhythm totally irregular?

Palpation of an irregularly irregular rhythm reliably indicates *atrial fibrillation*. For all other irregular patterns, an ECG is needed to identify the arrhythmia.

Respiratory Rate and Rhythm. Observe the *rate, rhythm, depth,* and *effort*

See Table 4-5, p. 74, Abnormalities in Rate and Rhythm of Breathing.

EXAMINATION TECHNIQUES   POSSIBLE FINDINGS

of breathing. Count the number of respirations in 1 minute either by visual inspection or by subtly listening over the patient's trachea with your stethoscope during examination of the head and neck or chest. Normally, adults take 14 to 20 breaths per minute in a quiet, regular pattern.

Temperature. Average *oral temperature*, usually 37°C (98.6°F), fluctuates considerably from the early morning to the late afternoon or evening. *Rectal temperatures are higher* than oral temperatures by about 0.4 to 0.5°C (0.7 to 0.9°F) but also vary.

Fever or pyrexia refers to an elevated body temperature. *Hyperpyrexia* refers to extreme elevation in temperature, above 41.1°C (106°F), while *hypothermia* refers to an abnormally low temperature, below 35°C (95°F) rectally.

In contrast, *axillary temperatures* are *lower* than oral temperatures by approximately 1° but take 5 to 10 minutes to register and are considered less accurate than other measurements.

Oral temperatures: Choose either glass or electronic thermometer.

Glass thermometer: Shake the thermometer down to 35°C (96°F) or below, insert it under the tongue, instruct the patient to close

Causes of *fever* include infection, trauma (such as surgery or crush injuries), malignancy, blood disorders (such as acute hemolytic

EXAMINATION TECHNIQUES

POSSIBLE FINDINGS

both lips, and wait 3 to 5 minutes. Then read the thermometer, reinsert for 1 minute, and read it again. Avoid breakage.

anemia), drug reactions, and immune disorders such as collagen vascular disease.

Electronic thermometer: Carefully place the disposable cover over the probe and insert the thermometer under the tongue for about 10 seconds.

Tympanic membrane temperature: Make sure the external auditory canal is free of cerumen. Position the probe in the canal. Wait 2 to 3 seconds until the digital reading appears. This method measures core body temperature, which is higher than the normal oral temperature by approximately 0.8°C (11.4°F).

The chief cause of *hypothermia* is exposure to cold. Other predisposing causes include reduced movement as in paralysis, interference with vasoconstriction as from sepsis or excess alcohol, starvation, hypothyroidism, and hypoglycemia. Older adults are especially suspectible to hypothermia and also less likely to develop fever.

Rectal thermometer: Ask the patient to lie on one side with the hip flexed. Select a rectal thermometer with a stubby tip, lubricate it, and insert it about 3 cm to 4 cm (1½ inches) into the anal canal, in a direction pointing to the umbilicus. Remove it after 3 minutes, then read. Alternatively, use an electronic thermometer after lubricating the probe cover. Wait about 10 seconds for the digital temperature recording to appear.

EXAMINATION TECHNIQUES

ACUTE AND CHRONIC PAIN

The experience of pain is complex and multifactorial. It involves sensory, emotional, and cognitive processing but may lack a specific physical etiology.

Chronic pain is defined in several ways: pain not associated with cancer or other medical conditions that persists for more than 3 to 6 months; pain lasting more than 1 month beyond the course of an acute illness or injury; or pain recurring at intervals of months or years. Chronic noncancer pain affects 5% to 33% of patients in primary care settings.

Adopt a comprehensive approach, carefully listening to the patient's description of the many features of pain and contributing factors. Accept the self-report, which experts state is the most reliable indicator of pain.

Location. Ask the patient to point to the pain. Lay terms may not be specific enough to localize the site of origin.

Severity. Use a consistent method to determine severity. Three scales are common: the Visual Analog

EXAMINATION TECHNIQUES

Scale, and two scales using ratings from 1 to 10—the Numeric Rating Scale and the Faces Pain Scale.

Associated Features. Ask the patient to describe the pain and how it started. Pursue the seven features of pain, as you would with any symptom.

Attempted Treatments, Medications, Related Illnesses, and Impact on Daily Activities. Be sure to ask about any treatments that the patient has tried, including medications, physical therapy, and alternative medicines. A comprehensive medication history helps you to identify drugs that interact with analgesics and reduce their efficacy.

Identify any comorbid conditions such as arthritis, diabetes, HIV/AIDS, substance abuse, sickle cell disease, or psychiatric disorders. These can significantly affect the patient's experience of pain.

Health Disparities. Be aware of the well-documented health disparities in pain treatment and delivery of care, which range from lower use of analgesics in emergency rooms for

EXAMINATION TECHNIQUES

African-American and Hispanic patients to disparities in use of analgesics for cancer, postoperative, and low back pain. Clinician stereotypes, language barriers, and unconscious clinician biases in decision making all contribute to these disparities. Critique your own communication style, seek information and best practice standards, and improve your techniques of patient education and empowerment.

RECORDING YOUR FINDINGS

Record the vital signs taken at the time of your examination. They are preferable to those taken earlier in the day by other providers. (Common abbreviations for blood pressure, heart rate, and respiratory rate are self-explanatory.)

Recording the Physical Examination— General Survey and Vital Signs

> "Mrs. Scott is a young, healthy-appearing woman, well-groomed, fit, and in good spirits. Height is 5′4″, weight 135 lbs, BP 120/80, HR 72 and regular, RR 16, temperature 37.5°C."
>
> **OR**
>
> "Mr. Jones is an elderly male who looks pale and chronically ill. He is alert, with good eye contact, but cannot speak more than two or three words at a time because of shortness of breath. He has intercostal muscle retraction when breathing and sits upright in bed. He is thin, with diffuse muscle wasting. Height is 6′2″, weight 175 lbs, BP 160/95, HR 108 and irregular, RR 32 and labored, temperature 101.2°F." (*Suggests COPD exacerbation*)

AIDS TO INTERPRETATION

TABLE 4-1 Eating Disorders and Excessively Low BMI

Anorexia Nervosa	Bulimia Nervosa
Refusal to maintain minimally normal body weight (or BMI above 17.5 kg/m²)	Repeated binge eating followed by self-induced vomiting, misuse of laxatives, diuretics, or other medications; fasting; or excessive exercise
Fear of appearing fat	Often with normal weight
Frequently starving but in denial; lacking insight	Overeating at least twice a week during 3-month period; large amounts of food consumed in short period (~2 hrs)
Often brought in by family members	
May present as failure to make expected weight gains in childhood or adolescence, amenorrhea in women, loss of libido or potency in men	Preoccupation with eating; craving and compulsion to eat; lack of control over eating; alternating with periods of starvation
Associated with depressive symptoms such as depressed mood, irritability, social withdrawal, insomnia, decreased libido	Dread of fatness but may be obese

Anorexia Nervosa (continued):

Additional features supporting diagnosis: self-induced vomiting or purging, excessive exercise, use of appetite suppressants and/or diuretics

Biologic complications
- *Neuroendocrine changes:* amenorrhea, hormonal alterations
- *Cardiovascular disorders:* bradycardia, hypotension, dysrhythmias, cardiomyopathy
- *Metabolic disorders:* hypokalemia, hypochloremic metabolic alkalosis, increased BUN, edema

Other: dry skin, dental caries, delayed gastric emptying, constipation, anemia, osteoporosis

Bulimia Nervosa (continued):

Subtypes of
- *Purging:* bulimic episodes accompanied by self-induced vomiting or use of laxatives, diuretics, or enemas
- *Nonpurging:* bulimic episodes accompanied by compensatory behavior such as fasting, exercise without purging

Biologic complications; see changes listed for anorexia nervosa.

(Sources: World Health Organization. The ICD-10 Classification of Mental and Behavioral Disorders: Diagnostic Criteria for Research. Geneva: World Health Organization, 1993; American Psychiatric Association. DSM-IV-TR: Diagnostic and Statistical Manual of Mental Disorders, 4th ed. Text Revision. Washington, DC: American Psychiatric Association, 2000. Halmi KA: Eating disorders: In: Kaplan HI, Sadock BJ, eds. Comprehensive Textbook of Psychiatry, 7th ed. Philadelphia: Lippincott Williams & Wilkins, 2000:1663–1676.)

TABLE 4-2 Nutrition Screening Checklist

I have an illness or condition that made me change the kind and/or amount of food I eat.	Yes (2 pts) _____
I eat fewer than 2 meals per day.	Yes (3 pts) _____
I eat few fruits or vegetables, or milk products.	Yes (2 pts) _____
I have 3 or more drinks of beer, liquor, or wine almost every day.	Yes (2 pts) _____
I have tooth or mouth problems that make it hard for me to eat.	Yes (2 pts) _____
I don't always have enough money to buy the food I need.	Yes (4 pts) _____
I eat alone most of the time.	Yes (1 pt) _____
I take 3 or more different prescribed or over-the-counter drugs each day.	Yes (1 pt) _____
Without wanting to, I have lost or gained 10 pounds in the last 6 months.	Yes (2 pts) _____
I am not always physically able to shop, cook, and/or feed myself.	Yes (2 pts) _____
	TOTAL _____

Instructions: Check "yes" for each condition that applies, then total the nutritional score. For total scores between 3 and 5 points (moderate risk) or ≥6 points (high risk), further evaluation is needed (especially for the elderly).

Source: American Academy of Family Physicians. The Nutrition Screening Initiative. Available at: www.aafp.org/PreBuilt/NSI_DETERMINE.pdf. Accessed January 23, 2008.

TABLE 4-3 Nutrition Counseling: Sources of Nutrients

Nutrient	Food Source
Calcium	Dairy foods such as yogurt, milk, and natural cheeses Breakfast cereal, fruit juice with calcium supplements Dark-green leafy vegetables such as collards, turnip greens
Iron	Shellfish Lean meat, dark turkey meat Cereals with iron supplements Spinach, peas, lentils Enriched and whole-grain bread
Folate	Cooked dried beans and peas Oranges, orange juice Dark-green leafy vegetables
Vitamin D	Milk (fortified) Eggs, butter, margarine Cereals (fortified)

(Source: Adapted from Dietary Guidelines Committee. 2000 Report. Nutrition and Your Health: Dietary Guidelines for Americans. Washington, DC: Agricultural Research Service, U.S. Department of Agriculture, 2000.)

TABLE 4-4	**Patients With Hypertension: Recommended Changes in Diet**
Dietary Change	**Food Source**
Increase foods high in potassium	Baked white or sweet potatoes, cooked greens such as spinach
	Bananas, plantains, many dried fruits, orange juice
Decrease foods high in sodium	Canned foods (soups, tuna fish)
	Pretzels, potato chips, pickles, olives
	Many processed foods (frozen dinners, ketchup, mustard)
	Batter-fried foods
	Table salt, including for cooking

(Source: Adapted from Dietary Guidelines Committee. 2000 Report. Nutrition and Your Health: Dietary Guidelines for Americans. Washington, DC: Agricultural Research Service, U.S. Department of Agriculture.)

Abnormalities in Rate and Rhythm of Breathing

TABLE 4-5

Inspiration Expiration

Time

Volume of air

Normal. In adults, 14 to 20 per minute; in infants, up to 44 per minute

Rapid Shallow Breathing (Tachypnea). Many causes, including restrictive lung disease, pleural chest pain, and an elevated diaphragm

Rapid Deep Breathing (Hyperpnea, Hyperventilation). Many causes, including exercise, anxiety, metabolic acidosis, brainstem injury. *Kussmaul breathing*, due to metabolic acidosis, is deep but rate may be fast, slow, or normal.

Slow Breathing. May be secondary to diabetic coma, drug-induced respiratory depression, increased intracranial pressure

Cheyne-Stokes Breathing. Rhythmically alternating periods of hyperpnea and apnea. In infants and the aged, may be normal during sleep; also accompanies brain damage, heart failure, uremia, drug-induced respiratory depression

Hyperpnea   Apnea

Ataxic (Biot's) Breathing. Unpredictable irregularity of depth and rate. Causes include brain damage and respiratory depression

Sighs

Sighing Breathing. Breathing punctuated by frequent sighs. When associated with other symptoms, it suggests the hyperventilation syndrome. Occasional sighs are normal.

Behavior and Mental Status

Empathic listening and close observation open a unique vista on the patient's outlook, concerns, and habits. Nevertheless, clinicians often miss clues of mental illness and harmful dysfunctional behaviors in patients. The prevalence of mental disorders in the U.S. population is 30%, yet only approximately 20% of affected patients receive treatment. Even for patients who obtain care, evidence suggests that adherence to treatment guidelines in primary care offices is less than 50%.

Often patients have more than one mental disorder, with symptoms that mirror medical illnesses. Clinicians are well-advised to look for depression or anxiety in patients with substance abuse, and to look for substance abuse in patients with depression or anxiety. "Difficult patients" are frequently those with multiple unexplained symptoms and underlying psychiatric conditions that are amenable to therapy. Without better "dual diagnosis," patient health, function, and quality of life are at risk.

MENTAL HEALTH DISORDERS AND UNEXPLAINED SYMPTOMS IN PRIMARY CARE SETTINGS

Mental Health Disorders in Primary Care

- Approximately 20% of primary care outpatients have mental disorders, but up to 50% to 75% of these disorders are undetected and untreated.
- Prevalence of mental disorders in primary care settings is roughly:
  - Anxiety—20%
  - Mood disorders including dysthymia and depressive and bipolar disorders—25%

(continued)

MENTAL HEALTH DISORDERS AND UNEXPLAINED SYMPTOMS IN PRIMARY CARE SETTINGS (CONTINUED)

- Depression—10%
- Somatoform disorder—10% to 15%
- Alcohol and substance abuse—15% to 20%

Explained and Unexplained Symptoms

- Physical symptoms account for approximately half of office visits.
- Roughly one-third of physical symptoms are unexplained; in 20% to 25% of patients, physical symptoms become chronic or recurring.
- In patients with *unexplained symptoms,* the prevalence of depression and anxiety exceeds 50% and increases with the total number of reported physical symptoms, making detection and "dual diagnosis" important clinical goals.

(Sources: Ansseau M, Dierick M, Buntinkxz F, et al. High prevalence of mental disorders in primary care. J Affect Disord 78(1):49–55, 2004; Kroenke K. The interface between physical and psychological symptoms. Primary Care Companion. J Clin Psychiatry, 5 (Suppl 7):11–18, 2003; Kroenke K. Patients presenting with somatic complaints: epidemiology, psychiatric comorbidity, and management. Int J Methods Psychiatr Res 12(1):34–43, 2003; Kroenke K, Sharpe M, Sykes R. Revising the classification of somatoform disorders: key questions and preliminary recommendations. Psychosomatics 48(4):277–285, 2007; Kroenke K, Spitzer RL, deGruy, et al. A symptom checklist for screen for somatoform disorders in primary care. Psychosomatics 39(3):263–272, 1998; Spitzer RL, Kroenke K, Williams JBW, et al. Validation and utility of a self-report version of PRIME-MD—the PHQ Primary Care Study. JAMA 282(18): 1737–1744, 1999; Staab JP, Datto CJ, Weinreig RM, et al. Detection and diagnosis of psychiatric disorders in primary medical care settings. Med Clin N Am 85(3):579–596, 2001.)

Unexplained conditions lasting beyond 6 weeks are increasingly recognized as common chronic disorders that should prompt screening for depression, anxiety, or both. Experts recommend brief screening questions with high sensitivity and specificity for patients at risk, followed by more detailed investigation when indicated. Several groups of patients warrant brief screening because of high rates of coexisting depression and anxiety.

PATIENT IDENTIFIERS FOR MENTAL HEALTH SCREENING

- Medically unexplained physical symptoms—more than half have a depressive or anxiety disorder
- Multiple physical or somatic symptoms or "high symptom count"
- High severity of the presenting somatic symptom
- Persisting pain
- Symptoms for more than 6 weeks
- Physician rating as a "difficult encounter"
- Recent stress
- Low self-rated health
- High use of health care services
- Substance abuse

(Source: Kroenke K. Patients presenting with somatic complaints: epidemiology, psychiatric comorbidity, and management. Int J Methods Psychiatr Res 12(1):34–43, 2003; Kroenke K. The interface between physical and psychological symptoms. Primary Care Companion. J Clin Psychiatry 5(Suppl 7):11–18, 2003.)

THE HEALTH HISTORY

Common or Concerning Symptoms

- Changes in attention, mood, or speech
- Changes in insight, orientation, or memory
- Anxiety, panic, ritualistic behavior, and phobias
- Delirium or dementia

Your assessment of mental status begins with the first words of the interview. As you gather the health history, you will quickly discern the patient's level of *alertness* and *orientation*, *mood*, *attention*, and *memory*. You will learn about the patient's *insight* and *judgment*, as well as any *recurring or unusual thoughts or perceptions*. For some, you will need to conduct a more formal evaluation of mental status.

Many of the terms used to describe the mental status examination are familiar to you from social conversation. Take the time to learn their precise meanings in the context of the formal evaluation of mental status (see next page).

Assess *level of consciousness*, general *appearance* and *mood*, and *ability to pay attention, remember, understand*, and *speak*.

See Table 5-2, Disorders of Mood, pp. 88–89.

Assess the patient's responses to illness and life circumstances, which often tell you about his or her *insight* and *judgment*. Test *orientation* and *memory*.

TERMINOLOGY: THE MENTAL STATUS EXAMINATION

Level of consciousness	Alertness or state of awareness of the environment
Attention	The ability to focus or concentrate over time on one task or activity
Memory	The process of registering or recording information. *Recent or short-term memory* covers minutes, hours, or days; *remote or long-term memory* refers to intervals of years.
Orientation	Awareness of personal identity, place, and time; requires both memory and attention
Perceptions	Sensory awareness of objects in the environment and their interrelationships; also refers to internal stimuli (e.g., dreams)
Thought processes	The logic, coherence, and relevance of the patient's thoughts, or *how* people think
Thought content	*What* the patient thinks about, including level of insight and judgment
Insight	Awareness that symptoms or disturbed behaviors are normal or abnormal
Judgment	Process of comparing and evaluating alternatives; reflects values that may or may not be based on reality and social conventions or norms

(continued)

TERMINOLOGY: THE MENTAL STATUS EXAMINATION (CONTINUED)	
Affect	An observable, usually episodic, feeling tone expressed through voice, facial expression, and demeanor
Mood	A more sustained emotion that may color a person's view of the world (mood is to affect as climate is to weather)
Language	A complex symbolic system for expressing, receiving, and comprehending words; essential for assessing other mental functions
Higher cognitive functions	Assessed by vocabulary, fund of information, abstract thinking, calculations, construction of objects with two or three dimensions

Explore any unusual thoughts, preoccupations, beliefs, or perceptions as they arise during the interview.

See Table 5-3, Anxiety Disorders, pp. 90–91, and Table 5-4, Selected Psychotic Disorders, p. 92.

All patients with documented or suspected brain lesions, psychiatric symptoms, or reports from family members of vague or changed behavioral symptoms need further systematic assessment.

See Table 20-1, Delirium and Dementia, pp. 424–425.

HEALTH PROMOTION AND COUNSELING

Important Topics for Health Promotion and Counseling

- Screening for depression and suicidality
- Screening for dementia

Depression. Lifetime prevalence of *major depression* meeting formal diagnostic criteria in the United States is approximately

16%, with an annual prevalence of approximately 6%. Primary care providers fail to diagnose major depression in up to 50% of affected patients, often missing early clues such as *low self-esteem, anhedonia* (lack of pleasure in daily activities), *sleep disorders,* and *difficulty concentrating* or *making decisions.* Failure to diagnose depression can have fatal consequences—suicide rates in patients with major depression are eight times higher than in the general population. Ask, "Over the past 2 weeks, have you felt down, depressed, or hopeless?" and "Over the past 2 weeks, have you felt little interest or pleasure in doing things?"

Suicide. Suicide rates are highest among men older than 85 years and are increasing among teenagers and young adults. More than half of patients committing suicide have visited their physicians in the prior month. More than 90% of suicide deaths occur in patients with depression or other mental health disorders or substance abuse. Risk factors include suicidal or homicidal ideation, intent, or plan; access to the means for suicide; current symptoms of psychosis or severe anxiety; any history of psychiatric illness (especially linked to a hospital admission); substance abuse; personality disorder; and prior history or family history of suicide. Patients with these risk factors should be immediately referred for psychiatric care and possibly hospitalization.

Alcohol and Substance Abuse. The interactions and comorbidity of alcohol and substance abuse with mental disorders and suicide are extensive. Alcohol, tobacco, and illicit drugs account for more illness, deaths, and disabilities than any other preventable condition. Lifetime prevalence of alcohol and illicit drug use in the United States is 13% and 3%. In recent U.S. surveys, 8% of those 12 years or older, or 19 million people, reported use of illicit drugs in the prior 30 days. An estimated 3% are dependent on or abuse illicit drugs; of these, 60% use marijuana. Because screening for alcohol and drug use is part of *every* patient history, information on screening is found in Chapter 3, Interviewing and the Health History.

TECHNIQUES OF EXAMINATION

Important Areas of Examination

- Appearance and behavior
- Speech and language
- Mood
- Thoughts and perceptions
- Cognition, including memory, attention, information and vocabulary, calculations, abstract thinking, and constructional ability

Observe patient's mental status throughout your interaction. **Test** specific functions if indicated during the interview or physical examination.

EXAMINATION TECHNIQUES   POSSIBLE FINDINGS

APPEARANCE AND BEHAVIOR

Assess the following:

- *Level of Consciousness.*
  Observe alertness and
  response to verbal and
  tactile stimuli.

  Normal consciousness,
  lethargy, obtundation, stupor,
  coma (see pp. 332–333)

- *Posture and Motor Behavior.*
  Observe pace, range,
  character, and appro-
  priateness of movements.

  Restlessness, agitation, bizarre
  postures, immobility,
  involuntary movements

- *Dress, Grooming, and
  Personal Hygiene*

  Fastidiousness, neglect

- *Facial Expressions.* **Assess**
  during rest and interaction.

  Anxiety, depression,
  elation, anger, responses
  to imaginary people or
  objects, withdrawal

- *Manner, Affect, and
  Relation to People and
  Things*

EXAMINATION TECHNIQUES   POSSIBLE FINDINGS

SPEECH AND LANGUAGE

Note quantity, rate, loudness, clarity, and fluency of speech. If indicated, test for aphasia.

Aphasia, dysphonia, dysarthria, changes with mood disorders

● Testing for Aphasia	
Word comprehension	Ask patient to follow a one-stage command, such as "Point to your nose." Try a two-stage command: "Point to your mouth, then your knee."
Repetition	Ask patient to repeat a phrase of one-syllable words (the most difficult repetition task): "No ifs, ands, or buts."
Naming	Ask patient to name the parts of a watch.
Reading comprehension	Ask patient to read a paragraph aloud.
Writing	Ask patient to write a sentence.

MOOD

Ask about the patient's spirits. **Note** nature, intensity, duration, and stability of any abnormal mood. If indicated, **assess** risk of suicide.

Happiness, elation, depression, anxiety, anger, indifference

THOUGHT AND PERCEPTIONS

Thought Processes. **Assess** logic, relevance, organization, and coherence.

Derailments, flight of ideas, incoherence, confabulation, blocking

Thought Content. **Ask** about and explore any unusual or unpleasant thoughts.

Obsessions, compulsions, delusions, feelings of unreality

EXAMINATION TECHNIQUES	POSSIBLE FINDINGS
Perceptions. **Ask** about any unusual perceptions (e.g., seeing or hearing things).	Illusions, hallucinations
Insight and Judgment. **Assess** patient's insight into the illness and level of judgment used in making decisions or plans.	Recognition or denial of mental cause of symptoms; bizarre, impulsive, or unrealistic judgment

COGNITIVE FUNCTIONS

If indicated, **assess:**

Orientation to time, place, and person	Disorientation

Attention

● *Digit span*—ability to repeat a series of numbers forward and then backward	Poor performance of digit span, serial 7s, and spelling backward are common in dementia and delirium but have other causes, too.
● *Serial 7s*—ability to subtract 7 repeatedly, starting with 100	
● *Spelling backward* of a five-letter word, such as W-O-R-L-D	
Remote Memory (e.g., birthdays, anniversaries, social security number, schools, jobs, wars)	Impaired in late stages of dementia
Recent Memory (e.g., events of the day)	Recent memory and new learning ability impaired in dementia, delirium, and amnestic disorders
New Learning Ability— ability to repeat three or four words after a few minutes of unrelated activity	

EXAMINATION TECHNIQUES   POSSIBLE FINDINGS

HIGHER COGNITIVE FUNCTIONS

If indicated, **assess:**

Information and Vocabulary. **Note** range and depth of patient's information, complexity of ideas expressed, and vocabulary used. For the fund of information, you also may ask names of presidents, other political figures, or large cities.

These attributes reflect intelligence, education, and cultural background. They are limited by mental retardation but are fairly well preserved in early dementia.

Calculating Abilities, such as addition, subtraction, and multiplication

Poor calculation in mental retardation and dementia

Abstract Thinking—ability to respond abstractly to questions about

Concrete responses (observable details rather than concepts) are common in mental retardation, dementia, and delirium. Responses are sometimes bizarre in schizophrenia.

● The meaning of *proverbs,* such as "A stitch in time saves nine"

● The *similarities* of beings or things, such as a cat and a mouse or a piano and a violin

Constructional Ability. **Ask** patient

Impaired ability common in dementia and with parietal lobe damage

● To copy figures such as circle, cross, diamond, and box, and two intersecting pentagons, or

● To draw a clock face with numbers and hands

EXAMINATION TECHNIQUES   POSSIBLE FINDINGS

SPECIAL TECHNIQUE

Mini-Mental State Examination (MMSE). This brief test
is useful in screening for cognitive dysfunction and dementia
and following their course over time. For more detailed
information regarding the MMSE, contact the Publisher,
Psychological Assessment Resources, Inc., 16204 North
Florida Avenue, Lutz, Florida 33549. Below are some sample
questions.

MMSE Sample Items

Orientation to Time
"What is the date?"

Registration
"Listen carefully; I am going to say three words. You say them
    back after I stop. Ready? Here they are . . .
HOUSE (pause), CAR (pause), LAKE (pause). Now repeat those
    words back o me." [Repeat up to five times, but score only
    the first trial.]

Naming
"What is this?" [Point to a pencil or pen.]

Reading
"Please read this and do what it says." [Show examinee the
    words on the stimulus form.]

CLOSE YOUR EYES

RECORDING YOUR FINDINGS

Recording the Examination—Mental Status

"*Mental Status:* The patient is alert, well-groomed, and cheerful. Speech is fluent and words are clear. Thought processes are coherent, insight is good. The patient is oriented to person, place, and time. Serial 7s accurate; recent and remote memory intact. Calculations intact."

OR

"*Mental Status:* The patient appears sad and fatigued; clothes are wrinkled. Speech is slow and words are mumbled. Thought processes are coherent but insight into current life reverses is limited. The patient is oriented to person, place, and time. Digit span, serial 7s, and calculations accurate but responses delayed. Clock drawing is good."

AIDS TO INTERPRETATION

TABLE 5-1   **Somatoform Disorders: Types and Approach**

Management Guidelines for Patients With Unexplained Medical Symptoms

General Aspects	Show empathy and understanding for the complaints and frustrating experiences the patient has had so far (e.g., explain that medically unexplained symptoms are common). Develop a good patient–physician relationship; try to be the "coordinator" of diagnostic procedures and care.
Diagnosis	Explore not only the history of complaints and former treatments, but impairment, (health) anxiety, psychosocial issues. Use screeners and self-report questionnaires as economic instruments for detection; use symptom diaries to assess course and influencing factors on symptoms. When the patient presents with a new symptom, examine the relevant organ system. Show the results of investigations to explain the absence of pathology and to give clear reassurance that there is no serious physical disease. Avoid unnecessary diagnostic tests or surgical procedures.
Treatment	Provide regularly scheduled visits (e.g., every 4-6 weeks), especially in the case of a history of very frequent health care utilization. Explain that treatment is coping, not curing (when pathology cannot be found or does not explain degree of complaints). Suggest coping strategies like regular physical activity, relaxation, distraction.
Referral	If referral is necessary to start psychotherapy or psychopharmacotherapy, prepare the patient for the treatment and reassure him/her that you will continue to be his/her "doctor."

(Source: Reif W, Martin A, Rauh E, et al. Evaluation of general practitioners' training: how to manage patients with unexplained physical symptoms. Psychosomatics 47(4):304-311, 2006.)

TABLE 5-2 Disorders of Mood

Major Depressive Episode	Manic Episode
At least five of the symptoms listed below (including one of the first two) must be present during the same 2-week period; they must represent a change from the person's previous state.	A distinct period of abnormally and persistently elevated, expansive, or irritable mood must be present for at least a week (any duration if hospitalization is necessary). During this time, at least three of the symptoms listed below have been persistent and significant. (Four symptoms are required if the mood is only irritable.)

* Depressed mood (may be an irritable mood in children and adolescents) most of the day, nearly every day
* Markedly diminished interest or pleasure in almost all activities most of the day, nearly every day
* Significant weight gain or loss (not dieting) or increased or decreased appetite nearly every day
* Insomnia or hypersomnia nearly every day
* Psychomotor agitation or retardation nearly every day
* Fatigue or loss of energy nearly every day
* Feelings of worthlessness or inappropriate guilt nearly every day
* Inability to think or concentrate or indecisiveness nearly every day
* Recurrent thoughts of death or suicide, or a specific plan for or attempt at suicide

* Inflated self-esteem or grandiosity
* Decreased need for sleep (feels rested after sleeping 3 hours)
* More talkative than usual or pressure to keep talking
* Flight of ideas or racing thoughts
* Distractibility
* Increased goal-directed activity (either socially at work or school, or sexually) or psychomotor agitation
* Excessive involvement in pleasurable high-risk activities (buying sprees, foolish business ventures, sexual indiscretions)

The symptoms cause significant distress or impair social, occupational, or

The disturbance is severe enough to impair social or occupational functions or

(table continues next page)

TABLE 5-2   Disorders of Mood (continued)

other important functions. In severe cases, hallucinations and delusions may occur.

relationships. It may necessitate hospitalization for the protection of self or others. In severe cases, hallucinations and delusions may occur.

Mixed Episode	Hypomanic Episode
A mixed episode, which must last at least 1 week, meets the criteria for both major and manic depressive episodes.	The mood and symptoms resemble those in a manic episode but are less impairing, do not require hospitalization, do not include hallucinations or delusions, and have a shorter minimum duration—4 days.

Dysthymic Disorder	Cyclothymic Episode
A depressed mood and symptoms for most of the day, for more days than not, over at least 2 years (1 year in children and adolescents). Freedom from symptoms lasts no more than 2 months at a time.	Numerous periods of hypomanic and depressive symptoms that last for at least 2 years (1 year in children and adolescents). Freedom from symptoms lasts no more than 2 months at a time.

(Tables 5-2, 5-3, and 5-4 are based, with permission, on the Diagnostic and Statistical Manual of Mental Disorders, Fourth ed., Text Revision [DSM IV-TR]. Washington, DC: American Psychiatric Association, 2000. For further details and criteria, the reader should consult this manual, its successor, or comprehensive textbooks of psychiatry.)

TABLE 5-3 Anxiety Disorders

Panic Disorder. Recurrent, unexpected panic attacks, at least one of which has been followed by a month or more of persistent concern about further attacks, worry over their implications or consequences, or a significant change in behavior in relation to the attacks.

A *panic attack* is a discrete period of intense fear or discomfort that develops abruptly and peaks within 10 minutes. It involves at least four of the following symptoms: (1) palpitations, pounding heart, or accelerated heart rate; (2) sweating; (3) trembling or shaking; (4) shortness of breath or a sense of smothering; (5) a feeling of choking; (6) chest pain or discomfort; (7) nausea or abdominal distress; (8) feeling dizzy, unsteady, lightheaded, or faint; (9) feelings of unreality or depersonalization; (10) fear of losing control or going crazy; (11) fear of dying; (12) paresthesias (numbness or tingling); and (13) chills or hot flushes.

Agoraphobia. Anxiety about being in places or situations where escape may be difficult or embarrassing or help for sudden symptoms unavailable. Such situations are avoided, require a companion, or cause marked anxiety.

Specific Phobia. A marked, persistent, and excessive or unreasonable fear that is cued by the presence or anticipation of a specific object or situation, such as dogs, injections, or flying. The person recognizes the fear as excessive or unreasonable, but exposure to the cue provokes immediate anxiety. Avoidance or fear impairs the person's normal routine, occupational or academic functioning, or social activities or relationships.

Social Phobia. A marked, persistent fear of one or more social or performance situations that involve exposure to unfamiliar people or to scrutiny by others. Those afflicted fear that they will act in embarrassing or humiliating ways, as by showing their anxiety. Exposure creates anxiety and possibly a panic attack, and the person avoids precipitating situations. He or she recognizes the fear as excessive or unreasonable. Normal functioning, social activities, or relationships are impaired.

Obsessive-Compulsive Disorder. Obsessions or compulsions that cause marked anxiety or distress. Although recognized as

(table continues next page)

TABLE 5-3 Anxiety Disorders (continued)

excessive or unreasonable, they are time consuming and interfere with the person's normal routine and relationships.

Acute Stress Disorder. Exposure to a traumatic event that involved actual or threatened death or serious injury to self or others, leading to intense fear, helplessness, or horror. During or immediately after this event, the person has at least three dissociative symptoms: (1) a subjective sense of numbing, detachment, or absence of emotional responsiveness; (2) a reduced awareness of surroundings, as in a daze; (3) feelings of unreality; (4) feelings of depersonalization; and (5) amnesia for an important part of the event. The event is persistently reexperienced, as in thoughts, images, dreams, illusions, and flashbacks. The person is anxious, shows increased arousal, and avoids stimuli that evoke memories of the event. Causes marked distress or impairs social, occupational, or other important functions. Symptoms occur within 4 weeks of the event and last from 2 days to 4 weeks.

Posttraumatic Stress Disorder. The event, fearful response, and persistent reexperiencing of the traumatic event resemble acute stress disorder. Hallucinations may occur. The person has increased arousal, tries to avoid stimuli related to the trauma, and has numbing of general responsiveness. Causes marked distress and impaired social or occupational function, and lasts for more than a month.

Generalized Anxiety Disorder. Lacks a specific traumatic event or focus for concern. Excessive anxiety and worry are hard to control and generalize to a number of events or activities. At least three of the following symptoms are associated: (1) feeling restless, keyed up, or on edge; (2) being easily fatigued; (3) difficulty in concentrating or mind going blank; (4) irritability; (5) muscle tension; and (6) difficulty in falling or staying asleep, or restless, unsatisfying sleep. Causes significant distress or impairs daily function.

TABLE 5-4 | **Selected Psychotic Disorder**

Schizophrenia. Impairs major functioning at work or school, in interpersonal relations, or in self-care. Performance of one or more of these functions must decrease for a significant time to a level markedly below prior achievement. Person displays at least two of the following for a significant part of 1 month: (1) delusions; (2) hallucinations; (3) disorganized speech; (4) grossly disorganized or catatonic behavior; and (5) negative symptoms such as a flat affect, alogia (lack of content in speech), or avolition (lack of interest, drive, and ability to set and pursue goals). Continuous signs of the disturbance must persist for at least 6 months.

Subtypes of this disorder include paranoid, disorganized, and catatonic schizophrenia.

Schizophreniform Disorder. Symptoms are similar to those of schizophrenia but last <6 months. Functional impairment need not be present.

Schizoaffective Disorder. Features both a major mood disturbance and schizophrenia. Mood disturbance (depressive, manic, or mixed) present during most of the illness and must, for a time, be concurrent with symptoms of schizophrenia and demonstrate delusions or hallucinations for at least 2 weeks without prominent mood symptoms.

Delusional Disorder. Nonbizarre delusions involve situations in real life, such as having a disease, and persists for at least a month. Functioning is not markedly impaired and behavior is not obviously odd or bizarre. Symptoms of schizophrenia, except for tactile and olfactory hallucinations, are not present.

Brief Psychotic Disorder. At least one of the following psychotic symptoms must be present: delusions, hallucinations, disordered speech such as frequent derailment or incoherence, or grossly disorganized or catatonic behavior. Disturbance lasts ≥1 day but <1 month, and person returns to prior functional level.

The Skin, Hair, and Nails

6

THE HEALTH HISTORY

Common or Concerning Symptoms

- Hair loss
- Rash
- Moles

HEALTH PROMOTION AND COUNSELING

Important Topics for Health Promotion and Counseling

- Risk factors for melanoma
- Avoidance of excessive sun exposure

Counsel patient to avoid unnecessary sun exposure and to use sunscreen with at least SPF-15. Teach the ABCD screen for dysplastic nevi/melanomas: **A**symmetry, irregular **B**orders, variation in **C**olor, and **D**iameter >6 mm. Survey skin at 3-year intervals for patients 20 to 40 years of age and annually for patients older than 40 years.

TECHNIQUES OF EXAMINATION

EXAMINATION TECHNIQUES	POSSIBLE FINDINGS

SKIN

Examine the entire skin surface under good lighting. **Inspect** and **palpate** each area.

Note:

● Color	Cyanosis, jaundice, carotenemia, changes in melanin
● Moisture	Dry, oily
● Temperature	Cool, warm
● Texture	Smooth, rough
● Mobility—ease with which a fold of skin can be moved	Decreased in edema
● Turgor—speed with which the fold returns into place	Decreased in dehydration

Note any lesions and their

● Anatomical location and distribution	Generalized, localized
● Patterns and shapes	Linear, clustered, dermatomal
● Type	Macule, papule, pustule, bulla, tumor
● Color	Red, white, brown, heliotrope

EXAMINATION TECHNIQUES	POSSIBLE FINDINGS

HAIR

Inspect and **palpate** the hair.

Note

● Quantity	Thin, thick
● Distribution	Patchy or total alopecia
● Texture	Fine, coarse

NAILS

Inspect and **palpate** the fingernails and toenails.

Note

● Color	Cyanosis, pallor
● Shape	Clubbing
● Any lesions	Paronychia, onycholysis

RECORDING YOUR FINDINGS

Recording the Physical Examination— The Skin, Hair, and Nails

"Color good. Skin warm and moist. Nails without clubbing or cyanosis. No suspicious nevi, rash, petechiae, or ecchymoses."

AIDS TO INTERPRETATION

TABLE 6-1 Color Changes in the Skin

Color/Mechanism	Selected Causes
Brown: Increased melanin (greater than a person's genetic norm)	Sun exposure Pregnancy (melasma) Addison's disease
Blue (cyanosis): Increased deoxyhemoglobin from hypoxia: • Peripheral • Central (arterial)	 Anxiety or cold environment Heart or lung disease
Abnormal hemoglobin	Methemoglobinemia, sulfhemoglobinemia
Red: Increased visibility of oxyhemoglobin from: • Dilated superficial blood vessels or increased blood flow in skin • Decreased use of oxygen in skin	 Fever, blushing, alcohol intake, local inflammation Cold exposure (e.g., cold ears)
Yellow: Increased bilirubin of jaundice (sclera looks yellow)	 Liver disease, hemolysis of red blood cells
Carotenemia (sclera does not look yellow)	Increased carotene intake from yellow fruits and vegetables
Pale: Decreased melanin	 Albinism, vitiligo, tinea versicolor
Decreased visibility of oxyhemoglobin from: • Decreased blood flow to skin • Decreased amount of oxyhemoglobin	 Syncope or shock Anemia
Edema (may mask skin pigments)	Nephrotic syndrome

TABLE 6-2 Primary Skin Lesions

Flat, Nonpalpable Lesions With Changes in Skin Color

Macule—Small flat spot, up to 1.0 cm

Examples: Hemangioma, vitiligo

Patch—Flat spot, 1.0 cm or larger
Example: Café-au-lait spot

Palpable Elevations: Solid Masses

Papule—Up to 1.0 cm
Example: An elevated nevus

Plaque—Elevated superficial lesion 1.0 cm or larger, often formed by coalescence of papules

(table continues next page)

TABLE 6-2 Primary Skin Lesions (continued)

Example: Psoriasis

Nodule—Marble-like lesion larger than 0.5 cm, often deeper and firmer than a papule
Example: Dermatofibroma

Cyst—Nodule filled with expressible material, either liquid or semisolid
Example: Epidermal inclusion cyst

Wheal—A somewhat irregular, relatively transient, superficial area of localized skin edema
Examples: Mosquito bite, hives (urticaria)

(table continues next page)

TABLE 6-2 Primary Skin Lesions (continued)

Palpable Elevations With Fluid-Filled Cavities

Vesicle—Up to 1.0 cm; filled with serous fluid

Example: Herpes simplex

Bulla—1.0 cm or larger; filled with serous fluid

Example: Insect bite

Pustule—Filled with pus

(table continues next page)

TABLE 6-2 Primary Skin Lesions (continued)

Examples: Acne, small pox (impetigo)

Burrow (scabies)—A minute, slightly raised tunnel in the epidermis, commonly found on the finger webs and on the sides of the fingers. It looks like a short (5–15 mm), linear or curved gray line and may end in a tiny vesicle. With a magnifying lens, look for the *burrow* of the mite that causes scabies.

TABLE 6-3 Secondary Skin Lesions

May arise from primary lesions, overtreatment, excess scratching

Scale—A thin flake of dead, exfoliated epidermis

Examples: Ichthyosis, dandruff, dry skin, psoriasis

(table continues next page)

| TABLE 6-3 | **Secondary Skin Lesions** (continued) |

Crust—The dried residue of skin exudates such as serum, pus, or blood
Example: Impetigo

Lichenification—Visible and palpable thickening of the epidermis and roughening of the skin with increased visibility of the normal skin furrows (often from chronic rubbing)
Example: Neurodermatitis

Scars—Connective tissue that arises from injury or disease
Example: Acne

Keloids—Hypertrophic scarring that extends beyond the borders of the initiating injury

(Sources of photos: *Hemangioma, Café-au-Lait Spot, Elevated Nevus, Psoriasis [bottom], Dermatofibroma, Herpes Simplex, Insect Bite [bottom], Impetigo, Lichenification*—Hall JC. Sauer's Manual of Skin Diseases, 9th ed. Philadelphia: Lippincott Williams & Wilkins, 2006; *Vitiligo, Psoriasis [top], Epidermal Inclusion Cyst, Urticaria, Insect Bite [top], Acne, Ichthyosis, Psoriasis, Acne Scar, Keloids*—Goodheart HP. Goodheart's Photoguide of Common Skin Disorders: Diagnosis and Management, 2nd ed. Philadelphia: Lippincott Williams & Wilkins, 2003; *Small Pox*—Ostler HB, Mailbach HI, Hoke AW, Schwab IR. Diseases of the Eye and Skin: A Color Atlas. Philadelphia: Lippincott Williams & Wilkins, 2004.)

TABLE 6-4 Secondary Skin Lesions—Depressed

Erosion—Nonscarring loss of the superficial epidermis; surface is moist but does not bleed
Example: Aphthous stomatitis, moist area after the rupture of a vesicle, as in chickenpox

Excoriation—Linear or punctate erosions caused by scratching
Example: Cat scratches

Fissure—A linear crack in the skin, often resulting from excessive dryness
Example: Athlete's foot

Ulcer—A deeper loss of epidermis and dermis; may bleed and scar
Examples: Stasis ulcer of venous insufficiency, syphilitic chancre

---

*These are secondary lesions (resulting from primary lesions).
(Sources of photos: *Erosion, Excoriation, Fissure*—Goodheart HP. Goodheart's Photoguide of Common Skin Disorders: Diagnosis and Management, 2nd ed. Philadelphia: Lippincott Williams & Wilkins, 2003; *Ulcer*—Hall JC. Sauer's Manual of Skin Diseases, 9th ed. Philadelphia: Lippincott Williams & Wilkins, 2006.)

TABLE 6-5 Vascular and Purpuric Lesions of the Skin

Lesion	Features
CHERRY ANGIOMA	**Appearance:** Bright or ruby red, may become brownish with age; 1–3 mm; round, flat, sometimes raised; may be surrounded by a pale halo **Distribution:** Found on trunk or extremities **Significance:** None; increase in size and number with aging
SPIDER ANGIOMA	**Appearance:** Fiery red; very small to 2 cm; central body, sometimes raised, radiating with erythema **Distribution:** Face, neck, arms, and upper trunk, but almost never below the waist **Significance:** Liver disease, pregnancy, vitamin B deficiency; normal in some people
SPIDER VEIN	**Appearance:** Bluish; varies from very small to several inches; may resemble a spider or be linear, irregular, or cascading **Distribution:** Most often on the legs, near veins; also on anterior chest **Significance:** Often accompanies increased pressure in the superficial veins, as in varicose veins
PETECHIA AND PURPURA	**Appearance:** Deep red or reddish purple; fades over time; 1–3 mm or larger; rounded, sometimes irregular, flat **Distribution:** Varies **Significance:** Blood outside the vessels; may suggest a bleeding disorder or, if petechiae, emboli to skin

(table continues next page)

TABLE 6-5	**Vascular and Purpuric Lesions of the Skin** (continued)

Lesion	Features
ECCHYMOSIS 	**Appearance:** Purple or purplish blue, fading to green, yellow, and brown over time; larger than petechiae; rounded, oval, or irregular **Distribution:** Varies **Significance:** Blood outside the vessels; often secondary to bruising or trauma; also seen in bleeding disorders

TABLE 6-6	**Skin Tumors**

Actinic Keratoses Superficial, flattened papules covered by a dry scale. Often multiple; may be round or irregular; pink, tan, or grayish. They appear on sun-exposed skin of older, fair-skinned persons. Though benign, 1 out of 1,000 per year develop into *squamous cell carcinoma* (suggested by rapid growth, induration, redness at the base, and ulceration). Typically on face and hands.

Seborrheic Keratoses Common, benign, yellowish to brown, raised lesions that feel slightly greasy and velvety or warty; have a "stuck-on" appearance. Typically multiple and symmetrically distributed on the trunk of older people, but also on the face and elsewhere.

(table continues next page)

TABLE 6-6 Skin Tumors (continued)

In blacks, may appear as small, deeply pigmented papules on cheeks and temples (dermatosis papulosa nigra).

Basal Cell Carcinoma Though malignant, grows slowly and seldom metastasizes. Most common in fair-skinned adults ≥ age 40; usually on the face. Initial translucent nodule spreads, leaving depressed center and firm elevated border. Telangiectatic vessels often visible.

Squamous Cell Carcinoma Usually on sun-exposed skin of fair-skinned adults ≥ age 60. May develop in an actinic keratosis. Usually grows more quickly than a basal cell carcinoma, is firmer, and looks redder. The face and the back of the hand are often affected.

Kaposi's Sarcoma in AIDS May appear in many forms: macules, papules, plaques, or nodules almost anywhere on the body. Lesions are often multiple and may involve internal structures.

TABLE 6-7 Characteristics of Nevi (Moles)

Normal

Diameter smaller than 6 mm
Symmetric; regular borders; even in
color

Malignant Melanoma: "ABCD"

Asymmetric

Borders irregular

Color varied
Diameter more than 6 mm

(Courtesy of American Cancer Society; American Academy of Dermatology)

TABLE 6-8 **Hair Loss**

Alopecia Areata
Clearly demarcated round or oval patches of hair loss, usually affecting young adults and children. There is no visible scaling or inflammation.

Trichotillomania
Hair loss from pulling, plucking, or twisting hair. Hair shafts are broken and of varying lengths. More common in children, often in settings of family or psychosocial stress.

(table continues next page)

TABLE 6-8 Hair Loss (continued)

Tinea Capitis ("Ringworm")
Round scaling patches of alopecia. Hairs are broken off close to the surface of the scalp. Usually caused by fungal infection from *tinea tonsurans*. Mimics seborrheic dermatitis.

(Sources of photos: *Alopecia Areata [top], Trichotillomania [top]*—Hall JC. Sauer's Manual of Skin Diseases, 9th ed. Philadelphia: Lippincott Williams & Wilkins, 2006; *Alopecia Areata [bottom], Tinea Capitis*—Goodheart HP. Goodheart's Photoguide of Common Skin Disorders: Diagnosis and Management, 2nd ed. Philadelphia: Lippincott Williams & Wilkins, 2003; *Trichotillomania [bottom]*—Ostler HB, Mailbach HI, Hoke AW, Schwab IR. Diseases of the Eye and Skin: A Color Atlas. Philadelphia: Lippincott Williams & Wilkins, 2004.)

TABLE 6-9 Fingernails

Clubbing	Dorsal phalanx rounded and bulbous; convexity of nail plate increased. Angle between plate and proximal nail fold increased to 180° or more. Proximal nail folds feel spongy. Many causes, including chronic hypoxia and lung cancer.
Paronychia	Inflammation of proximal and lateral nail folds, acute or chronic. Folds red, swollen, may be tender.

(table continues next page)

TABLE 6-9 **Fingernails (continued)**

Onycholysis

Painless separation of nail plate from nail bed, starting distally. Many causes.

Terry's Nails

Whitish with a distal band of reddish brown. Seen in aging and some chronic diseases.

Leukonychia

White spots caused by trauma. They grow out with nail(s).

Transverse White Lines

Curved white lines similar to curve of lunula. They follow an illness and grow out with nails.

The Head and Neck

7

THE HEALTH HISTORY

Common or Concerning Symptoms

• Headache	• Vertigo
• Change in vision	• Nosebleed, or epistaxis
• Double vision, or diplopia	• Sore throat, hoarseness
• Hearing loss, earache,	• Swollen glands
tinnitus	• Goiter

THE HEAD

Headache is a common symptom that always requires careful evaluation because a small fraction of headaches arise from life-threatening conditions. Elicit a full description of the headache and all seven attributes of the patient's pain (see p. 41).

See Table 7-1, Primary Headaches, p. 125, and Table 7-2, Secondary Headaches, pp. 126–127. *Tension* and *migraine headaches* are the most common recurring headaches.

Is the headache one-sided or bilateral? Steady or throbbing? Continuous or comes and goes? Ask the patient to *point to the area of pain or discomfort.* Assess *chronologic pattern* and *severity.*

Tension headaches often arise in the temporal areas; cluster headaches may be retro-orbital.

Changing or progressively severe headaches increase the likelihood of *tumor, abscess,* or other *mass lesion.* Extremely severe headaches suggest *subarachnoid hemorrhage* or *meningitis.*

Ask about associated symptoms. Inquire specifically about associated nausea and vomiting and neurologic symptoms such as change in vision or motor-sensory deficits.

Visual aura or scintillating scotomas may accompany *migraine.* Nausea and vomiting are common with migraine but also occur with *brain tumor* and *subarachnoid hemorrhage.*

Ask whether coughing, sneezing, or changing the position of the head has any effect (better, worse, or none) on the headache.

Such maneuvers may increase pain from brain tumor and acute sinusitis.

Ask about family history.

Family history is often positive in patients with migraine.

THE EYES

Ask "How is your vision?" and "Have you had any trouble with your eyes?" If the patient reports a change in vision, pursue the related details:

Gradual blurring, often from refractive errors; also in hyperglycemia.

• Is the onset sudden or gradual?

Sudden visual loss suggests *retinal detachment, vitreous hemorrhage,* or *occlusion of the central retinal artery.*

• Is the problem worse during close work or at distances?

Difficulty with close work suggests *hyperopia* (farsightedness) or *presbyopia* (aging vision); difficulty with distances suggests *myopia* (near-sightedness).

● Is there blurring of the entire field of vision or only parts? Is blurring central, peripheral, or only on one side?

Slow central loss in *nuclear cataract* and *macular degeneration*; peripheral loss in advanced *open-angle glaucoma*; one-sided loss in *hemianopsia* and quadrantic defects (p. 129).

● Has the patient seen lights flashing across the field of vision? Vitreous floaters?

These symptoms suggest detachment of vitreous from retina. Prompt eye consultation is indicated.

Ask about *pain* in or around the eyes, *redness,* and *excessive tearing* or *watering.*

Check for *diplopia,* or double vision.

Diplopia in brainstem or cerebellar lesions, also from weakness or paralysis of one or more extraocular muscles.

THE EARS

Ask "How is your hearing?"

See Table 7-8, Patterns of Hearing Loss, p. 135.

Does the patient have special difficulty understanding people as they talk? What difference does a noisy environment make?

Sensorineural loss leads to difficulty understanding speech, and complaints that others mumble; noisy environments worsen hearing. In *conductive loss,* noisy environments may help.

For complaints of *earache,* or *pain in the ear,* ask about associated fever, sore throat, cough, and concurrent upper respiratory infection.

Otitis externa if pain in the external ear; *otitis media* if pain associated with respiratory infection and in inner ear.

Tinnitus has no external stimulus—commonly, it manifests as a musical ringing or a rushing or roaring noise.

When associated with hearing loss and vertigo, tinnitus suggests *Ménière's disease.*

Ask about *vertigo,* the perception that the patient or the environment is rotating or spinning.

Vertigo in labrynthitis, CN VII lesions, brainstem lesions

THE NOSE AND SINUSES

Rhinorrhea, or drainage from the nose, frequently is associated with *nasal congestion.* Ask further about *sneezing,* watery eyes, and throat discomfort, and also *itching* in the eyes, nose, and throat.

Causes include viral infections, *allergic rhinitis* ("hay fever"), and *vasomotor rhinitis.* Itching favors an allergic cause.

For *epistaxis,* or bleeding from the nose, identify the source carefully—is bleeding from the nose or has the patient coughed up or vomited blood? Assess the site of bleeding, its severity, and associated symptoms.

Local causes of epistaxis include trauma (especially nose picking), inflammation, drying and crusting of the nasal mucosa, tumors, and foreign bodies.

THE MOUTH, THROAT, AND NECK

Sore throat is a frequent complaint. Ask about fever, swollen glands, and any associated cough.

Fever, pharyngeal exudates, and anterior cervical lymphadenopathy, especially without cough, suggest *streptococcal pharyngitis,* or "*strep throat*" (p. 139).

Hoarseness may arise from overuse of the voice, allergies, smoking, or inhaled irritants.

Also present in hypothyroidism, in laryngeal disease, or when extrapharyngeal lesions press on the laryngeal nerves

Assess thyroid function. Ask about *goiter, temperature intolerance,* and *sweating.*	With goiter, thyroid function may be increased, decreased, or normal. Cold intolerance in *hypothyroidism;* heat intolerance, palpitations, and involuntary weight loss in *hyperthyroidism*

HEALTH PROMOTION AND COUNSELING

Important Topics for Health Promotion and Counseling

- Changes in vision: cataracts, macular degeneration, glaucoma
- Hearing loss
- Oral health

Disorders of vision shift with age. Healthy young adults generally have refractive errors. Up to 25% of adults older than 65 years have refractive errors; *cataracts, macular degeneration,* and *glaucoma* also become more prevalent. Glaucoma is the leading cause of blindness in African-Americans and the second leading cause of blindness overall. Glaucoma causes gradual vision loss, with damage to the optic nerve, loss of visual fields, beginning usually at the periphery, and pallor and increasing size of the optic cup (enlarging to more than half the diameter of the optic disc).

More than one third of adults older than 65 years have *detectable hearing deficits.* Questionnaires and handheld audioscopes work well for periodic screening.

Be sure to promote *oral health:* up to half of all children 5 to 17 years of age have one to eight cavities, and the average U.S. adult has 10 to 17 decayed, missing, or filled teeth. More than half of all adults older than 65 years have no teeth! Inspect the oral cavity for decayed or loose teeth, inflammation of the gingiva, and signs of periodontal disease (bleeding, pus, receding gums, and bad breath). Counsel patients to use fluoride-containing toothpastes, brush, floss, and seek dental care at least annually.

TECHNIQUES OF EXAMINATION

EXAMINATION TECHNIQUES	POSSIBLE FINDINGS

 ## *THE HEAD*

Examine the

- Hair, including quantity, distribution, and texture — Coarse and sparse in *myxedema,* fine in *hyperthyroidism*

- Scalp, including lumps or lesions — *Pilar cysts, psoriasis,* pigmented nevi

- Skull, including size and contour — *Hydrocephalus,* skull depression from trauma

- Face, including symmetry and facial expression — Facial paralysis; flat affect of depression, moods such as anger, sadness

- Skin, including color, texture, hair distribution, and lesions — Pale, fine, hirsute, acne, skin cancer

THE EYES

Test visual acuity in each eye.   Diminished acuity

Assess visual fields, if indicated.   Hemianopsia, quadrantic defects in cerebrovascular accidents (CVAs)

Inspect the

- Position and alignment of eyes — Exophthalmos, strabismus

- Eyebrows — Seborrheic dermatitis

- Eyelids — Sty, chalazion, ectropion, ptosis, xanthelasma

- Lacrimal apparatus — Swollen lacrimal sac

EXAMINATION TECHNIQUES	POSSIBLE FINDINGS

- Conjunctiva and sclera

Red eye, jaundice

- Cornea, iris, and lens

Corneal opacity, cataract

Examine pupils for

- Size, shape, and symmetry

Miosis, mydriasis, anisocoria

- Reactions to light and if these are abnormal

Absent in paralysis of CN III

- The near reaction

Useful in tonic and Argyll Robertson pupils: slows in tonic pupil; absent in Argyll Robertson pupils of syphilis

THE NEAR REACTION

Assess the extraocular muscles by observing

- The corneal reflections from a midline light

Imbalance of extraocular muscles

- The six cardinal directions of gaze

Cranial nerve palsy, strabismus, nystagmus, lid lag of hyperthyroidism

Superior rectus (III)
Lateral rectus (VI)
Inferior rectus (III)

Inferior oblique (III)
Medial rectus (III)
Superior oblique (IV)

Superior rectus (III)
Lateral rectus (VI)
Inferior rectus (III)

- Convergence

Poor in hyperthyroidism

EXAMINATION TECHNIQUES	POSSIBLE FINDINGS

Inspect the fundi with an ophthalmoscope.

TIPS FOR USING THE OPHTHALMOSCOPE

- Darken the room. Turn the lens disc to the large round beam of white light. *Lower the brightness of the light beam* to make the examination more comfortable for the patient.
- Turn the lens disc to the 0 diopter (a diopter measures the power of a lens to converge or diverge light).
- Hold the ophthalmoscope *in your right hand* to examine *the patient's right eye;* hold it *in your left hand* to examine *the patient's left eye* to avoid bumping the patient's nose.
- Brace the ophthalmoscope firmly against the medial aspect of your bony orbit, with the handle tilted laterally at about 20°. Instruct the patient to look slightly up and over your shoulder at a point directly ahead on the wall.
- Place yourself about 15 inches away from the patient and *at an angle 15° lateral to the patient's line of vision.* Look for the orange glow in the pupil—the *red reflex.* Note any opacities interrupting the red reflex. No red reflex suggests an opacity of the lens (cataract) or possibly the vitreous.
- Place the thumb of your other hand across the patient's eyebrow. Keeping the light beam focused on the red reflex, move in at a 15° angle toward the pupil until you almost touch the patient's eyelashes. Adjust the position of your ophthalmoscope and angle of vision *as a unit* until you see the fundus.

Inspect the fundi for the following:

• Red reflex	Cataracts, artificial eye
• Optic disc	Papilledema, glaucomatous cupping, optic atrophy. See Table 7-5, Abnormalities of the Optic Disc, p. 132.

EXAMINATION TECHNIQUES   POSSIBLE FINDINGS

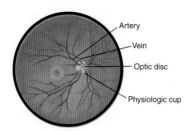

- Arteries, veins, and A–V crossings

  A–V nicking, copper wiring in hypertensive changes

- Adjacent retina (note any lesions)

  Hemorrhages, exudates, cotton-wool patches, microaneurysms, pigmentation

- Macular area

  Macular degeneration

- Anterior structures

  Vitreous floaters, cataracts

TIPS FOR EXAMINING THE OPTIC DISC AND THE RETINA

- *Locate the optic disc.* Look for the round yellowish-orange structure.
- Now, *bring the optic disc into sharp focus* by adjusting the lens of your ophthalmoscope.
- *Inspect the optic disc.* Note the following features:
  - *The sharpness or clarity of the disc outline*
  - *The color of the disc*
  - *The size of the physiologic cup* (an enlarged cup suggests chronic open-angle glaucoma)

(*continued*)

EXAMINATION TECHNIQUES   POSSIBLE FINDINGS

TIPS FOR EXAMINING THE OPTIC DISC AND THE RETINA (CONTINUED)

- *Venous pulsations* in the retinal veins as they emerge from the central portion of the disc (loss of venous pulsations in pathologic conditions such as head trauma, meningitis, or mass lesions may be an early sign of elevated intracranial pressure)
- *Inspect the retina.* Distinguish arteries from veins based on the features listed below.

	Arteries	Veins
Color	Light red	Dark red
Size	Smaller (⅔ to ⅘ the diameter of veins)	Larger
Light Reflex (reflection)	Bright	Inconspicuous or absent

- *Follow the vessels peripherally in each of four directions.*
- Inspect the *fovea* and surrounding *macula*. Macular degeneration types include *dry atrophic* (more common but less severe) and *wet exudative* (neovascular). Undigested cellular debris, called *drusen,* may be hard or soft.
- Assess for any *papilledema*.

THE EARS

Examine on each side:

THE AURICLE

Inspect the auricle.   Keloid, epidermoid cyst

If you suspect otitis:

- Move the auricle up and down, and press on the tragus.   Pain in otitis externa ("the tug test")

EXAMINATION TECHNIQUES	POSSIBLE FINDINGS

● Press firmly behind the ear.

Possible tenderness in otitis media and mastoiditis

THE EAR CANAL AND EARDRUM

Pull the auricle up, back, and slightly out.

Inspect, through an otoscope speculum:

● The canal

Cerumen; swelling and erythema in otitis externa

● The eardrum

Red bulging drum in acute otitis media; serous otitis media, tympanosclerosis, perforations. See Table 7-7, Abnormal Eardrum, p. 134.

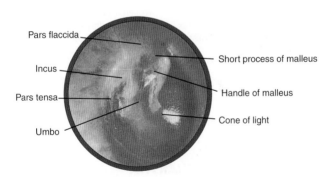

Pars flaccida
Incus
Pars tensa
Umbo
Short process of malleus
Handle of malleus
Cone of light

HEARING

Assess auditory acuity to whispered or spoken voice.

If hearing is diminished, use a 512-Hz tuning fork to:

These tests help distinguish between sensorineural and conduction hearing loss.

EXAMINATION TECHNIQUES	POSSIBLE FINDINGS
• Test *lateralization* (**Weber test**). Place vibrating and tuning fork on vertex of skull and check hearing.	See Table 7-8, Patterns of Hearing Loss, p. 135.
• Compare *air and bone conduction* (**Rinne test**). Place vibrating and tuning fork on mastoid bone, then remove and check hearing.	

THE NOSE AND SINUSES

Inspect the external nose.

Inspect, through a speculum, the

• Nasal mucosa that covers the septum and turbinates, noting its color and any swelling	Swollen and red in viral rhinitis, swollen and pale in allergic rhinitis; polyps; ulcer from cocaine use
• Nasal septum for position and integrity	Deviation, perforation

Palpate the frontal and maxillary sinuses.

Tender in acute sinusitis

THE MOUTH AND PHARYNX

Inspect the

• Lips	Cyanosis, pallor, cheilosis
• Oral mucosa	Canker sores
• Gums	Gingivitis, periodontal disease
• Teeth	Dental caries, tooth loss

EXAMINATION TECHNIQUES	POSSIBLE FINDINGS
• Roof of the mouth	Torus palatinus
• Tongue, including	See Table 7-10, Abnormalities of the Tongue, pp. 137–138.
Papillae	Glossitis
Symmetry	Deviation to one side from paralysis of CN XII from CVA
Any lesions	Cancer
• Floor of the mouth	Cancer
• Pharynx, including	See Table 7-11, Abnormalities of the Pharynx, p. 139.
Color or any exudate	Pharyngitis
Presence and size of tonsils	Tonsillitis, peritonsillar abscess
Symmetry of the soft palate as patient says "ah"	Soft palate fails to rise in paralysis of CN X from CVA

THE NECK

Inspect the neck.	Scars, masses, torticollis
Palpate the lymph nodes.	Cervical lymphadenopathy from inflammation, malignancy, HIV
Inspect and **palpate** the position of the trachea.	Deviated trachea from neck mass or pneumothorax
Inspect the thyroid gland:	
• At rest	Goiter, nodules. See Table 7-12, Abnormalities of the Thyroid Gland, p. 140.
• As patient swallows water	

EXAMINATION TECHNIQUES | POSSIBLE FINDINGS

From behind patient, **palpate** the thyroid gland, including the isthmus and the lateral lobes:

Goiter, nodules, tenderness of thyroiditis

- At rest

- As patient swallows water

After examining the thyroid gland from behind the patient, you may proceed to musculoskeletal examination of the neck and upper back and check for costovertebral angle tenderness.

RECORDING YOUR FINDINGS

Recording the Physical Examination—The Head, Eyes, Ears, Nose, and Throat (HEENT)

HEENT: Head—Skull is normocephalic/atraumatic (NC/AT). Hair with average texture. *Eyes*—Visual acuity 20/20 bilaterally. Sclera white; conjunctiva pink. Pupils constrict 4 mm to 2 mm, equally round and reactive to light and accommodations. Disc margins sharp; no hemorrhages or exudates; no arteriolar narrowing. *Ears*—Acuity good to whispered voice. Tympanic membranes (TMs) with good cone of light. Weber midline. AC > BC. *Nose*—Nasal mucosa pink, septum midline; no sinus tenderness. *Throat (or Mouth)*—Oral mucosa pink; dentition good; pharynx without exudates. *Neck*—Trachea midline. Neck supple; thyroid isthmus palpable, lobes not felt. *Lymph Nodes*—No cervical, axillary, epitrochlear, inguinal adenopathy.

AIDS TO INTERPRETATION

TABLE 7-1 Primary Headaches

Problem	Common Characteristics	Associated Symptoms, With Provoking and Relieving Factors
Tension	**Location:** Variable **Quality:** Pressing or tightening pain; mild to moderate intensity **Onset:** Gradual **Duration:** Minutes to days	Sometimes photophobia, phonophobia; nausea absent ↑ by sustained muscle tension, as in driving or typing ↓ possibly by massage, relaxation
Migraine • *With aura* • *Without aura* • *Variants*	**Location:** Unilateral in ~70%; bifrontal or global in ~30% **Quality:** Throbbing or aching, variable in severity **Onset:** Fairly rapid, reaching a peak in 1–2 hrs **Duration:** 4–72 hrs	Nausea, vomiting, photophobia, phonophobia, visual auras (flickering zigzagging lines), motor auras affecting hand or arm, sensory auras (numbness, tingling usually precede headache) ↑ by alcohol, certain foods, or tension, noise, bright light. More common premenstrually. ↓ by quiet dark room, sleep
Cluster	**Location:** Unilateral, usually behind or around the eye **Quality:** Deep, continuous, severe **Onset:** Abrupt, peaks within minutes **Duration:** Up to 3 hrs	Lacrimation, rhinorrhea, miosis, ptosis, eyelid edema, conjunctival infection ↑ sensitivity to alcohol during some episodes

TABLE 7-2 Secondary Headaches

Problem	Common Characteristics	Associated Symptoms, With Provoking and Relieving Factors
Analgesic Rebound	**Location:** Previous headache pattern **Quality:** Variable **Onset:** Variable **Duration:** Depends on prior headache pattern	Depends on prior headache pattern ↑ by fever, carbon monoxide, hypoxia, withdrawal of caffeine, other headache triggers ↓ —depends on cause
Headaches From Eye Disorders Errors of Refraction (farsightedness and astigmatism, but not nearsightedness)	**Location:** Around and over the eyes; may radiate to the occipital area **Quality:** Steady, aching, dull **Onset:** Gradual **Duration:** Variable	Eye fatigue, "sandy" sensation in eyes, redness of the conjunctiva ↑ by prolonged use of the eyes, particularly for close work ↓ by rest of the eyes
Acute Glaucoma	**Location:** In and around one eye **Quality:** Steady, aching, often severe **Onset:** Often rapid **Duration:** Variable, may depend on treatment	Diminished vision, sometimes nausea and vomiting ↑ —sometimes by drops that dilate the pupils
Headache from Sinusitis	**Location:** Usually above eye (frontal sinus) or over maxillary sinus	Local tenderness, nasal congestion, discharge, and fever ↑ by coughing, sneezing, or jarring the head

(table continues next page)

TABLE 7-2 Secondary Headaches (continued)

Problem	Common Characteristics	Associated Symptoms, With Provoking and Relieving Factors
	Quality: Aching or throbbing, variable in severity; consider possible migraine **Onset:** Variable **Duration:** Often several hours at a time, recurring over days or longer	↓ by nasal decongestants, antibiotics
Meningitis	**Location:** Generalized **Quality:** Steady or throbbing, very severe **Onset:** Fairly rapid **Duration:** Variable, usually days	Fever, stiff neck
Subarachnoid Hemorrhage	**Location:** Generalized **Quality:** Severe, "the worst of my life" **Onset:** Usually abrupt; prodromal symptoms may occur **Duration:** Variable, usually days	Nausea, vomiting, possibly loss of consciousness, neck pain
Brain Tumor	**Location:** Varies with the location of the tumor **Quality:** Aching, steady, variable in intensity	↑ by coughing, sneezing, or sudden movements of the head

(table continues next page)

TABLE 7-2 Secondary Headaches (continued)

Problem	Common Characteristics	Associated Symptoms, With Provoking and Relieving Factors
	Onset: Variable **Duration:** Often brief	
Cranial Neuralgias: Trigeminal Neuralgia (CN V)	**Location:** Cheek, jaws, lips, or gums; trigeminal nerve divisions 2 and 3 >1 **Quality:** Shocklike, stabbing, burning, severe **Onset:** Abrupt, paroxysmal **Duration:** Each jab lasts seconds but recurs at intervals of seconds or minutes	Exhaustion from recurrent pain ↑ by touching certain areas of the lower face or mouth; chewing, talking, brushing teeth
Giant Cell (Temporal) Arteritis	**Location:** Near the involved artery, often the temporal, also the occipital; age-related **Quality:** Throbbing, generalized, persistent, often severe **Onset:** Gradual or rapid **Duration:** Variable	Tenderness of the adjacent scalp; fever (in ~50%), fatigue, weight loss; new headache (~60%), jaw claudication (~50%), visual loss or blindness (~15%–20%), polymyalgia rheumatica (~50%) ↑ by movement of neck and shoulders

(table continues next page)

TABLE 7-2 Secondary Headaches (continued)

Problem	Common Characteristics	Associated Symptoms, With Provoking and Relieving Factors
Post-traumatic Headache	**Location:** Injured area, but not necessarily **Quality:** Generalized, dull, aching, constant **Onset:** Within hours to 1–2 days of the injury **Duration:** Weeks, months, or even years	Poor concentration, problems with memory, vertigo, irritability, restlessness, fatigue ↑ by mental and physical exertion, straining, stooping, emotional excitement, alcohol ↓ by rest

TABLE 7-3 Visual Field Defects

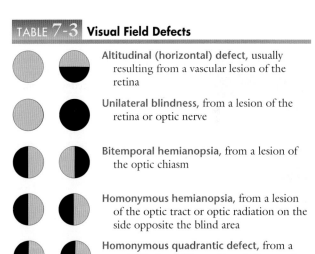

Altitudinal (horizontal) defect, usually resulting from a vascular lesion of the retina

Unilateral blindness, from a lesion of the retina or optic nerve

Bitemporal hemianopsia, from a lesion of the optic chiasm

Homonymous hemianopsia, from a lesion of the optic tract or optic radiation on the side opposite the blind area

Homonymous quadrantic defect, from a partial lesion of the optic radiation on the side opposite the blind area

LEFT   **RIGHT**

(*from patient's viewpoint*)

TABLE 7-4 **Physical Findings in and Around the Eye**

Eyelids

Ptosis. A drooping upper eyelid that narrows the palpebral fissure from a muscle or nerve disorder

Ectropion. Outward turning of the margin of the lower lid, exposing the palpebral conjunctiva

Entropion. Inward turning of the lid margin, causing irritation of the cornea or conjunctiva

In and Around the Eye

Pinguecula. Harmless yellowish nodule in the bulbar conjunctiva on either side of the iris; associated with aging

Episcleritis. A localized ocular redness from inflammation of the episcleral vessels

(table continues next page)

TABLE 7-4 **Physical Findings in and Around the Eye** (continued)

Sty. A pimple-like infection around a hair follicle near the lid margin

Chalazion. A beady nodule in either eyelid caused by a chronically inflamed meibomian gland

TABLE 7-5 Abnormalities of the Optic Disc

	Process	Appearance
Normal	Tiny disc vessels give normal color to the disc.	Disc is yellowish orange to creamy pink. Disc vessels are tiny. Disc margins are sharp (except perhaps nasally).
Papilledema	Venous stasis leads to engorgement and swelling.	Disc is pink, hyperemic. Disc vessels are more visible, more numerous, and curve over the borders of the disc. Disc is swollen, with margins blurred.
Glaucomatous Cupping	Increased pressure within the eye leads to increased cupping (backward depression of the disc) and atrophy.	The base of the enlarged cup is pale.
Optic Atrophy	Death of optic nerve fibers leads to loss of the tiny disc vessels.	Disc is white. Disc vessels are absent.

TABLE 7-6 Diabetic Retinopathy

Nonproliferative Retinopathy, Moderately Severe	Note tiny red dots or microaneurysms, also the ring of hard exudates (white spots) located superotemporally. Retinal thickening or edema in the area of hard exudates can impair visual acuity if it extends to center of macula (detection requires specialized stereoscopic examination).
Nonproliferative Retinopathy, Severe	In superior temporal quadrant, note large retinal hemorrhage between two cotton-wool patches, beading of the retinal vein just above, and tiny tortuous retinal vessels above superior temporal artery, termed *intraretinal microvascular abnormalities.*
Proliferative Retinopathy, With Neovascularization	Note new preretinal vessels arising on disc and extending across disc margins. Visual acuity is currently normal, but risk of severe visual loss is high. (Photocoagulation can reduce this risk ≥50%.)
Proliferative Retinopathy, Advanced	Same eye as above, but 2 yrs later and without treatment. Neovascularization has increased, now with fibrous proliferations, distortion of macula, and reduced visual acuity.

(Source: Early Treatment Diabetic Retinopathy Study Research Group. Courtesy of M. F. Davis, MD, University of Wisconsin, Madison.)

TABLE 7-7 **Abnormal Eardrum**

Perforation

Hole in the eardrum that may be central or marginal
Usually from *otitis media* or trauma

Tympanosclerosis

A chalky white patch
Scar of an old otitis media; of little or no clinical consequence

Serous Effusion

Amber fluid behind the eardrum, with or without air bubbles
Associated with viral upper respiratory infections or sudden changes in atmospheric pressure (diving, flying)

Acute Otitis Media

Red, bulging drum, loss of landmarks
Associated with bacterial infection

TABLE 7-8 Patterns of Hearing Loss

	Conductive Loss	Sensorineural Loss
Impaired understanding of words	Minor	Often troublesome
Effect of noisy environment	May help	Increases the hearing difficulty
Usual age of onset	Childhood, young adulthood	Middle and old age
Ear canal and drum	Often a visible abnormality	Problem not visible
Weber test (in unilateral hearing loss)	Lateralizes to the impaired ear	Lateralizes to the good ear
Rinne test	BC > AC or BC = AC	AC > BC
Causes include	Plugged ear canal, *otitis media,* immobile or perforated drum, otosclerosis, foreign body	Sustained loud noise, drugs, inner ear infections, trauma, hereditary disorder, aging

TABLE 7-9 Abnormalities of the Lips

Angular cheilitis. Softening and cracking of the angles of the mouth

Herpes simplex. Painful vesicles, followed by crusting; also called **cold sore** or **fever blister**

Angioedema. Diffuse, tense, subcutaneous swelling, usually allergic in cause

Hereditary hemorrhagic telangiectasia. Red spots, significant because of associated bleeding from nose and GI tract

Peutz-Jeghers syndrome. Brown spots of the lips and buccal mucosa, significant because of their association with intestinal polyposis

Syphilitic chancre. A firm lesion that ulcerates and may crust

Carcinoma of the lip. A thickened plaque or irregular nodule that may ulcerate or crust; malignant

TABLE 7-10 Abnormalities of the Tongue

Geographic tongue. Scattered areas in which the papillae are lost, giving a maplike appearance; harmless

Hairy tongue. Results from elongated papillae that may look yellowish, brown, or black; harmless

Fissured tongue. May appear with aging; harmless

Smooth tongue. Results from loss of papillae, caused by vitamin B or iron deficiency or possibly anticancer drugs

Candida infection. May show a thick, white coat, which, when scraped off, leaves a raw red surface; tongue may also be red; antibiotics, corticosteroids, AIDS may predispose

Hairy leukoplakia. White raised, feathery areas, usually on sides of tongue. Seen in HIV/AIDS

(table continues next page)

TABLE 7-10 Abnormalities of the Tongue (continued)

 Varicose veins. Dark round spots in the undersurface of the tongue, associated with aging; also called **caviar lesions**

 Aphthous ulcer (canker sore). Painful, small, whitish ulcer with a red halo; heals in 7–10 days

 Mucous patch of syphilis. Slightly raised, oval lesion, covered by a grayish membrane

 Carcinoma of the tongue or floor of the mouth. A malignancy that should be considered in any nodule or nonhealing ulcer at the base or edges of the mouth

TABLE 7-11   Abnormalities of the Pharynx

Pharyngitis, mild to moderate. Note redness and vascularity of the pillars and uvula.

Pharyngitis, diffuse. Note redness is diffuse and intense. Cause may be viral or, if patient has fever, bacterial. If patient has no fever, exudate, or cervical lymphadenopathy, viral infection is more likely.

Exudative pharyngitis. A sore red throat with patches of white exudate on the tonsils is associated with streptococcal pharyngitis and some viral illnesses.

Diphtheria. An acute infection caused by *Corynebacterium diphtheriae.* The throat is dull red, and a gray exudate appears on the uvula, pharynx, and tongue.

Koplik's spots. These small white specks that resemble grains of salt on a red background are an early sign of measles.

TABLE 7-12 Abnormalities of the Thyroid Gland

Diffuse enlargement. May result from Graves' disease, Hashimoto's thyroiditis, endemic goiter (iodine deficiency), or sporadic goiter

Multinodular goiter. An enlargement with two or more identifiable nodules, usually metabolic in cause

Single nodule. May result from a cyst, a benign tumor, or cancer of the thyroid, or may be one palpable nodule in a clinically unrecognized multinodular goiter

The Thorax and Lungs

Common or Concerning Symptoms

- Chest pain
- Shortness of breath (dyspnea)
- Wheezing
- Cough
- Blood-streaked sputum (hemoptysis)

Complaints of *chest pain* or *chest discomfort* raise the specter of heart disease but often arise from conditions in the thorax and lungs. For this important symptom, keep the possible causes below in mind. Also see Table 8-1, Chest Pain, pp. 152–153.

- The myocardium   Angina pectoris, myocardial infarction

- The pericardium   Pericarditis

- The aorta   Dissecting aortic aneurysm

- The trachea and large bronchi   Bronchitis

- The parietal pleura   Pericarditis, pneumonia

- The chest wall, including the musculoskeletal system and skin   Costochondritis, herpes zoster

- The esophagus

Reflux esophagitis, esophageal spasm

- Extrathoracic structures such as the neck, gallbladder, stomach

Cervical arthritis, biliary colic, gastritis

For patients who are *short of breath*, focus on such *pulmonary complaints* as

- dyspnea and wheezing

See Table 8-2, Dyspnea, pp. 154–155.

- cough and hemoptysis

See Table 8-3, Cough and Hemoptysis, pp. 156–159.

HEALTH PROMOTION AND COUNSELING

Despite declines in smoking over the past several decades, ~23% of Americans still smoke.* Regularly counsel all adults, pregnant women, parents, and adolescents who smoke to stop. Include "the five **A's**":

- **A**sk about smoking at each visit,

- **A**dvise patients to quit in regular, clear, personalized messages.

- **A**ssess patient readiness to quit.

- **A**ssist patients to set stop dates and provide educational materials for self-help.

- **A**rrange for follow-up visits to monitor and support progress.

Provide flu shots and pneumonia vaccine in target groups.

---

*Centers for Disease Control (CDC). At A Glance. Targeting tobacco use: The nation's leading cause of death, 2004. Available at: www.cdc.gov/nccdphp/aag/pdf/aag_osh2004.pdf. Accessed September 11, 2007.

TECHNIQUES OF EXAMINATION

EXAMINATION TECHNIQUES   POSSIBLE FINDINGS

SURVEY OF THORAX

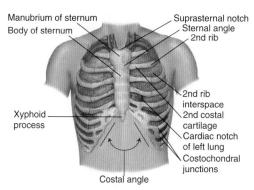

Manubrium of sternum — Suprasternal notch
Body of sternum — Sternal angle
2nd rib
2nd rib interspace
2nd costal cartilage
Xyphoid process — Cardiac notch of left lung
Costochondral junctions
Costal angle

EXAMINATION TECHNIQUES	POSSIBLE FINDINGS
Inspect the thorax and its respiratory movements. **Note:**	
• Rate, rhythm, depth, and effort of breathing	Tachypnea, hyperpnea, Cheyne–Stokes breathing
• Inspiratory retraction of the supraclavicular areas	Occurs in chronic obstructive pulmonary disease (COPD), asthma, upper airway obstruction
• Inspiratory contraction of the sternomastoids	Indicates severe breathing difficulty
Observe shape of patient's chest.	Normal or barrel chest (see Table 8-4, Deformities of the Thorax, pp. 159–160)
Listen to patient's breathing for	
• Rate and rhythm of breathing	14–16 breaths/minute in adults (see Chapter 4, pp. 64–65)

EXAMINATION TECHNIQUES	POSSIBLE FINDINGS

● Stridor

Stridor in upper airway obstruction from foreign body or epiglottitis

● Wheezes

Expiratory wheezing in asthma and COPD

THE POSTERIOR CHEST

Inspect the chest for

● Deformities or asymmetry

Kyphoscoliosis

● Abnormal inspiratory retraction of the interspaces

Retraction in airway obstruction

● Impairment or unilateral lag in respiratory movement

Disease of the underlying lung or pleura, phrenic nerve palsy

Palpate the chest for

● Tender areas

Fractured ribs

● Assessment of visible abnormalities

Masses, sinus tracts

● Chest expansion

Impairment, both sides in COPD and restrictive lung disease

EXAMINATION TECHNIQUES

POSSIBLE FINDINGS

- Tactile fremitus as the patient says "aa" or "blue moon"

Local or generalized decrease or increase

Percuss the chest in the areas illustrated, comparing one side with the other at each level, using the side-to-side "ladder pattern."

Dullness when fluid or solid tissue replaces normally air-filled lung; *hyperresonance* in emphysema or pneumothorax

⬤ Percussion Notes		
	Relative Intensity, Pitch, and Duration	**Examples**
Flatness	Soft/high/short	Large pleural effusion
Dullness	Medium/medium/ medium	Lobar pneumonia
Resonance	Loud/low/long	Normal lung, simple chronic bronchitis
Hyperresonance	Louder/lower/ longer	Emphysema, pneumothorax
Tympany	Loud/high (timbre is musical)	Large pneumothorax

EXAMINATION TECHNIQUES

POSSIBLE FINDINGS

Percuss level of diaphragmatic dullness on each side and **estimate** diaphragmatic descent after patient takes full inspiration.

Pleural effusion or a *paralyzed diaphragm* raises level of dullness.

Location and sequence of percussion

Resonant

Level of diaphragm

Dull

Listen to chest with stethoscope in the "ladder" pattern, again comparing sides.

See Table 8-5, Physical Findings in Selected Chest Disorders, p. 161.

● Evaluate the breath sounds.

Vesicular, bronchovesicular, or bronchial breath sounds; decreased breath sounds from decreased airflow

● Note any adventitious (added) sounds.

Crackles (fine and coarse) and continuous sounds (wheezes and rhonchi)

Observe their qualities, place in the respiratory cycle, and location on the chest wall. Do they clear with deep breathing or coughing?

● Breath Sounds

	Duration	Intensity and Pitch of Expiratory Sound	Example Locations
Vesicular	Insp > exp	Soft/low	Most of the lungs
Bronchovesicular	Insp = exp	Medium/ medium	1st and 2nd interspaces, interscapular area
Bronchial	Exp > insp	Loud/high	Over the manubrium; lobar pneumonia
Tracheal	Insp = exp	Very loud/ high	Over the trachea

Duration is indicated by the length of the line, intensity by the width of the line, and pitch by the slope of the line.

● Adventitious or Added Breath Sounds

Crackles (or Rales)	Wheezes and Rhonchi
● Discontinuous	● Continuous
● Intermittent, nonmusical, and brief	● ≥250 msec, musical, prolonged (but not necessarily persisting throughout the respiratory cycle)
	● Like dashes in time
● Like dots in time	● *Wheezes:* Relatively high-pitched (≥400 Hz) with hissing or shrill quality
● *Fine crackles:* Soft, high-pitched, very brief (5–10 msec)	
	WWWWW
● *Coarse crackles:* Somewhat louder, lower in pitch, brief (20–30 msec)	● *Rhonchi:* Relatively low-pitched (≤200 Hz) with snoring quality
● ● ● ● ●	ᶺᴧᴧᴧ

EXAMINATION TECHNIQUES   POSSIBLE FINDINGS

Assess transmitted voice
sounds if you have heard
bronchial breath sounds
in abnormal places. Ask
patient to

- Say "99" and "ee."   Bronchophony and egophony

- Whisper "99" or "1, 2, 3."   Whispered pectoriloquy

⬤ Transmitted Voice Sounds

Through Normally Air-Filled Lung	**Through Airless Lung***
Spoken words muffled and indistinct	Spoken words louder, clearer (*bronchophony*)
Spoken "ee" heard as "ee"	Spoken "ee" heard as "ay" (*egophony*)
Whispered words faint and indistinct, if heard at all	Whispered words louder, clearer (*whispered pectoriloquy*)
Usually accompanied by vesicular breath sounds and normal tactile fremitus	Usually accompanied by bronchial or bronchovesicular breath sounds and increased tactile fremitus

*As in lobar pneumonia and toward the top of a large pleural effusion

---

While the patient is still sitting, you may inspect
the breasts and examine the axillary and epitrochlear
lymph nodes, and examine the temporomandibular
joint and the musculoskeletal system of the upper
extremities.

EXAMINATION TECHNIQUES   POSSIBLE FINDINGS

THE ANTERIOR CHEST

Midsternal line

Midclavicular line

Anterior axillary line

Anterior axillary line

Midaxillary line

Posterior axillary line

ANTERIOR VIEW   **RIGHT ANTERIOR OBLIQUE VIEW**

Inspect the chest for

● Deformities or asymmetry	Pectus excavatum
● Intercostal retraction	From obstructed airways
● Impaired or lagging respiratory movement	Disease of the underlying lung or pleura, phrenic nerve palsy

Palpate the chest for

● Tender areas	Tender pectoral muscles, costochondritis
● Assessment of visible abnormalities	Flail chest
● Respiratory expansion	
● Tactile fremitus	

Percuss the chest in the areas illustrated.

Normal cardiac dullness may disappear in emphysema.

EXAMINATION TECHNIQUES | POSSIBLE FINDINGS

Listen to the chest with stethoscope. **Note:**

- Breath sounds

- Adventitious sounds

- If indicated, transmitted voice sounds

SPECIAL TECHNIQUES

ASSESSMENT OF PULMONARY FUNCTION

Walk with patient down the hall or up a flight of stairs. Observe rate, effort, and sound of breathing, and inquire about symptoms.

Older adults walking 8 feet in <3 seconds are less likely to be disabled than those taking >5–6 seconds.

FORCED EXPIRATORY TIME

Ask patient to take a deep breath in and then breathe out as quickly and completely as possible, with mouth open. Listen over trachea with diaphragm of stethoscope, and time audible expiration. Try to get three consistent readings, allowing rests as needed.

If the patient understands and cooperates well, a forced expiratory time of 6 to 8 strongly suggests COPD.

EXAMINATION TECHNIQUES

RECORDING YOUR FINDINGS

Recording the Physical Examination—
The Thorax and Lungs

"Thorax is symmetric with good expansion. Lungs resonant. Breath sounds vesicular; no rales, wheezes, or rhonchi. Diaphragms descend 4 cm bilaterally."

OR

"Thorax symmetric with moderate kyphosis and increased anteroposterior (AP) diameter, decreased expansion. Lungs are hyperresonant. Breath sounds distant with delayed expiratory phase and scattered expiratory wheezes. Fremitus decreased; no bronchophony, egophony, or whispered pectoriloquy. Diaphragms descend 2 cm bilaterally."

(Suggests COPD)

AIDS TO INTERPRETATION

TABLE 8-1 Chest Pain

Problem and Location	Quality, Severity, Timing, and Associated Symptoms
Cardiovascular	
Angina Pectoris Retrosternal or across the anterior chest, sometimes radiating to the shoulders, arms, neck, lower jaw, or upper abdomen	**Quality:** Pressing, squeezing, tight, heavy, occasionally burning **Severity:** Mild to moderate, sometimes perceived as discomfort rather than pain **Timing:** Usually 1–3 min but up to 10 min; prolonged episodes up to 20 min **Associated Symptoms:** Sometimes dyspnea, nausea, swelling
Myocardial Infarction Same as in angina	**Quality:** Same as in angina **Severity:** Often but not always a severe pain **Timing:** 20 min to several hours **Associated Symptoms:** Nausea, vomiting, sweating, weakness
Pericarditis *Precordial:* May radiate to the tip of the shoulder and to the neck	**Quality:** Sharp, knifelike **Severity:** Often severe **Timing:** Persistent **Associated Symptoms:** Of the underlying illness; relieved by leaning forward
Retrosternal	**Quality:** Crushing **Severity:** Severe **Timing:** Persistent **Associated Symptoms:** Of the underlying illness
Dissecting Aortic Aneurysm Anterior chest, radiating to the neck, back, or abdomen	**Quality:** Ripping, tearing **Severity:** Very severe **Timing:** Abrupt onset, early peak, persistent for hours or more **Associated Symptoms:** Syncope, hemiplegia, paraplegia

(table continues next page)

TABLE 8-1 Chest Pain (continued)	
Problem and Location	**Quality, Severity, Timing, and Associated Symptoms**

Pulmonary

Tracheobronchitis
Upper sternal or on either side of the sternum

Quality: Burning
Severity: Mild to moderate
Timing: Variable
Associated Symptoms: Cough

Pleural Pain
Chest wall overlying the process

Quality: Sharp, knifelike
Severity: Often severe
Timing: Persistent
Associated Symptoms: Of the underlying illness

Gastrointestinal and Other

Reflex Esophagitis
Retrosternal, may radiate to the back

Quality: Burning, may be squeezing
Severity: Mild to severe
Timing: Variable
Associated Symptoms: Sometimes regurgitation, dysphagia

Diffuse Esophageal Spasm
Retrosternal, may radiate to the back, arms, and jaw

Quality: Usually squeezing
Severity: Mild to severe
Timing: Variable
Associated Symptoms: Dysphagia

Chest Wall Pain
Often below the left breast or along the costal cartilages; also elsewhere

Quality: Stabbing, sticking, or dull aching
Severity: Variable
Timing: Fleeting to hours or days
Associated Symptoms: Often local tenderness

Anxiety/Panic Attack

TABLE 8-2 **Dyspnea**

Problem	Timing	Provoking and Relieving Factors
Left-sided Heart Failure (*left ventricular failure or mitral stenosis*)	Dyspnea may progress slowly or suddenly, as in acute pulmonary edema	↑ by exertion, lying down ↓ by rest, sitting up, though dyspnea may become persistent **Associated Symptoms:** Often cough, orthopnea, paroxysmal nocturnal dyspnea, sometimes wheezing
Chronic Bronchitis (*may be seen with COPD*)	Chronic productive cough followed by slowly progressive dyspnea	↑ by exertion, inhaled irritants, respiratory infections ↓ by expectoration, rest though dyspnea may become persistent **Associated Symptoms:** Chronic productive cough, recurrent respiratory infections; wheezing possible
Chronic Obstructive Pulmonary Disease (COPD)	Slowly progressive; relatively mild cough later	↑ by exertion ↓ by rest, though dyspnea may become persistent **Associated Symptoms:** Cough with scant mucoid sputum
Asthma	Acute episodes, then symptom-free periods; nocturnal episodes common	↑ by allergens, irritants, respiratory infections, exercise, emotion ↓ by separation from aggravating factors **Associated Symptoms:** Wheezing, cough, tightness in chest

(table continues next page)

TABLE 8-2 Dyspnea (continued)		

Problem	Timing	Provoking and Relieving Factors
Acute Pulmonary Embolism	Sudden onset of dyspnea	**Associated Symptoms:** Often none; retrosternal oppressive pain if occlusion is massive; pleuritic pain, cough, and hemoptysis may follow an embolism if pulmonary infarction ensues; symptoms of anxiety
Pneumonia	Acute illness; timing varies with causative agent	**Associated Symptoms:** Pleuritic pain, cough, sputum, fever, though not necessarily present
Diffuse Interstitial Lung Diseases (*sarcoidosis, neoplasms, asbestosis, idiopathic pulmonary fibrosis*)	Progressive; varies in rate of development depending on cause	↑ by exertion ↓ by rest, though dyspnea may become persistent **Associated Symptoms:** Often weakness, fatigue; cough less common than in other lung diseases
Spontaneous Pneumothorax	Sudden onset of dyspnea	**Associated Symptoms:** Pleuritic pain, cough

TABLE 8-3 Cough and Hemoptysis

Problem	Cough, Sputum, Associated Symptoms, and Setting
Acute Inflammation	
Laryngitis	**Cough and Sputum:** Dry, or with variable amounts of sputum **Associated Symptoms and Setting:** Acute, fairly minor illness with hoarseness. May be associated with viral nasopharyngitis
Tracheobronchitis	**Cough and Sputum:** Dry or productive of sputum **Associated Symptoms and Setting:** An acute, often viral illness, with burning retrosternal discomfort
Mycoplasma and Viral Pneumonias	**Cough:** Dry and hacking **Sputum:** Often mucoid **Associated Symptoms and Setting:** An acute febrile illness, often with malaise, headache, and possibly dyspnea
Bacterial Pneumonias	**Cough and Sputum:** With *pneumococcal infection*, mucoid or purulent; may be blood streaked, diffusely pinkish, or rusty. With *Klebsiella*, similar to pneumococcal, or sticky red and jelly-like. **Associated Symptoms and Setting:** An acute illness with chills, high fever, dyspnea, and chest pain; often preceded by acute upper respiratory infection. *Klebsiella* often in older alcoholic men.

(table continues next page)

TABLE 8-3 Cough and Hemoptysis (continued)

Problem	Cough, Sputum, Associated Symptoms, and Setting
Chronic Inflammation	
Postnasal Drip	**Cough:** Chronic **Sputum:** Mucoid or mucopurulent **Associated Symptoms and Setting:** Repeated attempts to clear the throat. Postnasal drip, discharge in posterior pharynx. Associated with chronic rhinitis, with or without sinusitis
Chronic Bronchitis	**Cough:** Chronic **Sputum:** Mucoid to purulent; may be blood streaked or even bloody **Associated Symptoms and Setting:** Often long-standing cigarette smoking. Recurrent superimposed infections; often wheezing and dyspnea.
Bronchiectasis	**Cough:** Chronic **Sputum:** Purulent, often copious and foul smelling; may be blood streaked or bloody **Associated Symptoms and Setting:** Recurrent bronchopulmonary infections common; sinusitis may coexist
Pulmonary Tuberculosis	**Cough and Sputum:** Dry, mucoid or purulent; may be blood streaked or bloody **Associated Symptoms and Setting:** Early, no symptoms. Later, anorexia, weight loss, fatigue, fever, and night sweats.
Lung Abscess	**Cough and Sputum:** Purulent and foul smelling; may be bloody **Associated Symptoms and Setting:** A febrile illness. Often poor dental hygiene and a prior episode of impaired consciousness

(table continues next page)

TABLE 8-3 Cough and Hemoptysis (continued)

Problem	Cough, Sputum, Associated Symptoms, and Setting
Asthma	**Cough and Sputum:** Thick and mucoid, especially near end of an attack **Associated Symptoms and Setting:** Episodic wheezing and dyspnea, but cough may occur alone. Often a history of allergy
Gastroesophageal Reflux	**Cough and Sputum:** Chronic, especially at night or early morning **Associated Symptoms and Setting:** Wheezing, especially at night (often mistaken for asthma), early morning hoarseness, repeated attempts to clear throat. Often with history of heartburn and regurgitation
Neoplasm *Lung Cancer*	**Cough:** Dry to productive **Sputum:** May be blood streaked or bloody **Associated Symptoms and Setting:** Usually a long history of cigarette smoking
Cardiovascular Disorders *Left Ventricular Failure or Mitral Stenosis*	**Cough:** Often dry, especially on exertion or at night **Sputum:** May progress to pink and frothy, as in pulmonary edema, or to frank hemoptysis **Associated Symptoms and Setting:** Dyspnea, orthopnea, paroxysmal nocturnal dyspnea
Pulmonary Embolus	**Cough:** Dry to productive **Sputum:** May be dark, bright red, or mixed with blood

(table continues next page)

TABLE 8-3   Cough and Hemoptysis (continued)

Problem	Cough, Sputum, Associated Symptoms, and Setting
	Associated Symptoms and Setting: Dyspnea, anxiety, chest pain, fever; factors that predispose to deep venous thrombosis
Irritating Particles, Chemicals, or Gases	**Cough and Sputum:** Variable. There may be a latent period between exposure and symptoms.
	Associated Symptoms and Setting: Exposure to irritants; eye, nose, and throat symptoms

TABLE 8-4   Deformities of the Thorax

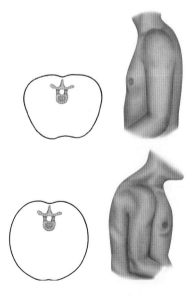

Cross-Section of Thorax Normal Adult
The thorax is wider than it is deep; lateral diameter is greater than anteroposterior (A-P) diameter.

Barrel Chest
Has increased A-P diameter, seen in normal infants and normal aging; also in COPD.

(table continues next page)

TABLE 8-4 Deformities of the Thorax (continued)

Traumatic Flail Chest
If multiple ribs are fractured, can see paradoxical movements of the thorax. Descent of the diaphragm decreases intrathoracic pressure on inspiration. The injured area may cave inward; on expiration, it moves outward.

— Expiration
— Inspiration

Funnel Chest (*Pectus Excavatum*)
Depression in the lower portion of the sternum. Related compression of the heart and great vessels may cause murmurs.

Cross-Section of Thorax Pigeon Chest (*Pectus Carinatum*)
Sternum is displaced anteriorly, increasing the A-P diameter; costal cartilages adjacent to the protruding sternum are depressed.

Depressed costal cartilages

Anteriorly displaced sternum

Thoracic Kyphoscoliosis
Abnormal spinal curvatures and vertebral rotation deform the chest, making interpretation of lung findings difficult.

Spinal convexity to the right (patient bending forward)

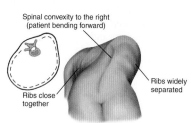

Ribs widely separated

Ribs close together

TABLE 8-5 Physical Findings in Selected Chest Disorders

	Trachea	Percussion Note	Breath Sounds	Transmitted Voice Sounds	Adventitious Sounds
Chronic Bronchitis	Midline	Resonant	Normal	Normal	None, or wheezes, rhonchi, crackles
Left Heart Failure (early)	Midline	Resonant	Normal	Normal	Late inspiratory crackles in lower lungs; possible wheezes
Consolidation*	Midline	Dull	Bronchial	Increased†	Late inspiratory crackles
Atelectasis (Lobar)	May be shifted *toward* involved side	Dull	Usually absent	Usually absent	None
Pleural Effusion (large)	May be shifted *away*	Dull	Decreased to absent	Decreased to absent	Usually none, possible pleural rub
Pneumothorax	May be shifted *away*	Hyperresonant or tympanitic	Decreased to absent	Decreased to absent	Possible pleural rub
COPD	Midline	Hyperresonant	Decreased to absent	Decreased	None unless bronchitis also
Asthma	Midline	Resonant to hyperresonant	May be obscured by wheezes	Decreased	Wheezes, perhaps crackles

*As in lobar pneumonia, pulmonary edema, or pulmonary hemorrhage

†With increased tactile fremitus, bronchophony, egophony, whispered pectoriloquy

The Cardiovascular System

Common or Concerning Symptoms

- Chest pain
- Palpitations
- Shortness of breath: dyspnea, orthopnea, or paroxysmal nocturnal dyspnea
- Swelling or edema

As you assess reports of *chest pain or discomfort,* keep serious adverse events in mind, such as *angina pectoris, myocardial infarction,* or even a *dissecting aortic aneurysm.* Ask also about palpitations, orthopnea, paroxysmal nocturnal dyspnea (PND), and edema.

- *Palpitations* are an unpleasant awareness of the heart beat.

- *Shortness of breath* may represent dyspnea, orthopnea, or PND.

  - *Dyspnea* is an uncomfortable awareness of breathing that is inappropriate for a given level of exertion.

  - *Orthopnea* is dyspnea that occurs when the patient is lying down and improves when the patient sits up. It suggests *left ventricular heart failure* or *mitral stenosis;* it also may accompany *obstructive pulmonary disease.*

  - *PND* describes episodes of sudden dyspnea and orthopnea that awaken the patient from sleep, usually 1 to 2 hours after going to bed, prompting the patient to sit up, stand up, or go to a window for air.

- *Edema* refers to the accumulation of excessive fluid in the interstitial tissue spaces; it appears as swelling. *Dependent edema* appears in the feet and lower legs when sitting or in the sacrum when bedridden.

HEALTH PROMOTION AND COUNSELING

Important Topics for Health Promotion and Counseling

- Screening for hypertension
- Screening for coronary heart disease and stroke
- Screening for dyslipidemias
- Promoting lifestyle modification and risk factor reduction

Cardiovascular disease is the leading cause of death for both men and women in the United States. *Primary prevention,* in those without evidence of cardiovascular disease, and *secondary prevention,* in those with known cardiovascular events (e.g., angina), remain important clinical priorities. Use education and counseling to help your patients maintain optimal levels of blood pressure, cholesterol, weight, and exercise and to reduce risk factors for cardiovascular disease and stroke.

Screening for Hypertension.   The U.S. Preventive Services Task Force recommends *screening adults 18 years or older for high blood pressure.* The Seventh Report of the Joint National Committee on Prevention, Detection, Evaluation, and Treatment of High Blood Pressure (JNC 7) has issued a simpler and more stringent blood pressure classification (see table on p. 63). Note that:

- Normal blood pressure is defined as less than 120/80 mm Hg. Lifestyle interventions should begin when blood pressure is ≥120–139/80–89, termed **prehypertension.**

- Adoption of healthy lifestyles by all people is considered indispensable.

Screening for Coronary Heart Disease and Stroke. The
American Heart Association (AHA) recommends *risk factor
screening* beginning at age 20 years and *global absolute
coronary heart disease (CHD) risk estimation* for all adults
40 years or older.

● Risk Assessment for Adults Beginning at Age 20 Years

Risk Factor	Screening Frequency
Family history of CHD	Update regularly
Smoking status Diet Alcohol intake Physical activity	At each routine visit
Blood pressure Body mass index (BMI) Waist circumference Pulse (to detect atrial fibrillation)	At each routine visit (at least every 2 years)
Fasting lipoprotein profile	At least every 5 years
Fasting glucose	If risk factors for hyperlipidemia or diabetes present, every 2 years

---

GLOBAL RISK ESTIMATION FOR 10-YEAR RISK OF CHD FOR ADULTS 40 YEARS OR OLDER

Establish multiple risk score for CHD based on age, sex,
smoking status, systolic (and sometimes diastolic) blood pressure, total (and sometimes LDL) cholesterol, HDL cholesterol,
and diabetes.

For calculation of global CHD risk, use the risk calculators
found at either of the Web sites below (or other equations):

www.americanheart.org/presenter.jhtml?identifier=
3003499

http://hin.nhlbi.nih.gov/atpiii/calculator.asp?usertype=prof

Screening for Dyslipidemias. LDL is the primary target of cholesterol-lowering therapy. Ten-year risk categories are as follows:

- *High risk* (10-year risk >20%): established CHD and CHD risk equivalents

- *Moderately high risk* (10-year risk 10% to 20%): multiple or 2+ risk factors

- *Low risk* (10-year risk <10%): 0 to 1 risk factor

For high-risk people, the recommended LDL goal is less than 70 mg/dL and intensive lipid therapy is a *therapeutic option*. A summary table of LDL goals based on risk is below.

● Updated Adult Treatment Panel III Guidelines		
10-Year Risk Category	**LDL Goal**	**Consider Drug Therapy**
High risk (>20%)	<100 mg/dL *Optional goal:* <70 mg/dL	≥100 mg/dL (<100 mg/dL: consider drug options, including further 30% to 40% reduction in LDL)
Moderately high risk (10%–20%)	<130 mg/dL *Optional goal:* <100 mg/dL	≥130 mg/dL (100–129 mg/dL: consider drug options to achieve goal of <100 mg/dL)
Moderate risk (<10%)	<130 mg/dL	≥160 mg/dL
Lower risk (0 to 1 risk factor)	<160 mg/dL	>190 mg/dL (160–189 mg/dL: drug therapy *optional*)

(Source: Adapted from National Cholesterol Education Panel Report. Implications of recent clinical trials for the National Cholesterol Education Program Adult Treatment Panel III Guidelines. Grundy SM, Cleeman JI, Merz NB, et al., for the Coordinating Committee of the National Cholesterol Education Program. Circulation 119:227–239, 2004.)

For definitions of risk factors, CHD events, and CHD risk equivalents (such as diabetes or peripheral vascular disease), refer to *Bates' Guide to Physical Examination and History Taking*, 10th edition, Chapter 9.

Promoting Lifestyle Modification and Risk Factor Reduction.
The JNC 7 and AHA encourage well-studied effective lifestyle modification and risk interventions to prevent hypertension, CHD, and stroke.

LIFESTYLE MODIFICATIONS FOR CARDIOVASCULAR HEALTH

- Optimal weight (BMI of 18.5–24.9 kg/m²)
- Salt intake less than 6 g/day of sodium chloride or 2.4 g/day of sodium
- Regular aerobic exercise (e.g., brisk walking) for at least 30 min/day, most days of the week
- Moderate alcohol consumption of two or fewer drinks per day for men and one drink or fewer per day for women
- Diet rich in fruits, vegetables, and low-fat dairy products with reduced saturated and total fat
- Dietary intake of >3,500 mg of potassium
- Optimal blood pressure control (see pp. 56–57)
- Lipid management
- Diabetes management so that fasting glucose level is below 110 mg/dL and HgA1C is less than 7%
- Complete smoking cessation
- Conversion of atrial fibrillation to normal sinus rhythm or, if chronic, anticoagulation

---

Chapter 4 discusses healthy eating habits and dietary counseling in more detail. Remember to assess BMI and to evaluate the patient's eating habits and weight patterns in the family. To reduce risk for CHD, counsel patients to pursue aerobic exercise for at least 30 minutes on most days of the week. Spur motivation by emphasizing the immediate benefits to health and well-being.

TECHNIQUES OF EXAMINATION

EXAMINATION TECHNIQUES   POSSIBLE FINDINGS

HEART RATE AND BLOOD PRESSURE

If not already done, measure the radial or apical pulse.

Estimate systolic blood pressure by palpation and **add** 30 mm Hg. Use this sum as the target for further cuff inflations.

This step helps you to detect an auscultatory gap and avoid recording an inappropriately low systolic blood pressure.

Measure blood pressure with a sphygmomanometer. If indicated, **recheck** it.

Orthostatic (postural) hypotension with position change from supine to standing, SBP↓ ≥20 mm Hg; HR↑ ≥20 beats/min

JUGULAR VEINS

Identify *jugular venous pulsations* and their highest point in the neck. Start with head of the bed at 30°; adjust angle of the bed as necessary.

Study the waves of venous pulsation. Note the *a* wave of atrial contraction and the *v* wave of venous filling.

Absent *a* waves in *atrial fibrillation;* prominent *v* waves in *tricuspid regurgitation.*

Measure *jugular venous pressure* (JVP)—the vertical distance between this highest point and the sternal angle, normally less than 3–4 cm.

Elevated JVP in right-sided heart failure; decreased JVP in hypovolemia from dehydration or gastrointestinal bleeding

CAROTID PULSE

Assess the amplitude and contour of the carotid upstroke.

A *delayed* upstroke in *aortic stenosis;* a *bounding* upstroke in *aortic insufficiency*

Listen for bruits.

Carotid bruits suggest atherosclerotic narrowing.

THE HEART

● Sequence of the Cardiac Examination	
Patient Position	**Examination**
Supine, with the head elevated 30°	Inspect and palpate the precordium: the 2nd interspaces; the right ventricle; and the left ventricle, including the apical impulse (diameter, location, amplitude, duration).
Left lateral decubitus	Palpate the apical impulse if not previously detected. Listen at the apex with the *bell of the stethoscope for low-pitched extra sounds* (S₃, opening snap, diastolic rumble of mitral stenosis).
Supine, with the head elevated 30°	Listen at the 2nd right and left interspaces, along the left sternal border, and across to the apex with the diaphragm. Listen with the bell at the right sternal border for tricuspid murmurs and sounds.
Sitting, leaning forward, after full exhalation	Listen along the left sternal border and at the apex for the soft decrescendo diastolic murmur of *aortic insufficiency.*

EXAMINATION TECHNIQUES   POSSIBLE FINDINGS

INSPECTION AND PALPATION

Inspect and **palpate** the
anterior chest for heaves,
lifts, or thrills.

Identify the *apical impulse.*
Turn patient to left as
necessary. **Note:**

● Location of impulse

Displaced to left in
pregnancy

● Diameter

Increased diameter,
amplitude, and duration
in left ventricular dilatation
from *congestive heart failure*
(CHF) or *ischemic
cardiomyopathy*

● Amplitude—usually
tapping

Sustained in left ventricular
hypertrophy; *diffuse* in CHF

● Duration

Feel for a right ventricular
impulse in left parasternal
and epigastric areas.

Prominent impulses
suggest right ventricular
enlargement.

Palpate left and right
second interspaces close to
sternum. **Note** any thrills in
these areas.

Pulsations of great vessels;
accentuated S_2; thrills of *aortic*
or *pulmonic stenosis*

EXAMINATION TECHNIQUES	POSSIBLE FINDINGS

AUSCULTATION

Listen to heart by "inching" your stethoscope from the base to the apex (or apex to base) in the areas illustrated.

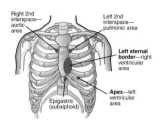

Right 2nd interspace—aortic area

Left 2nd interspace—pulmonic area

Left sternal border—right ventricular area

Apex—left ventricular area

Epigastric (subxiphoid)

Use the *diaphragm* in the areas illustrated above for relatively *high-pitched sounds* like S_1, S_2.

Also murmurs of *aortic and mitral regurgitation; pericardial friction rubs*

Use the *bell* for *low-pitched sounds* at the lower left sternal border and apex.

S_3, S_4, murmur of *mitral stenosis*

Listen at each area for:

See Table 9-1, Heart Sounds, p. 176; Table 9-2, Variations in the First Heart Sound (S_1), p. 177; Table 9-3, Variations in the Second Heart Sound (S_2), pp. 178–179.

- S_1

- S_2. Is splitting normal in left 2nd and 3rd interspaces?

Physiologic (inspiratory) or pathologic (expiratory) splitting

- Extra sounds in systole

Systolic clicks

- Extra sounds in diastole

S_3, S_4

- Systolic murmurs

Midsystolic, pansystolic, late systolic murmurs

- Diastolic murmurs

Early, mid-, or late diastolic murmurs

EXAMINATION TECHNIQUES | POSSIBLE FINDINGS

ASSESSING AND DESCRIBING MURMURS

Identify, if murmurs are present, their

- Timing in the cardiac cycle (systole, diastole)

See Table 9-4, Heart Murmurs, p. 180.

- Shape

Plateau, crescendo, decrescendo

A *crescendo–decrescendo murmur* first rises in intensity, then falls.

A *plateau murmur* has the same intensity throughout.

A *crescendo murmur* grows louder.

A *decrescendo murmur* grows softer.

- Location of maximal intensity

- Radiation

- Pitch

High, medium, low

- Quality

Blowing, harsh, musical, rumbling

- Intensity on a 6-point scale

See "Gradations of Murmurs" on next page.

✂ **Listen** at the apex with patient turned toward left side for low-pitched sounds.

Left-sided S_3, S_4, and diastolic murmur of *mitral stenosis*

EXAMINATION TECHNIQUES   POSSIBLE FINDINGS

♪ **Listen** down left sternal border to the apex as patient sits, leaning forward, with breath held after exhalation.

Diastolic decrescendo murmur of *aortic regurgitation*

● Gradations of Murmurs	
Grade	**Description**
Grade 1	Very faint, heard only after listener has "tuned in"; may not be heard in all positions
Grade 2	Quiet, but heard immediately after placing the stethoscope on the chest
Grade 3	Moderately loud
Grade 4	Loud, with palpable thrill
Grade 5	Very loud, with thrill. May be heard when the stethoscope is partly off the chest
Grade 6	Very loud, with thrill. May be heard with stethoscope entirely off the chest

EXAMINATION TECHNIQUES   POSSIBLE FINDINGS

SPECIAL TECHNIQUES

PULSUS ALTERNANS

Feel pulse for alternation in amplitude. Lower pressure of blood pressure cuff slowly to systolic level while you listen with stethoscope over brachial artery.

Alternating amplitude of pulse or sudden doubling of Korotkoff sounds indicates *pulsus alternans*—a sign of left ventricular heart failure.

PARADOXICAL PULSE

Lower pressure of blood pressure cuff slowly and note two pressure levels: (1) where Korotkoff sounds are first heard and (2) where they first persist through the respiratory cycle. These levels are normally not more than 3–4 mm Hg apart.

A drop of greater than 10 mm Hg during inspiration signifies a paradoxical pulse. Consider obstructive pulmonary disease, pericardial tamponade, or constrictive pericarditis.

AIDS TO IDENTIFY SYSTOLIC MURMURS

Valsalva Maneuver

Ask patient to strain down.

In suspected *mitral valve prolapse (MVP),* listen to the timing of click and murmur.

Ventricular filling decreases, the systolic click of MVP is earlier, and the murmur lengthens.

To distinguish *aortic stenosis (AS)* from *hypertrophic cardiomyopathy (HC),* listen to the intensity of the murmur.

In AS, the murmur decreases; in HC, it often increases.

EXAMINATION TECHNIQUES

POSSIBLE FINDINGS

 Squatting and Standing

In suspected *MVP,* listen for the click and murmur in both positions.

Squatting increases ventricular filling and delays the click and murmur. Standing reverses the changes.

Try to distinguish *AS* from *HC* by listening to the murmur in both positions.

Squatting increases murmur of AS and decreases murmur of HC. Standing reverses the changes.

RECORDING YOUR FINDINGS

Recording the Physical Examination— The Cardiovascular Examination

"The jugular venous pulse (JVP) is 3 cm above the sternal angle with the head of the bed elevated to 30°. Carotid upstrokes are brisk, without bruits. The point of maximal impulse (PMI) is tapping, 7 cm lateral to the midsternal line in the 5th intercostal space. Crisp S_1 and S_2. At the base, S_2 is greater than S_1 and physiologically split, with $A_2 > P_2$. At the apex, S_1 is greater than S_2 and constant. No murmurs or extra sounds."

OR

"The JVP is 5 cm above the sternal angle with the head of the bed elevated to 50°. Carotid upstrokes are brisk; a bruit is heard over the left carotid artery. The PMI is diffuse, 3 cm in diameter, palpated at the anterior axillary line in the 5th and 6th intercostal spaces. S_1 and S_2 are soft. S_3 present at the apex. High-pitched, harsh 2/6 holosystolic murmur best heard at the apex, radiating to the axilla. No S_4 or diastolic murmurs." *(Suggests CHF with possible left carotid occlusion and mitral regurgitation)*

AIDS TO INTERPRETATION

TABLE 9-1 Heart Sounds

Finding	Possible Causes
S_1 accentuated	Tachycardia, states of high cardiac output; mitral stenosis
S_1 diminished	First-degree heart block; reduced left ventricular contractility; immobile mitral valve, as in mitral regurgitation
Systolic clicks(s)	Mitral valve prolapse
S_2 accentuated in right 2nd interspace	Systemic hypertension, dilated aortic root
S_2 diminished or absent in right 2nd interspace	Immobile aortic valve, as in calcific aortic stenosis
P_2 accentuated	Pulmonary hypertension, dilated pulmonary artery, atrial septal defect
P_2 diminished or absent	Aging, pulmonic stenosis
Opening snap	Mitral stenosis
S_3	Physiologic (usually in children and young adults); volume overload of ventricle, as in mitral regurgitation or congestive heart failure
S_4	Excellent physical conditioning (trained athletes); resistance to ventricular filling because of decreased compliance, left ventricular hypertrophy from pressure overload, as in hypertensive heart disease, aortic stenosis

TABLE 9-2 Variations in the First Heart Sound (S₁)

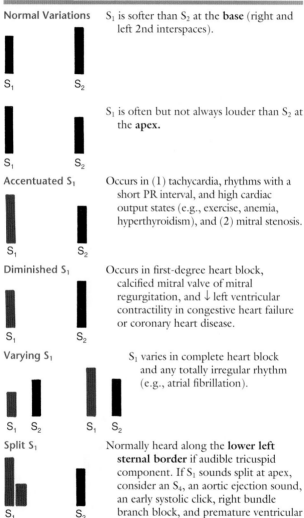

Normal Variations — S_1 is softer than S_2 at the **base** (right and left 2nd interspaces).

S_1 is often but not always louder than S_2 at the **apex.**

Accentuated S_1 — Occurs in (1) tachycardia, rhythms with a short PR interval, and high cardiac output states (e.g., exercise, anemia, hyperthyroidism), and (2) mitral stenosis.

Diminished S_1 — Occurs in first-degree heart block, calcified mitral valve of mitral regurgitation, and ↓ left ventricular contractility in congestive heart failure or coronary heart disease.

Varying S_1 — S_1 varies in complete heart block and any totally irregular rhythm (e.g., atrial fibrillation).

Split S_1 — Normally heard along the **lower left sternal border** if audible tricuspid component. If S_1 sounds split at apex, consider an S_4, an aortic ejection sound, an early systolic click, right bundle branch block, and premature ventricular contractions.

TABLE 9-3 Variations in the Second Heart Sound (S₂)

Inspiration	Expiration

Physiologic Splitting

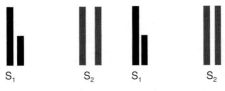

Heard in the 2nd or 3rd left interspace: the pulmonic component of S₂ is usually too faint to be heard at the apex or aortic area, where S₂ is single and derived from aortic valve closure alone. Accentuated by inspiration; usually disappears on exertion.

Pathologic Splitting

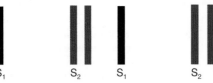

Wide splitting of S₂ persists throughout respiration; from delayed closure of the pulmonic valve (e.g., by pulmonic stenosis or right bundle branch block); also from early closure of the aortic valve, as in mitral regurgitation.

Fixed Splitting

Does not vary with respiration, as in atrial septal defect, right ventricular failure.

(table continues next page)

TABLE 9-3	**Variations in the Second Heart Sound (S_2)** (continued)

Inspiration	Expiration

Paradoxical or Reversed Splitting

P_2 A_2

S_1 S_2 S_1 S_2

Appears on expiration and disappears on inspiration. Closure of
the aortic valve is abnormally delayed, so A_2 follows P_2 on
expiration, as in left bundle branch block.

More on A_2 and P_2

Increased Intensity of A_2, Second Right Interspace (where
only A_2 can usually be heard) occurs in systemic hypertension
because of the increased pressure. It also occurs when the aortic
root is dilated, probably because the aortic valve is then closer
to the chest wall.

Decreased or Absent A_2, Second Right Interspace is noted in
calcific aortic stenosis because of immobility of the valve. If A_2
is inaudible, no splitting is heard.

Increased Intensity of P_2. When P_2 is equal to or louder than
A_2, pulmonary hypertension may be suspected. Other causes
include a dilated pulmonary artery and an atrial septal defect.
Splitting of the second heart sound that is heard widely, even
at the apex and the right base, indicates an accentuated P_2.

Decreased or Absent P_2 is most commonly due to the increased
anteroposterior diameter of the chest associated with aging. It
can also result from pulmonic stenosis. If P_2 is inaudible, no
splitting is heard.

TABLE 9-4 Heart Murmurs

	Likely Causes
Midsystolic S_1 S_2	Innocent murmurs (no valve abnormality) Physiologic murmurs (from ↑ flow across a semilunar valve, as in pregnancy, fever, anemia) Aortic stenosis Murmurs that mimic aortic stenosis—aortic sclerosis, bicuspid aortic valve, dilated aorta, and pathologically ↑ systolic flow across aortic valve Hypertrophic cardiomyopathy Pulmonic stenosis
Pansystolic S_1 S_2	Mitral regurgitation Tricuspid regurgitation Ventricular septal defect
Late Systolic S_1 C S_2	Mitral valve prolapse, often with click (C)
Early Diastolic S_1 S_2 S_1	Aortic regurgitation
Middiastolic and Presystolic S_1 S_2 OS S_1	Mitral stenosis—note opening snap (OS)
Continuous Murmurs and Sounds S_1 S_2 S_1	Patent ductus arteriosus—harsh, machinery-like
S_1 S_2 S_1	Pericardial friction rub—a scratchy sound with 1–3 components
S_1 S_2 S_1	Venous hum—continuous, above midclavicles, loudest in diastole

The Breasts and Axillae

Common or Concerning Symptoms

- Breast lump or mass
- Breast pain or discomfort
- Nipple discharge

Ask, "Do you examine your breasts?" . . . "How often?" Ask about any discomfort, pain, or lumps in the breasts. Also ask about any discharge from the nipples, change in breast contour, dimpling, swelling, or puckering of the skin over the breasts.

HEALTH PROMOTION AND COUNSELING

Important Topics for Health Promotion and Counseling

- Palpable masses of the breast
- Assessing risk factors for breast cancer
- Breast cancer screening
- Breast self-examination (BSE)

Palpable Masses of the Breast.   Breast masses show marked variation in etiology, from fibroadenomas and cysts seen in younger women, to abscess or mastitis, to primary breast cancer. All breast masses warrant careful evaluation, and definitive diagnostic measures should be pursued.

Assessing Risk Factors for Breast Cancer.   Although 70% of affected women have no known predisposing factors, definite

● Palpable Masses of the Breast

Age	Common Lesion	Characteristics
15–25	Fibroadenoma	Usually fine, round, mobile, nontender
25–50	Cysts	Usually soft to firm, round, mobile; often tender
	Fibrocystic changes	Nodular, ropelike
	Cancer	Irregular, stellate, firm, not clearly delineated from surrounding tissue
50 or older	Cancer until proven otherwise	As above
Pregnancy/ lactation	Lactating adenomas, cysts, mastitis, and cancer	As above

(Adapted from Schultz MZ, Ward BA, Reiss M. Breast diseases. In: Noble J, Greene HL, Levinson W, et al., eds: Primary Care Medicine, 2nd ed. St. Louis: Mosby, 1996. See also Venet L, Strax P, Venet W, et al. Cancer 28(6):1546–1551, 1971.)

risk factors are well established. Use the Breast Cancer Risk Assessment Tool of the National Cancer Institute (http://brca.nci.nih/gov/brc/start/htm) or other available clinical models, such as the Gail model, to individualize risk factor assessment for your patients. Ask women beginning in their 20s about any family history of breast or ovarian cancer, or both, on the maternal or paternal side, to help assess risk of BRCA1 or BRCA2 gene mutation. See Table 10-1, Breast Cancer: Factors That Increase Relative Risk, p. 190.

Breast Cancer Screening. The American Cancer Society recommends:

- *Clinical breast examination* (CBE) by a health care professional every 3 years for women between 20 and 39 years of age, and annually after 40 years of age

- Yearly *mammography* for women 40 years of age and older. For women at increased risk, many clinicians advise initiating screening mammography between ages 30 and 40, then every 2 to 3 years until 50 years of age.

- Regular breast self-examination (BSE) to help promote health awareness

TECHNIQUES OF EXAMINATION

EXAMINATION TECHNIQUES   POSSIBLE FINDINGS

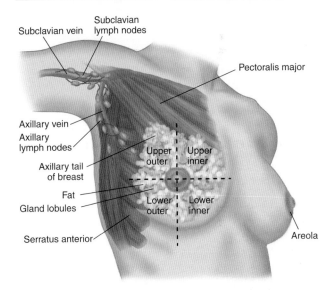

THE FEMALE BREAST

Inspect the breasts in four positions.

Note:

- Size and symmetry   Development, asymmetry

- Contour   Flattening, dimpling

EXAMINATION TECHNIQUES	POSSIBLE FINDINGS

- Appearance of the skin

Edema (peau d'orange) in breast cancer

ARMS AT SIDES

ARMS OVER HEAD

HANDS PRESSED AGAINST HIPS

LEANING FORWARD

Inspect the nipples.

- Compare their size, shape, and direction of pointing.

Inversion, retraction, deviation

- Note any rashes, ulcerations, or discharge.

Paget's disease of the nipple, galactorrhea

○— **Palpate** the breasts, including augmented breasts. Breast tissue should be flattened and the patient supine. Palpate a rectangular area extending from the clavicle to the inframammary fold or bra line, and from the midsternal line to the posterior axillary line and well into the axilla for the tail of Spence.

EXAMINATION TECHNIQUES	POSSIBLE FINDINGS

Note:

- Consistency

  Physiologic nodularity

- Tenderness

  Infection, premenstrual tenderness

- Nodules. If present, **note** *location, size, shape, consistency, delimitation, tenderness,* and *mobility.*

  Cyst, fibroadenoma, cancer

Use *vertical strip pattern* (currently the best validated technique) or a circular or wedge pattern. Palpate in *small, concentric circles.*

- For *the lateral portion of the breast,* ask the patient to roll onto the opposite hip, place her hand on her forehead, but keep shoulders pressed against the bed or examining table.

- For *the medial portion of the breast,* ask the patient to lie with her shoulders flat against the bed or examining table, place her hand at her neck, and lift up her elbow until it is even with her shoulder.

Palpate each nipple.

Thickening in cancer

Palpate and inspect along the incision lines of mastectomy.

Local recurrences of breast cancer.

EXAMINATION TECHNIQUES   POSSIBLE FINDINGS

THE MALE BREAST

Inspect and **palpate** the nipple and areola.

Gynecomastia, mass suspicious for cancer, fat

AXILLAE

Inspect for rashes, infection, and pigmentation.

Hidradenitis suppurativa, acanthosis nigricans

Palpate the axillary nodes, including the central, pectoral, lateral, and subscapular groups.

Lymphadenopathy

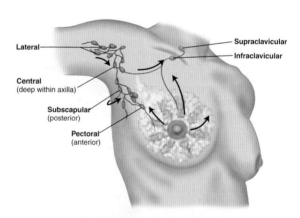

ARROWS INDICATE DIRECTION OF LYMPH FLOW

SPECIAL TECHNIQUE

○— BREAST DISCHARGE

Compress the areola in a spoke-like pattern around the nipple. Watch for discharge.

Type and source of discharge may be identified

BREAST SELF-EXAMINATION

PATIENT INSTRUCTIONS FOR THE BREAST SELF-EXAMINATION (BSE)

Supine

1. Lie down with a pillow under your right shoulder. Place your right arm behind your head.
2. Use the finger pads of the three middle fingers on your left hand to feel for lumps in the right breast. The finger pads are the top third of each finger.
3. Press firmly enough to know how your breast feels. A firm ridge in the lower curve of each breast is normal. If you're not sure how hard to press, talk with your health care provider, or try to copy the way the doctor or nurse does it.
4. Press firmly on the breast in an up-and-down or "strip" pattern. You can also use a circular or wedge pattern, but be sure to use the same pattern every time. Check the entire breast area, and remember how your breast feels from month to month.
5. Repeat the examination on your left breast, using the finger pads of the right hand.
6. If you find any changes, see your doctor right away.

(continued)

PATIENT INSTRUCTIONS FOR THE
BREAST SELF-EXAMINATION (BSE) (CONTINUED)

Standing

1. Repeat the examination of both breasts while standing, with one arm behind your head. The upright position makes it easier to check the upper outer part of the breasts (toward your armpit). This is where about half of breast cancers are found. You may want to do the upright part of the BSE while you are in the shower. Your soapy hands will make it easy to check how your breasts

feel as they glide over the wet skin.
2. For added safety, you might want to check your breasts by standing in front of a mirror right after your BSE each month. See if there are any changes in the way your breasts look, such as dimpling of the skin, changes in the nipple, redness, or swelling.
3. If you find any changes, see your doctor right away.

(Adapted from the American Cancer Society, www.cancer.org. Accessed October 24, 2007.)

RECORDING YOUR FINDINGS

Recording the Physical Examination—
Breasts and Axillae

> "Breasts symmetric and smooth, without masses. Nipples without discharge." (Axillary adenopathy usually included after Neck in section on Lymph Nodes; see p. 123.)
>
> **OR**
>
> "Breasts pendulous with diffuse fibrocystic changes. Single firm 1 × 1 cm mass, mobile and nontender, with overlying peau d'orange appearance in right breast, upper outer quadrant at 11 o'clock, 2 cm from the nipple."
>
> *(Suggests possible breast cancer)*

AIDS TO INTERPRETATION

TABLE 10-1	**Breast Cancer in Women: Factors That Increase Relative Risk**
Relative Risk	**Factor**
>4.0	• Female • Age (65+ versus <65 years, although risk increases across all ages until age 80) • Certain inherited genetic mutations for breast cancer (BRCA1 and/or BRCA2) • Two or more first-degree relatives with breast cancer diagnosed at an early age • Personal history of breast cancer • High breast tissue density • Biopsy-confirmed atypical hyperplasia
2.1–4.0	• One first-degree relative with breast cancer • High-dose radiation to chest • High bone density (postmenopausal)

(table continues next page)

TABLE 10-1	**Breast Cancer in Women: Factors That Increase Relative Risk** (continued)

Relative Risk	Factor
1.1–2.0 Factors that affect circulating hormones	• Late age at first full-term pregnancy (>30 years) • Early menarche (<12 years) • Late menopause (>55 years) • No full-term pregnancies • Never breast-fed a child • Recent oral contraceptive use • Recent and long-term use of hormone replacement therapy • Obesity (postmenopausal)
Other factors	• Personal history of endometrium, ovary, or colon cancer • Alcohol consumption • Height (tall) • High socioeconomic status • Jewish heritage

(Source: American Cancer Society. Breast Cancer Facts and Figures 2007–2008, p. 10. Available at: www.cancer.org/downloads/STT/BCFF-Final.pdf. Accessed October 20, 2007.)

TABLE 10-2 Visible Signs of Breast Cancer

Retraction Signs

Fibrosis from breast cancer produces retraction signs: dimpling, changes in contour, and retraction or deviation of the nipple. Other causes of retraction include fat necrosis and mammary duct ectasia.

Skin Dimpling

Abnormal Contours

Look for any variation in the normal convexity of each breast, and compare one side with the other.

Nipple Retraction and Deviation

A retracted nipple is flattened or pulled inward. It may also be broadened and feel thickened. The nipple may deviate, or point in a different direction, typically toward the underlying cancer.

(table continues next page)

TABLE 10-2 Visible Signs of Breast Cancer (continued)

Edema of the Skin
From lymphatic blockade,
appearing as thickened skin
with enlarged pores—the so-
called *peau d'orange* (orange
peel) *sign*.

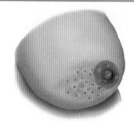

Paget's Disease of the Nipple
An uncommon form of breast
cancer that usually starts as a
scaly, eczema-like lesion. The
skin may also weep, crust, or
erode. A breast mass may be
present. Suspect Paget's
disease in any persisting
dermatitis of the nipple and
areola.

Dermatitis of
areola

Erosion of
nipple

The Abdomen

Common or Concerning Symptoms

Gastrointestinal Disorders	**Urinary and Renal Disorders**
• Abdominal pain, acute and chronic	• Suprapubic pain
• Indigestion, nausea, vomiting including blood, loss of appetite, early satiety	• Dysuria, urgency, or frequency
• Dysphagia and/or odynophagia	• Hesitancy, decreased stream in males
• Change in bowel function	• Polyuria or nocturia
• Diarrhea, constipation	• Urinary incontinence
• Jaundice	• Hematuria
	• Kidney or flank pain
	• Ureteral colic

PATTERNS AND MECHANISMS OF ABDOMINAL PAIN

Be familiar with three broad categories:

Visceral pain—occurs when hollow abdominal organs such as the intestine or biliary tree contract unusually forcefully or are distended or stretched.

Visceral pain in the right upper quadrant (RUQ) from liver distention against its capsule in *alcoholic hepatitis*

- May be difficult to localize

- Varies in quality; may be gnawing, burning, cramping, or aching

- When severe, may be associated with sweating, pallor, nausea, vomiting, restlessness.

Parietal pain—from inflammation of the parietal peritoneum

- Steady, aching

- Usually more severe

- Usually more precisely localized over the involved structure than visceral pain

Visceral periumbilical pain in *early acute appendicitis* from distention of inflamed appendix gradually changes to parietal pain in the right lower quadrant (RLQ) from inflammation of the adjacent parietal peritoneum.

Referred pain—occurs in more distant sites innervated at approximately the same spinal levels as the disordered structure.

Pain of duodenal or pancreatic origin may be referred to the back; pain from the biliary tree—to the right shoulder or right posterior chest.

Pain from the chest, spine, or pelvis may be referred to the abdomen.

Pain from *pleurisy* or *acute myocardial infarction* may be referred to the upper abdomen.

THE GASTROINTESTINAL TRACT

Ask patients to *describe the abdominal pain in their own words,* especially timing of the pain (acute or chronic); then ask them to *point to the pain.*

Pursue important details: "Where does the pain start?"

"Does it radiate or travel?"
"What is the pain like?"
"How severe is it?" "How
about on a scale of 1 to 10?"
"What makes it better or
worse?"

Elicit any *symptoms
associated with the pain,* such
as fever or chills; ask their
sequence.

***Upper Abdominal Pain or
Discomfort.*** Ask about
chronic or recurrent upper
abdominal discomfort, or
dyspepsia. Related symptoms
include bloating, nausea,
upper abdominal fullness,
and heartburn.

Find out just what your
patient means. Possibilities
include:

• Bloating from excessive
  gas, especially with
  frequent belching,
  abdominal distention, or
  flatus, the passage of gas
  by rectum

• *Nausea and vomiting*

• Unpleasant *abdominal
  fullness* after normal
  meals or *early satiety*,
  the inability to eat a
  full meal

Consider diabetic gastroparesis,
anticholinergic drugs, gastric
outlet obstruction, gastric
cancer. Early satiety may
signify *hepatitis.*

• *Heartburn*

Suggests *gastroesophageal
reflux disease (GERD)*

*Lower Abdominal Pain
or Discomfort*

If acute, is the pain sharp and continuous or intermittent and cramping?	Right lower quadrant (RLQ) pain, or pain migrating from periumbilical region in *appendicitis;* in women with RLQ pain, possible *pelvic inflammatory disease, ectopic pregnancy* Left lower quadrant (LLQ) pain in *diverticulitis*
If chronic, is there a change in bowel habits? Alternating diarrhea and constipation?	*Colon cancer; irritable bowel syndrome*

Other GI Symptoms

• Anorexia	Liver disease, pregnancy, diabetic ketoacidosis, adrenal insufficiency, uremia, anorexia nervosa
• Dysphagia or difficulty swallowing	Of solids and liquids: usually neuromuscular disorders affecting motility If only solids, consider structural conditions like Zenker's diverticulum, Schatzki's ring, stricture, neoplasm
• Odynophagia, or painful swallowing	Radiation; caustic ingestion, infection from *cytomegalovirus,* herpes simplex, HIV
• Diarrhea, acute (<2 weeks) and chronic	Acute infection (viral, salmonella, shigella, etc.); chronic in *Crohn's disease,* ulcerative colitis; if oily (*steatorrhea*)—pancreatic insufficiency. See Table 11-1.

• Constipation	Medications, especially anticholinergic agents and opioids; colon cancer
• Melena, or black tarry stools	GI bleed
• Jaundice from increased levels of bilirubin; intrahepatic jaundice can be *hepatocellular*, from damage to the hepatocytes, or *cholestatic*, from impaired excretion caused by damaged hepatocytes or intra-hepatic bile ducts	Impaired excretion of conjugated bilirubin in *viral hepatitis, cirrhosis, primary biliary cirrhosis,* drug-induced cholestasis
Extrahepatic jaundice from obstructed extrahepatic bile ducts, commonly the cystic and common bile ducts	
Ask about the *color of the urine and stool.*	Dark urine from increased conjugated bilirubin in serum excreted in urine; acholic clay-colored stool when excretion of bilirubin into intestine is obstructed

RISK FACTORS FOR LIVER DISEASE

- *Hepatitis A:* Travel or meals in areas with poor sanitation, ingestion of contaminated water or foodstuffs
- *Hepatitis B:* Parenteral or mucous membrane exposure to infectious body fluids such as blood, serum, semen, and saliva, especially through sexual contact with an infected partner or use of shared needles for injection drug use
- *Hepatitis C:* Illicit intravenous drug use or blood transfusion
- *Alcoholic hepatitis* or *alcoholic cirrhosis:* Interview the patient carefully about alcohol use

(continued)

RISK FACTORS FOR LIVER DISEASE (CONTINUED)

- *Toxic liver damage* from medications, industrial solvents, or environmental toxins
- *Extrahepatic biliary obstruction:* Resulting from gallbladder disease or surgery
- *Hereditary disorders* in the Family History

THE URINARY TRACT

Ask about *pain on urination,* usually a burning sensation, sometimes termed *dysuria* (also refers to difficulty voiding).

Bladder infection

Also, consider bladder stones, foreign bodies, tumors, and *acute prostatitis*. In women, internal burning in *urethritis,* external burning in *vulvovaginitis*

Other associated symptoms include

- *Urgency,* an unusually intense and immediate desire to void

May lead to urge incontinence

- *Urinary frequency,* or abnormally frequent voiding

- Fever or chills; blood in the urine

- Any pain in the abdomen, flank, or back

Dull, steady pain in *pyelonephritis;* severe colicky pain in ureteral obstruction from renal stone

In men *hesitancy* in starting the urine stream, *straining to void, reduced caliber and force of the urine stream,* or *dribbling* as they complete voiding

Prostatitis, urethritis

Assess any:

• *Polyuria,* a significant increase in 24-hour urine volume	*Diabetes mellitus, diabetes insipidus*
• *Nocturia,* urinary frequency at night	Bladder obstruction
• *Urinary incontinence,* involuntary loss of urine	See Table 11-2, Urinary Incontinence, pp. 211–212.
• From coughing, sneezing, lifting	*Stress incontinence* (poor urethral sphincter tone)
• From urge to void	*Urge incontinence* (detrusor overactivity)
• From bladder fullness with leaking but incomplete emptying	*Overflow incontinence* (anatomic obstruction, impaired neural innervation to bladder)

HEALTH PROMOTION AND COUNSELING

Important Topics for Health Promotion and Counseling

> • Screening for alcohol abuse
> • Risk factors for hepatitis A, B, and C
> • Screening for colon cancer

Assessing *use of alcohol* is an important clinician responsibility. Focus on detection, counseling, and, for significant impairment, specific treatment recommendations. Use the four CAGE questions to screen for alcohol dependence or abuse in all adolescents and adults, including pregnant women (see Chap. 3, p. 41). Brief counseling interventions have been shown to reduce alcohol consumption by 13% to 34% over 6 to 12 months.

Protective measures against *infectious hepatitis* include counseling about transmission:

• *Hepatitis A:* Transmission is fecal–oral. Illness occurs approximately 30 days after exposure. Hepatitis A vaccine is recommended for travelers to endemic areas; food handlers; military personnel; caretakers of children; Native Americans and Alaska Natives; selected health care, sanitation, and laboratory workers; homosexual men; and injection drug users.

- *Hepatitis B:* Transmission occurs during contact with infected body fluids, such as blood, semen, saliva, and vaginal secretions. Infection increases risk of fulminant hepatitis, chronic infection, and subsequent cirrhosis and hepatocellular carcinoma. Provide counseling and serologic screening for patients at risk. Hepatitis B vaccine is recommended for all young adults not previously immunized, injection drug users and their sexual partners, people at risk for sexually transmitted diseases, travelers to endemic areas, recipients of blood products as in hemodialysis, and health care workers with frequent exposure to blood products. Many of these groups also should be screened for HIV infection, especially pregnant women at their first prenatal visit.

- *Hepatitis C:* Hepatitis C, now the most common form, is spread by blood exposure and is associated with injection drug use. No vaccine is available.

For colorectal cancer, screen for risk factors, namely family history of colonic polyps, history of colorectal cancer or adenoma in a first-degree relative, and personal history of ulcerative colitis, adenomatous polyps, or prior diagnosis of endometrial, ovarian, or breast cancer. For men and women at average risk, the American Cancer Society recommends *one* of the following beginning at age 50:

- Fecal occult blood test (FOBT) annually
- Flexible sigmoidoscopy every 5 years
- Annual FOBT plus flexible sigmoidoscopy every 5 years
- Double contrast barium enema every 5 years
- Colonoscopy every 10 years

Detection rates for colorectal cancer and insertion depths of endoscopy are roughly as follows: 25% to 30% at 20 cm; 50% to 55% at 35 cm; 40% to 65% at 40 cm to 50 cm. Full colonoscopy or air contrast barium enema detects 80% to 95% of colorectal cancers.

TECHNIQUES OF EXAMINATION

EXAMINATION TECHNIQUES   POSSIBLE FINDINGS

THE ABDOMEN

○— **Inspect** the abdomen, including

- Skin   Scars, striae, veins

- Umbilicus   Hernia, inflammation

- Contours for shape,   Bulging flanks, suprapubic
  symmetry, enlarged organs   bulge, large liver or spleen,
  or masses   tumors

- Any peristaltic waves   GI obstruction

- Any pulsations   Increased in aortic aneurysm

Auscultate the abdomen for

- Bowel sounds   Increased or decreased motility

- Bruits   Bruit of renal artery stenosis

- Friction rubs   Liver tumor, splenic infarct

● Bowel Sounds and Bruits

Change	Seen With
Increased bowel sounds	Diarrhea Early intestinal obstruction
Decreased, then absent bowel sounds	Adynamic ileus Peritonitis
High-pitched tinkling bowel sounds	Intestinal fluid Air under tension in a dilated bowel

(continued)

EXAMINATION TECHNIQUES   POSSIBLE FINDINGS

● Bowel Sounds and Bruits (continued)

Change	Seen With
High-pitched rushing bowel sounds with cramping	Intestinal obstruction
Hepatic bruit	Carcinoma of the liver Alcoholic hepatitis
Arterial bruits	Partial obstruction of the aorta or renal arteries

Aorta
Renal artery
Iliac artery
Femoral artery

Percuss the abdomen for patterns of tympany and dullness.

Ascites, GI obstruction, pregnant uterus, ovarian tumor

Palpate all quadrants of the abdomen

See Table 11-3.

● Lightly for guarding, rebound, and tenderness

Firm, boardlike abdominal wall suggests peritoneal inflammation. *Guarding* occurs when the patient flinches, grimaces, or reports pain during palpation.

Rebound tenderness from peritoneal inflammation; pain is greater when you withdraw

EXAMINATION TECHNIQUES	POSSIBLE FINDINGS

your hand than when you
press down. Press slowly on
a tender area, then quickly
"let go."

● Deeply for masses or
tenderness

Tumors, a distended viscus

THE LIVER

Percuss span of liver dullness
in the midclavicular line
(MCL).

Hepatomegaly

4–8 cm in
midsternal line

6–12 cm
in right
midclavicular
line

} Normal liver spans

Feel the liver edge, if
possible, as patient
breathes in.

Firm edge of cirrhosis

Measure its distance from
the costal margin in the
MCL.

Increased in hepatomegaly—
may be missed (as below) by
starting palpation too high in
the RUQ

EXAMINATION TECHNIQUES	POSSIBLE FINDINGS

Note any tenderness or masses.

Tender liver of hepatitis or congestive heart failure; tumor mass

THE SPLEEN

Percuss across left lower anterior chest, noting change from tympany to dullness.

Try to **feel** spleen with the patient

Splenomegaly

- Supine

- ○⟶ Lying on the right side with legs flexed at hips and knees

EXAMINATION TECHNIQUES   POSSIBLE FINDINGS

THE KIDNEYS

○— Try to **palpate** each kidney.

Enlargement from cysts, cancer, hydronephrosis

⌐ **Check** for costovertebral angle (CVA) tenderness.

Tender in kidney infection

THE AORTA

○— **Palpate** the aorta's pulsations. In older people, **estimate** its width.

Periumbilical mass with expansile pulsations ≥3 cm in diameter in abdominal aortic aneurysm. Assess further due to risk of rupture.

EXAMINATION TECHNIQUES   POSSIBLE FINDINGS

ASSESSING ASCITES

∘— / ∘⊸ **Palpate** for shifting dullness. Map areas of tympany and dullness with patient supine, then lying on side (see below).

Ascitic fluid usually shifts to dependent side, changing the margin of dullness (see below)

Tympany

Dullness

Tympany

Dullness

∘— Check for a fluid wave. Ask patient or an assistant to press edges of both hands into midline of abdomen. Tap one side and feel for a wave transmitted to the other side.

A palpable wave suggests but does not prove ascites.

EXAMINATION TECHNIQUES

POSSIBLE FINDINGS

⊶ **Ballotte** an organ or
mass in an ascitic
abdomen. Place your
stiffened and straightened
fingers on the abdomen,
briefly jab them toward the
structure, and try to touch
its surface.

Your hand, quickly displacing
the fluid, stops abruptly as it
touches the solid surface.

ASSESSING POSSIBLE APPENDICITIS

Ask:

In *classic appendicitis:*

"Where did the pain begin?"

Near the umbilicus

"Where is it now?"

Right lower quadrant (RLQ)

Ask patient to cough.
"Where does it hurt?"

RLQ

Palpate for local tenderness.

RLQ tenderness

Palpate for muscular rigidity.

RLQ rigidity

Perform a rectal examination
and, in women, a pelvic
examination (see Chaps. 14
and 15).

Local tenderness, especially if
appendix is retrocecal

● *Rovsing's sign:* Press
deeply and evenly in the
left lower quadrant. Then
quickly withdraw your
fingers.

Pain in the *right* lower
quadrant during *left*-
sided pressure suggests
appendicitis (a *positive*
Rovsing's sign).

● *Psoas sign:* Place your hand
just above the patient's
right knee. Ask the patient
to raise that thigh against
your hand. Or, ask the

Pain from irritation of the
psoas muscle suggests an
inflamed appendix (a *positive*
psoas sign).

EXAMINATION TECHNIQUES   POSSIBLE FINDINGS

patient to turn onto the
left side. Then extend the
patient's right leg at the hip
to stretch the psoas muscle.

- *Obturator sign:* Flex the
patient's right thigh at the
hip, with the knee bent, and
rotate the leg internally at
the hip, which stretches the
internal obturator muscle.

Right hypogastric pain in a
positive obturator sign,
suggesting irritation of the
obturator muscle by an
inflamed appendix.

ASSESSING POSSIBLE ACUTE CHOLECYSTITIS

Auscultate, percuss, and
palpate the abdomen for
tenderness.

Bowel sounds may be active or
decreased; tympany may
increase with an ileus; RUQ
tenderness.

Assess for *Murphy's sign.*
Hook your thumb under the
right costal margin at edge
of rectus muscle, and ask
patient to take a deep breath.

Sharp tenderness and a sudden
stop in inspiratory effort
constitute a *positive* Murphy's
sign.

RECORDING YOUR FINDINGS

Recording the Physical Examination—The Abdomen

"Abdomen is protuberant with active bowel sounds. It is
soft and nontender; no masses or hepatosplenomegaly.
Liver span is 7 cm and in the right MCL; edge is smooth
and palpable 1 cm below the right costal margin. Spleen
and kidneys not felt. No CVA tenderness."

OR

"Abdomen is flat. No bowel sounds heard. It is firm and
boardlike, with increased tenderness, guarding, and
rebound in the right midquadrant. Liver percusses to 7 cm
in the MCL; edge not felt. Spleen and kidneys not felt. No
palpable mass. No. CVA tenderness." *(Suggests peritonitis
from possible appendicitis; see pp. 207–208.)*

AIDS TO INTERPRETATION

TABLE 11-1 Diarrhea

Problem/Process	Characteristics of Stool
Acute Diarrhea	
Secretory Infections	
Infection by viruses; preformed bacterial toxins such as *Staphylococcus aureus, Clostridium perfringens,* toxigenic *Escherichia coli; Vibrio cholerae, Cryptosporidium, Giardia lamblia*	Watery, without blood, pus, or mucus
Inflammatory Infections	
Colonization or invasion of intestinal mucosa as in nontyphoid *Salmonella, Shigella, Yersinia, Campylobacter,* enteropathic *E. coli, Entamoeba histolytica*	Loose to watery, often with blood, pus, or mucus
Drug-induced Diarrhea	
Action of many drugs, such as magnesium-containing antacids, antibiotics, antineoplastic agents, and laxatives	Loose to watery
Chronic Diarrhea	
Diarrheal Syndromes	
• Irritable bowel syndrome: A disorder of bowel motility with alternating diarrhea and constipation	Loose; may show mucus but no blood. Small, hard stools with constipation
• Cancer of the sigmoid colon: Partial obstruction by a malignant neoplasm	May be blood streaked

(table continues next page)

TABLE 11-1 **Diarrhea** (continued)	
Problem/Process	**Characteristics of Stool**
Inflammatory Bowel Disease	
• *Ulcerative colitis:* inflammation and ulceration of the mucosa and submucosa of the rectum and colon	From soft to watery, often containing blood
• *Crohn's disease* of the small bowel (regional enteritis) or colon (granulomatous colitis): chronic inflammation of the bowel wall, typically involving the terminal ileum, proximal colon, or both	Small, soft to loose or watery, usually free of gross blood (enteritis) or with less bleeding than ulcerative colitis (colitis)
Voluminous Diarrheas	
• Malabsorption syndromes: Defective absorption of fat, including fat-soluble vitamins, with steatorrhea (excessive excretion of fat) as in pancreatic insufficiency, bile salt deficiency, bacterial overgrowth	Typically bulky, soft, light yellow to gray, mushy, greasy or oily, and sometimes frothy; particularly foul smelling; usually floats in the toilet
• Osmotic diarrheas	
• Lactose intolerance: Deficiency in intestinal lactase	Watery diarrhea of large volume
• Abuse of osmotic purgatives: Laxative habit, often surreptitious	Watery diarrhea of large volume
• Secretory diarrheas from bacterial infection, secreting villous adenoma, fat or bile salt malabsorption, hormone-mediated conditions (gastrin in Zollinger–Ellison syndrome, vasoactive intestinal peptide [VIP]): Process is variable	Watery diarrhea of large volume

TABLE 11-2 Urinary Incontinence

Problem	Mechanisms
Stress Incontinence: Urethral sphincter weakened. Transient increases in intra-abdominal pressure raise bladder pressure to levels exceeding urethral resistance. Leads to voiding *small amounts* during laughing, coughing, and sneezing.	In women, weakness of the pelvic floor with inadequate muscular support of the bladder and proximal urethra and a change in the angle between the bladder and the urethra from childbirth, surgery, and local conditions affecting the internal urethral sphincter, such as postmenopausal atrophy of the mucosa and urethral infection In men, prostatic surgery
Urge Incontinence: Detrusor contractions are stronger than normal and overcome normal urethral resistance. Bladder is typically small. Results in voiding *moderate amounts,* urgency, frequency, and nocturia.	• Decreased cortical inhibition of detrusor contractions, as in stroke, brain tumor, dementia, and lesions of the spinal cord above the sacral level • Hyperexcitability of sensory pathways, as in bladder infection, tumor, and fecal impaction • Deconditioning of voiding reflexes, caused by frequent voluntary voiding at low bladder volumes
Overflow Incontinence: Detrusor contractions are insufficient to overcome urethral resistance. Bladder is typically large, even after an effort to void, leading to *continuous dribbling.*	• Obstruction of the bladder outlet, as by benign prostatic hyperplasia or tumor

(table continues next page)

TABLE 11-2 Urinary Incontinence (continued)

Problem	Mechanisms
	• Weakness of detrusor muscle associated with peripheral nerve disease at the sacral level
	• Impaired bladder sensation that interrupts the reflex arc, as in diabetic neuropathy
Functional Incontinence: Inability to get to the toilet in time because of impaired health or environmental conditions	Problems in mobility from weakness, arthritis, poor vision, other conditions; environmental factors such as unfamiliar setting, distant bathroom facilities, bed rails, physical restraints
Incontinence Secondary to Medications: Drugs may contribute to any type of incontinence listed.	Sedatives, tranquilizers, anticholinergics, sympathetic blockers, potent diuretics

TABLE 11-3 Abdominal Tenderness

Visceral Tenderness	Peritoneal Tenderness

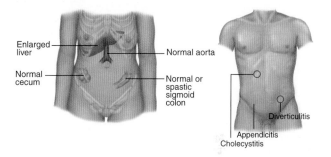

Tenderness From Disease in the Chest and Pelvis

Acute Pleurisy	*Acute Salpingitis*

Unilateral or bilateral, upper or lower abdomen

The Peripheral Vascular System

Common or Concerning Symptoms

- Pain in the arms or legs
- Intermittent claudication
- Cold, numbness, pallor in the legs, hair loss
- Color change in fingertips or toes in cold weather
- Swelling in calves, legs, or feet
- Swelling with redness or tenderness

Ask about any *pain in the arms and legs.*

Is there *intermittent claudication,* exercise-induced pain that is absent at rest, makes the patient stop exertion, and abates within about 10 minutes? Ask "Have you ever had any pain or cramping in your legs when you walk or exercise?" "How far can you walk without stopping to rest?" and "Does pain improve with rest?"

Peripheral arterial disease (PAD) can cause symptomatic limb ischemia with exertion; distinguish this from spinal stenosis, which produces leg pain with exertion that may be reduced by leaning forward (stretching the spinal cord in the narrowed vertebral canal) and less readily relieved by rest.

Ask also about *coldness, numbness,* or *pallor* in legs or feet or *hair loss* over the anterior tibial surfaces.

Hair loss over the anterior tibiae in PAD. "Dry" or brown-black ulcers from gangrene may ensue.

Because patients have few symptoms, identify background risk factors—tobacco abuse, hypertension, diabetes, hyperlipidemia, and history of myocardial infarction or stroke.

Only approximately 10% of affected patients have the classic symptoms of exertional calf pain relieved by rest.

"Do your fingertips or toes ever change color in cold weather or when you handle cold objects?"

Digital ischemic changes from arterial spasm cause blanching, followed by cyanosis and then rubor with cold exposure and rewarming in *Raynaud's phenomenon or disease*

Ask about *swelling of feet and legs,* or any ulcers on lower legs, often near the ankles from peripheral vascular disease.

Calf swelling in deep venous thrombosis; hyperpigmentation, edema, and possible cyanosis, especially when legs are dependent, in *venous stasis ulcers;* swelling with redness and tenderness in *cellulitis*

HEALTH PROMOTION AND COUNSELING

Important Topics for Health Promotion and Counseling

- Screening for peripheral arterial disease (PAD); the ankle-brachial index
- Screening for renal artery disease
- Screening for abdominal aortic aneurysm

Screening for Peripheral Arterial Disease (PAD). PAD involves the femoral and popliteal arteries most commonly, followed by the tibial and peroneal arteries. PAD affects from 12% to 29% of community populations; despite significant association with cardiovascular and cerebrovascular disease, PAD often is underdiagnosed in office practices. Most patients with PAD have either no symptoms or a range of *nonspecific leg symptoms*, such as *aching, cramping, numbness,* or *fatigue.*

Screen patients for PAD risk factors, such as tobacco abuse, elevated cholesterol, diabetes, age older than 70 years, hypertension, or atherosclerotic coronary, carotid, or renal artery disease. Pursue aggressive risk factor intervention. Consider use of the ankle-brachial index (ABI), a highly accurate test for detecting stenoses of 50% or more in major vessels of the legs.

A wide range of interventions is available to reduce both onset and progression of PAD, including meticulous foot care and well-fitting shoes, tobacco cessation, treatment of hyperlipidemia, optimal control and treatment of diabetes and hypertension, use of antiplatelet agents, graded exercise, and, if needed, surgical revascularization. Patients with ABIs in the lowest category have a 20% to 25% annual risk for death.

Screening for Renal Artery Disease. The American College of Cardiology and the American Heart Association recommend diagnostic studies for renal artery disease, usually beginning with ultrasound, in patients with the following conditions: hypertension before 30 years; severe hypertension (see p. 63) after 55 years; accelerated, resistant, or malignant hypertension; new worsening of renal function or worsening after use of an angiotensin-converting enzyme inhibitor or an angiotensin-receptor blocking agent; an unexplained small kidney; or sudden unexplained pulmonary edema, especially in the setting of worsening renal function. Symptoms arise from these conditions rather than directly from atherosclerotic changes in the renal artery.

Screening for Abdominal Aortic Aneurysm (AAA). An AAA is present when the infrarenal aortic diameter exceeds 3.0 cm. Rupture and mortality rates dramatically increase for AAAs exceeding 5.5 cm in diameter. The strongest risk factor for rupture is excess aortic diameter. Additional risk factors are smoking, age older than 65 years, family history, coronary artery disease, PAD, hypertension, and elevated cholesterol level. Because symptoms are rare, and screening is now shown to reduce mortality by approximately 40%, the U.S. Preventive Services Task Force recommends one-time screening by ultrasound in men between 65 and 75 years old with a history of "ever smoking," defined as more than 100 cigarettes in a lifetime.

TECHNIQUES OF EXAMINATION

EXAMINATION TECHNIQUES   POSSIBLE FINDINGS

ARMS

Inspect for

• Size and symmetry, any swelling	Lymphedema, venous obstruction
• Venous pattern	Venous obstruction
• Color and texture of skin and nails	*Raynaud's disease*

Palpate and grade the pulses:

● Grading Arterial Pulses	
3+	Bounding
2+	Brisk, expected (normal)
1+	Diminished, weaker than expected
0	Absent, unable to palpate

EXAMINATION TECHNIQUES	POSSIBLE FINDINGS

- Radial

Bounding radial, carotid, and femoral pulses in *aortic insufficiency*

Lost in *thromboangiitis obliterans* or *acute arterial occlusion*

- Brachial

Feel for the epitrochlear nodes.

Lymphadenopathy from local cut, infection

○— *LEGS*

Inspect for

- Size and symmetry, any swelling in thigh or calf

Venous insufficiency, lymphedema; deep venous thrombosis

- Venous pattern

Varicose veins

- Color and texture of skin

Pallor, rubor, cyanosis; erythema, warmth in *cellulitis, thrombophlebitis*

EXAMINATION TECHNIQUES	POSSIBLE FINDINGS

● Hair distribution

Loss in arterial insufficiency

Check for pitting edema.

Dependent edema, congestive heart failure, hypoalbuminemia, nephrotic syndrome

Palpate the calves.

Tenderness in deep venous thrombosis (though tenderness often not present)

Palpate and grade the pulses:

Loss of pulses in acute arterial occlusion and arteriosclerosis obliterans

● Femoral

● Popliteal

● Dorsalis pedis

EXAMINATION TECHNIQUES	POSSIBLE FINDINGS

● Posterior tibial

Palpate the inguinal lymph nodes:

Lymphadenopathy in genital infections, lymphoma, AIDs

● Horizontal group

● Vertical group

Horizontal Femoral artery group
Femoral vein
Vertical group
Great saphenous vein

Ask patient to stand, and reinspect the venous pattern.

Varicose veins

EXAMINATION TECHNIQUES POSSIBLE FINDINGS

SPECIAL TECHNIQUES

EVALUATING ARTERIAL SUPPLY TO THE HAND

Feel ulnar pulse, if possible. Perform an **Allen test**.

Persisting pallor of palm indicates occlusion of the released artery or its distal branches.

1. Ask patient to make a tight fist, palm up. Occlude both radial and ulnar arteries with your thumb.

2. Ask patient to open hand into a relaxed, slightly flexed position.

3. Release your pressure over one artery.

4. Palm should flush within 3 to 5 seconds. Repeat, releasing other artery.

EXAMINATION TECHNIQUES	POSSIBLE FINDINGS

o—/ **POSTURAL COLOR CHANGES OF CHRONIC ARTERIAL INSUFFICIENCY**

Raise both legs to 60° for about 1 minute. Then ask patient to sit up with legs dangling down. Note time required for (1) return of pinkness (normally 10 seconds) and (2) filling of veins on feet and ankles (normally about 15 seconds).

Marked pallor of feet on elevation, delayed color return and venous filling, and rubor of dependent feet suggest arterial insufficiency.

RECORDING YOUR FINDINGS

Recording the Physical Examination— The Peripheral Vascular System

"Extremities are warm and without edema. No varicosities or stasis changes. Calves are supple and nontender. No femoral or abdominal bruits. Brachial, radial, femoral, popliteal, dorsalis pedis (DP), and posterior tibial (PT) pulses are 2+ and symmetric."

OR

"Extremities are pale below the midcalf, with notable hair loss. Rubor noted when legs dependent but no edema or ulceration. Bilateral femoral bruits; no abdominal bruits heard. Brachial and radial pulses 2+; femoral, popliteal, DP, and PT pulses 1+." (Alternatively, pulses can be recorded as below.)

	Radial	Brachial	Femoral	Popliteal	Dorsalis Pedis	Posterior Tibial
RT	2+	2+	1+	1+	1+	1+
LT	2+	2+	1+	1+	1+	1+

(Suggests atherosclerotic PAD)

AIDS TO INTERPRETATION

| TABLE 12-1 | Chronic Insufficiency of Arteries and Veins |

Condition	Characteristics
Chronic Arterial Insufficiency Rubor Ischemic ulcer	Intermittent claudication progressing to pain at rest. Decreased or absent pulses. Pale, especially on elevation; dusky red on dependency. Cool. No or mild edema, which may develop on lowering the leg to relieve pain. Thin, shiny, atrophic skin, with hair loss over foot and toes and thickened, ridged nails. Possible ulceration on toes or points of trauma on feet. Potential gangrene.
Chronic Venous Insufficiency 	No pain to aching pain on dependency. Normal pulses, though may be hard to feel because of edema. Color normal or cyanotic on dependency; petechiae or brown pigment may develop. Often marked edema. Stasis dermatitis, possible thickening of skin, and narrowing of leg as scarring develops. Potential ulceration at sides of ankles. No gangrene.

TABLE 12-2 Common Ulcers of the Feet and Ankles

Ulcer	Characteristics
Arterial Insufficiency	Located on toes, feet, or possible areas of trauma. No callus or excess pigment. May be atrophic. Pain often severe, unless masked by neuropathy. Possible gangrene. Decreased pulses, trophic changes, pallor of foot on elevation, dusky rubor on dependency.
Chronic Venous Insufficiency	Located on inner or outer ankle. Pigmented, sometimes fibrotic. Pain not severe. No gangrene. Edema, pigmentation, stasis dermatitis, and possibly cyanosis of feet on dependency.
Neuropathic Ulcer	Located on pressure points in areas with diminished sensation, as in diabetic neuropathy. Skin calloused. No pain (which may cause ulcer to go unnoticed). Usually no gangrene. Decreased sensation, absent ankle jerks.

TABLE 12-3 Using the Ankle–Brachial Index

Instructions for Measuring the Ankle–Brachial Index (ABI)*

1. Patient should rest supine in a warm room for at least 10 minutes before testing.

Doppler

Brachial artery

2. Place blood pressure cuffs on both arms and ankles as illustrated, then apply ultrasound gel over brachial, dorsalis pedis, and posterior tibial arteries.
3. Measure systolic pressures in the arms
   - Use Doppler to locate brachial pulse
   - Inflate cuff 20 mm Hg above last audible pulse
   - Deflate cuff slowly and record pressure at which pulse becomes audible
   - Obtain 2 measures in each arm and record the average as the brachial pressure in that arm

Dorsalis pedis (DP) artery

Doppler

Doppler

Posterior tibial (PT) artery

4. Measure systolic pressures in ankles
   - Use Doppler to locate dorsalis pedis pulse
   - Inflate cuff 20 mm Hg above last audible pulse

(table continues next page)

TABLE 12-3   Using the Ankle–Brachial Index (continued)

Instructions for Measuring the Ankle–Brachial Index (ABI)*

- Deflate cuff slowly and record pressure at which pulse becomes audible
- Obtain 2 measures in each ankle and record the average as the dorsalis pedis pressure in that leg
- Repeat above steps for posterior tibial arteries
5. Calculate ABI

$$\text{Right ABI} = \frac{\text{highest right average ankle pressure (DP or PT)}}{\text{highest average arm pressure (right or left)}}$$

$$\text{Left ABI} = \frac{\text{highest left average ankle pressure (DP or PT)}}{\text{highest average arm pressure (right or left)}}$$

Interpretation of Ankle–Brachial Index*

Ankle–Brachial Index Result	Clinical Interpretation
>0.90 (with a range of 0.90 to 1.30)	Normal lower extremity blood flow
<0.89 to >0.60	Mild PAD
<0.59 to >0.40	Moderate PAD
<0.39	Severe PAD

(*Source: Laine C, Goldman D, Wilson JF. In the clinic: peripheral arterial disease. Ann Int Med 146(5):ITC 3-1, 2007.)

Male Genitalia and Hernias

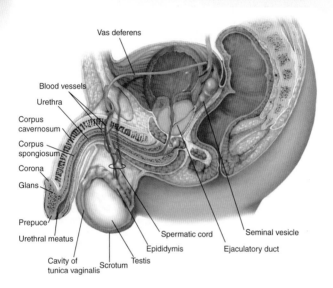

Vas deferens

Blood vessels

Urethra

Corpus cavernosum

Corpus spongiosum

Corona

Glans

Prepuce

Urethral meatus

Cavity of tunica vaginalis

Scrotum

Testis

Epididymis

Spermatic cord

Seminal vesicle

Ejaculatory duct

THE HEALTH HISTORY

Common or Concerning Symptoms

- Sexual preference and sexual response
- Penile discharge or lesions
- Scrotal pain, swelling, or lesions

Explain your concern for the patient's sexual health. Pose questions in a neutral and nonjudgmental way.

● "What is your relationship status? Tell me about your sexual preference."

● "How is sexual function for you?" "Are you satisfied with your sexual life?" "What about your ability to perform sexually?"

To assess *libido*, or desire: "Have you maintained an interest in sex?"	Decreased interest from psychogenic causes such as depression, endocrine dysfunction, or side effects of medications
For the *arousal* phase: "Can you achieve and maintain an erection?"	Erectile dysfunction from psychogenic causes, especially if early morning erection is preserved; also from decreased testosterone, decreased blood flow in hypogastric arterial system, impaired neural innervation
If *ejaculation* is premature or early: "About how long does intercourse last?" "Do you climax too soon?" For reduced or absent ejaculation: "Do you find that you cannot have orgasm even though you can have an erection?" "Does the problem involve the pleasurable sensation of *orgasm*, the ejaculation of seminal fluid, or both?"	Premature ejaculation is common, especially in young men. Less common is reduced or absent ejaculation affecting middle-aged or older men. Possible causes are medications, surgery, neurologic deficits, or lack of androgen. Lack of orgasm with intact ejaculation is usually psychogenic.

To assess possible infection from sexually transmitted diseases (STDs), ask about any *discharge from the penis.*

Penile discharge in *gonococcal* (usually yellow) and *nongonococcal* (clear or white) *urethritis*

Inquire about *sores or growths on the penis* and any *pain or swelling in the scrotum.*

See Table 13-1, Abnormalities of the Penis and Scrotum (p. 236), and Table 13-2, Sexually Transmitted Diseases of Male Genitalia (p. 237).

STDs may involve other parts of the body. Ask about practices of oral and anal sex and any related sore throat, oral itching or pain, diarrhea, or rectal bleeding.

Rash in disseminated gonococcal infection

HEALTH PROMOTION AND COUNSELING

Important Topics for Health Promotion and Counseling

- Prevention of STDs and HIV
- Testicular self-examination

Prevention of STDs and HIV Infection. Focus on patient education about STDs and HIV, early detection of infection during history taking and physical examination, and identification and treatment of infected partners. Identify the patient's sexual orientation, the number of sexual partners in the past month, and any history of STDs. Also query use of alcohol and drugs, particularly injection drugs. Counsel patients at risk about limiting the number of partners, using condoms, and establishing regular medical care for treatment of STDs and HIV infection.

Counseling and testing for HIV are recommended for: all people at increased risk for infection with HIV, STDs, or both; men with male partners; past or present injection drug users; men and women having unprotected sex with multiple partners; sex workers; any past or present partners of people with HIV infection, bisexual practices, or injection drug use; and patients with a history of transfusion between 1978 and 1985.

Testicular Self-examination.   Encourage men, especially those between 15 and 35 years of age, to perform monthly testicular self-examinations.

TECHNIQUES OF EXAMINATION

EXAMINATION TECHNIQUES   POSSIBLE FINDINGS

MALE GENITALIA

Wear gloves. The patient may be standing or supine.

THE PENIS

○—/ ♀   **Inspect** the

- Development of the penis   Sexual maturation, lice
  and the skin and hair at its
  base

- Prepuce   *Phimosis*

- Glans   *Balanitis, chancre, herpes,*
                             warts, cancer

- Urethral meatus   *Hypospadias,* discharge of
                             urethritis

Palpate

- Any visible lesions   *Chancre,* cancer

- The shaft   Urethral stricture or cancer

EXAMINATION TECHNIQUES   POSSIBLE FINDINGS

THE SCROTUM AND ITS CONTENTS

Inspect

- Contours of scrotum   Hernia, *hydrocele, cryptorchidism*

- Skin of scrotum   Rashes

Palpate each

- Testis, noting any

  - Lumps   Testicular carcinoma

  - Tenderness   Orchitis, torsion of the
  spermatic cord, strangulated
  inguinal hernia

- Epididymis   Epididymitis, cyst

- Spermatic cord and
  adjacent areas   Varicocele if multiple tortuous
  veins; if cystic structure, may
  be a hydrocele

EXAMINATION TECHNIQUES	POSSIBLE FINDINGS

HERNIAS

Patient is usually standing.

Inspect inguinal and femoral areas as patient strains down.

Inguinal and femoral hernias

Palpate external inguinal ring through scrotal skin and ask patient to strain down.

Indirect and direct inguinal hernias

Inguinal ligament

External inguinal ring

SPECIAL TECHNIQUE

THE TESTICULAR SELF-EXAMINATION

> ## PATIENT INSTRUCTIONS FOR THE TESTICULAR SELF-EXAMINATION
>
> This examination is best performed after a warm bath or shower. The heat relaxes the scrotum and makes it easier to find anything unusual.
>
> - Standing in front of a mirror, check for any swelling on the skin of the scrotum.
> - Examine each testicle with both hands. Cup the index and middle fingers under the testicle and place the thumbs on top.
> - Roll the testicle gently between the thumbs and fingers. One testicle may be larger than the other . . . that's normal, but be concerned about any lump or area of pain.
>
> *(continued)*

PATIENT INSTRUCTIONS FOR THE
TESTICULAR SELF-EXAMINATION (CONTINUED)

● Find the epididymis. This is a soft, tubelike structure at the back of the testicle that collects and carries sperm, not an abnormal lump.

● If you find any lump, don't wait. See your doctor. The lump may just be an infection, but if it is cancer, it will spread unless stopped by treatment.

(Source: Medline Plus. U.S. National Library of Medicine and National Institutes of Health. Medical Encyclopedia—Testicular self-examination. Available at: www.nlm.nih.gov/medlineplus/ency/article/003909.htm. Accessed June 8, 2007.)

RECORDING YOUR FINDINGS

Recording the Physical Examination—
Male Genitalia and Hernias

"Circumcised male. No penile discharge or lesions. No scrotal swelling or discoloration. Testes descended bilaterally, smooth, without masses. Epididymis nontender. No inguinal or femoral hernias."

OR

"Uncircumcised male; prepuce easily retractible. No penile discharge or lesions. No scrotal swelling or discoloration. Testes descended bilaterally; right testicle smooth; 1 × 1 cm firm nodule on left lateral testicle. It is fixed and nontender. Epididymis nontender. No inguinal or femoral hernias."

(Suspicious for testicular carcinoma, the most common form of cancer in men between 15 and 35 years of age)

AIDS TO INTERPRETATION

TABLE 13-1 Abnormalities of the Penis and Scrotum

Hypospadias
A congenital displacement of the urethral meatus to the inferior surface of the penis. A groove extends from the actual urethral meatus to its normal location on the tip of the glans.

Scrotal Edema
Pitting edema may make the scrotal skin taut; seen in congestive heart failure or nephrotic syndrome.

Peyronie's Disease
Palpable, nontender, hard plaques are found just beneath the skin, usually along the dorsum of the penis. The patient complains of crooked, painful erections.

Fingers can get above mass

Hydrocele
A nontender, fluid-filled mass within the tunica vaginalis. It transilluminates, and the examining fingers can get above the mass within the scrotum.

Carcinoma of the Penis
An indurated nodule or ulcer that is usually nontender. Limited almost completely to men who are not circumcised, it may be masked by the prepuce. Any persistent penile sore is suspicious.

Fingers cannot get above mass

Scrotal Hernia
Usually an *indirect inguinal hernia* that comes through the external inguinal ring, so the examining fingers cannot get above it within the scrotum.

TABLE 13-2 Sexually Transmitted Diseases of Male Genitalia

Genital Warts (condylomata acuminata)

- *Appearance:* Single or multiple papules or plaques of variable shapes; may be round, acuminate (or pointed), or thin and slender. May be raised, flat, or cauliflower-like (verrucous).
- *Causative organism: Human papillomavirus (HPV)*, usually from subtypes 6, 11; carcinogenic subtypes rare, approximately 5–10% of all anogenital warts. *Incubation:* weeks to months; infected contact may have no visible warts.
- Can arise on penis, scrotum, groin, thighs, anus; usually asymptomatic, occasionally cause itching and pain.
- May disappear without treatment.

Genital Herpes Simplex

- *Appearance:* Small scattered or grouped vesicles, 1–3 mm in size, on glans or shaft of penis. Appear as erosions if vesicular membrane breaks.
- *Causative organism:* Usually *Herpes simplex virus 2* (90%), a double-stranded DNA virus. *Incubation:* 2 to 7 days after exposure.
- Primary episode may be asymptomatic; recurrence usually less painful, of shorter duration.
- Associated with fever, malaise, headache, arthralgias; local pain and edema, lymphadenopathy.
- Need to distinguish from genital herpes zoster (usually in older patients with dermatomal distribution); candidiasis.

Primary Syphilis

- *Appearance:* Small red papule that becomes a *chancre*, or *painless* erosion up to 2 cm in diameter. Base of chancre is clean, red, smooth, and glistening; borders are raised and indurated. Chancre heals within 3–8 weeks.
- *Causative organism: Treponema pallidum*, a spirochete. *Incubation:* 9 to 90 days after exposure.
- May develop inguinal lymphadenopathy within 7 days; lymph nodes are rubbery, nontender, mobile.
- 20–30% of patients develop secondary syphilis while chancre still present (suggests co-infection with HIV).
- Distinguish from: genital herpes simplex, chancroid, granuloma inguinale from *Klebsiella granulomatis* (rare in U.S.; 4 variants, so difficult to identify).

Chancroid

- *Appearance:* Red papule or pustule initially, then forms a *painful* deep ulcer with ragged non-indurated margins; contains necrotic exudate, has a friable base.
- *Causative organism: Haemophilus ducreyi*, an anaerobic bacillus. *Incubation:* 3 to 7 days after exposure.
- Painful inguinal adenopathy; suppurative bobos in 25% of patients.
- Need to distinguish from: primary syphilis; genital herpes simplex; lymphomogranuloma venerium; granuloma inguinale from *Klebsiella granulomatis* (both rare in U.S.).

TABLE **13-3** **Abnormalities of the Testes**

Cryptorchidism
Testis is atrophied and may lie in the inguinal canal or the abdomen, resulting in an unfilled scrotum. As above, there is no palpable left testis or epididymis. Cryptorchidism markedly raises the risk for testicular cancer.

Small Testis
In adults, testicular length is usually ≤3.5 cm. Small, firm testes seen in *Klinefelter's syndrome,* usually ≤2 cm. Small, soft testes suggesting atrophy seen in cirrhosis, myotonic dystrophy, use of estrogens, and hypopituitarism; may also follow orchitis.

Acute Orchitis
The testis is acutely inflamed, painful, tender, and swollen. It may be difficult to distinguish from the epididymis. The scrotum may be reddened. Seen in mumps and other viral infections; usually unilateral.

Early

Late

Tumor of the Testis
Usually appears as a painless nodule. Any nodule within the testis warrants investigation for malignancy.

As a testicular neoplasm grows and spreads, it may seem to replace the entire organ. The testicle characteristically feels heavier than normal.

TABLE 13-4 Abnormalities of the Epididymis and Spermatic Cord

Acute Epididymitis

An acutely inflamed epididymis is tender and swollen and may be difficult to distinguish from the testis. The scrotum may be reddened and the vas deferens inflamed. It occurs chiefly in adults. Coexisting urinary tract infection or prostatitis supports the diagnosis.

Spermatocele and Cyst of the Epididymis

A painless, movable cystic mass just above the testis suggests a spermatocele or an epididymal cyst. Both transilluminate. The former contains sperm, and the latter does not, but they are clinically indistinguishable.

Varicocele

Varicocele refers to varicose veins of the spermatic cord, usually found on the left. It feels like a soft "bag of worms" separate from the testis, and slowly collapses when the scrotum is elevated in the supine patient.

Torsion of the Spermatic Cord

Twisting of the testicle on its spermatic cord produces an acutely painful and swollen organ that is retracted upward in the scrotum, which becomes red and edematous. There is no associated urinary infection. It is a surgical emergency because of obstructed circulation.

TABLE 13-5 Hernias in the Groin

Indirect Inguinal

Most common hernia at all ages, both sexes. Originates above inguinal ligament and often passes into scrotum. *May touch examiner's fingertip in inguinal canal.*

Direct Inguinal

Less common than indirect hernia, usually occurs in men older than 40 years. Originates above inguinal ligament near external inguinal ring and *rarely enters scrotum. May bulge anteriorly, touching side of examiner's finger.*

Femoral

Least common hernia, more common in women than in men. Originates below inguinal ligament, more lateral than inguinal hernia. *Never enters scrotum.*

Female Genitalia

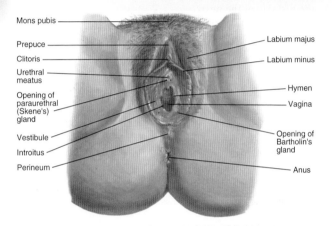

Mons pubis

Prepuce

Clitoris

Urethral meatus

Opening of paraurethral (Skene's) gland

Vestibule

Introitus

Perineum

Labium majus

Labium minus

Hymen

Vagina

Opening of Bartholin's gland

Anus

THE HEALTH HISTORY

Common Concerns

- Menarche, menstruation, menopause, postmenopausal bleeding
- Pregnancy
- Vulvovaginal symptoms
- Sexual preference and sexual response

For the *menstrual history,* ask the patient when her menstrual periods began (age at menarche).

The interval from previous periods can signal possible pregnancy or menstrual irregularities.

When did her last period start, and the one before that? What is the interval between periods, from the first day of one to the first day of the next? Are menses regular or irregular? How long do they last? How heavy is the flow?

In amenorrhea from *pregnancy, common early symptoms* are tenderness, tingling, or increased size of breasts; urinary frequency; nausea and vomiting; easy fatigability; and feelings that the baby is moving (usually noted at about 20 weeks).

Amenorrhea followed by heavy bleeding in threatened abortion or dysfunctional uterine bleeding

Dysmenorrhea, or painful menses, is common.

Primary dysmenorrhea from increased prostaglandin production; secondary dysmenorrhea from *endometriosis, pelvic inflammatory disease,* endometrial polyps

Amenorrhea is the absence of periods. Failure to begin periods is called *primary amenorrhea,* while cessation of established periods is termed *secondary amenorrhea.*

Secondary amenorrhea from low body weight from causes such as malnutrition, *anorexia nervosa,* stress, chronic illness, and hypothalamic–pituitary–ovarian dysfunction

Menopause, the absence of menses for 12 consecutive months, usually occurs between 48 and 55 years. Associated symptoms include hot flashes, flushing, sweating, and sleep disturbances.

Postmenopausal bleeding, or bleeding occurring 6 months after menses have stopped, raises the question of endometrial cancer, hormone replacement therapy, or uterine or cervical polyps.

For *vaginal discharge* and local *itching,* inquire about amount, color, consistency, and odor of discharge.

See Table 14-1, Lesions of the Vulva, pp. 251–252; and Table 14-4, Vaginal Discharge, p. 255.

To assess sexual function, start with general nonjudgmental questions like "How is sex for you?" or "Are you having any problems with sex?"

Direct questions help you assess each phase of the sexual response: desire, arousal, and orgasm.

Ask also about *dyspareunia,* or discomfort or pain during intercourse.

Superficial pain suggests local inflammation, atrophic vaginitis, or inadequate lubrication; deeper pain may result from pelvic disorders or pressure on a normal ovary.

For *sexually transmitted diseases* (STDs), identify sexual preference (male, female, or both) and the number of sexual partners in the previous month. Ask if the patient has concerns about HIV infection, desires HIV testing, or has current or past partners at risk.

In women, some STDs do not produce symptoms, but do pose as risk of infertility.

HEALTH PROMOTION AND COUNSELING

Important Topics for Health Promotion and Counseling

- Cervical cancer screening; Pap smear and HPV infection
- Options for family planning
- STDs and HIV
- Changes in menopause

Cervical Cancer Screening and HPV Infection.   Observe the guidelines from the American College of Obstetricians and Gynecologists (ACOG) in 2003 for *Pap smear* screening in different age groups:

- **First screen:** 3 years after first sexual intercourse or by age 21, whichever comes first

- **Women up to 30 years:** Annual screening

- **Women 30 years or older:**

  - Screen every 2 to 3 years if three consecutive annual cervical cytology results are negative or if combined cervical cytology testing and high-risk human papillomavirus (HPV) testing are negative

  - Screen more frequently in patients with positive Pap or high-risk HPV test; HIV infection; immunosuppression; DES exposure in utero; prior history of cervical cancer

- **Women with hysterectomy:** Discontinue routine screening **if** the cervix was removed for benign reasons and there is no history of abnormal or cancerous cell growth. If the woman has such a history, screen annually, and discontinue screening if three consecutive vaginal cytology tests are negative.

- **Older women:** Base continued screening on clinical assessment of individual health and ability to monitor the patient.

The most important risk factor for cervical cancer is human papillomavirus (HPV) infection from HPV strains 16, 18, 6, or 11. The HPV vaccine prevents HPV 16 and 18 infection when given *before* sexual exposure.

Options for Family Planning. Counsel women, particularly adolescents, about the *timing of ovulation,* which occurs midway in the regular menstrual cycle. Discuss methods for contraception and their effectiveness: natural (periodic abstinence, withdrawal, lactation); barrier (condom, diaphragm, cervical cap); implantable (intrauterine device, subdermal implant); pharmacologic (spermicide, oral contraceptives, subdermal implant of levonorgestrel, estrogen/progesterone injectables and patch, vaginal ring); and surgical (tubal ligation).

STDs and HIV. *For STDs and HIV,* assess risk factors by taking a careful sexual history and counseling patients about spread of disease and ways to reduce high-risk practices. Test women younger than 24 years and pregnant women for chlamydia; in women at increased risk and pregnant women, test for gonorrhea, syphilis, and HIV.

Menopause. Be familiar with the psychological and physiologic changes of *menopause.* Help the patient to weigh the benefits and risks of treatment, taking into account the personal and family history of cardiovascular disease and osteoporosis.

TECHNIQUES OF EXAMINATION

TIPS FOR THE SUCCESSFUL PELVIC EXAMINATION

The Patient	*The Examiner*
• Avoids intercourse, douching, or use of vaginal suppositories for 24 to 48 hours before examination	• Obtains permission
	• Explains each step of the examination in advance; selects chaperone
	• Drapes patient from mid-abdomen to knees; depresses drape between knees to provide eye contact with patient
• Empties bladder before examination	• Avoids unexpected or sudden movements
• Lies supine, with head and shoulders elevated, arms at sides or folded across chest to enhance eye contact and reduce tightening of abdominal muscles	• Chooses a speculum that is the correct size
	• Warms speculum with tap water
	• Wears gloves
	• Monitors comfort of the examination by watching the patient's face
	• Uses excellent but gentle technique, especially when inserting the speculum

Male examiners should be accompanied by female assistants. Female examiners should be assisted whenever possible.

EXAMINATION TECHNIQUES	POSSIBLE FINDINGS

EXTERNAL GENITALIA

Observe pubic hair to assess sexual maturity.

Normal or *delayed puberty*

Examine the external genitalia.

• Labia

Inflammation

EXAMINATION TECHNIQUES	POSSIBLE FINDINGS

- Clitoris

  Enlarged in masculinization

- Urethral orifice

  Urethral caruncle

- Introitus

  Imperforate hymen

Palpate for enlargement or tenderness of Bartholin's glands.

Bartholin's gland infection

Milk the urethra for discharge, if indicated.

Discharge of urethritis

INTERNAL GENITALIA AND PAP SMEAR

Locate the cervix with a gloved and water-lubricated index finger.

Assess support of vaginal outlet by asking patient to strain down.

Cystocele, cystourethrocele, rectocele

Enlarge the introitus by pressing its posterior margin downward.

Insert a water-lubricated speculum of suitable size, starting with speculum held obliquely.

ENTRY ANGLE

EXAMINATION TECHNIQUES	POSSIBLE FINDINGS

Rotate the speculum, open it, and inspect cervix.

Observe

- Position

Cervix faces forward if uterus is retroverted.

- Color

Purplish in pregnancy

- Epithelial surface

Squamous and columnar epithelium

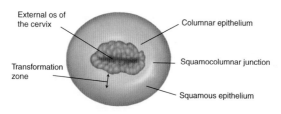

External os of the cervix

Columnar epithelium

Transformation zone

Squamocolumnar junction

Squamous epithelium

- Any discharge or bleeding

Discharge from os in mucopurulent cervicitis from chlamydia or gonorrhea

- Any ulcers, nodules, or masses

Herpes, polyp, cancer

Obtain specimens for cytology (Pap smears) with

Early cancer before it is clinically evident

- An endocervical spatula or brush (except in pregnant women), to scrape the ectocervix

- Or, if the woman is not pregnant, a cervical broom for a combined specimen (also used for Thin Prep)

EXAMINATION TECHNIQUES	POSSIBLE FINDINGS

Inspect the vaginal mucosa as you withdraw the speculum.

Bluish color and deep rugae in pregnancy; vaginal cancer

Palpate, by means of a bimanual examination,

* The cervix and fornices

Pain on moving cervix in *pelvic inflammatory disease*

* The uterus

Pregnancy, myomas; soft isthmus in early pregnancy

* Right and left adnexa (ovaries)

Ovarian masses, salpingitis, tubal pregnancy

Assess strength of pelvic muscles. With your vaginal fingers clear of the cervix, ask patient to tighten her muscles around your fingers as hard and long as she can.

A firm squeeze that compresses your fingers, moves them up and inward, and lasts more than 3 seconds is full strength.

EXAMINATION TECHNIQUES   POSSIBLE FINDINGS

When indicated,
perform a rectovaginal
examination (see p. 264).

Retroverted
uterus

SPECIAL TECHNIQUE

HERNIAS

Ask the woman to strain down,
as you palpate for a bulge in

● The femoral canal   Femoral hernia

● The labia majora up to just   Indirect inguinal hernia
   lateral to the pubic tubercle

RECORDING YOUR FINDINGS

Recording the Physical Examination—Female Genitalia

"No inguinal adenopathy. External genitalia without
erythema, lesions, or masses. Vaginal mucosa pink. Cervix
parous, pink, and without discharge. Uterus anterior,
midline, smooth, and not enlarged. No adnexal tenderness.
Pap smear obtained. Rectovaginal wall intact. Rectal vault
without masses. Stool brown and hemoccult negative."

OR

"Bilateral shotty inguinal adenopathy. External genitalia
without erythema or lesions. Vaginal mucosa and cervix
coated with thin, white, homogenous discharge with mild
fishy odor. After swabbing cervix, no discharge visible in
cervical os. Uterus midline; no adnexal masses. Rectal vault
without masses. Stool brown and hemoccult negative."
(Suggests bacterial vaginosis)

AIDS TO INTERPRETATION

TABLE 14-1 Lesions of the Vulva

Epidermoid Cyst

Cystic nodule in skin

A small, firm, round cystic nodule in the labia suggests an *epidermoid cyst*. They are sometimes yellowish in color. Look for the dark punctum marking the blocked opening of the gland.

Venereal Wart
(Condyloma Acuminatum)

Warts

Warty lesions on the labia and within the vestibule suggest *condylomata acuminata* from infection with human papillomavirus.

Genital Herpes

Shallow ulcers on red bases

Shallow, small, painful ulcers on red bases suggest a herpes infection. Initial infection may be extensive, as illustrated here. Recurrent infections are usually confined to a small local patch.

(table continues next page)

TABLE 14-1 Lesions of the Vulva (continued)

Syphilitic Chancre

A firm, painless ulcer suggests the chancre of *primary syphilis.* Because most chancres in women develop internally, they often go undetected.

Secondary Syphilis
(Condyloma Latum)

Flat, gray papules

Slightly raised, round or oval flat-topped papules covered by a gray exudate suggest *condylomata lata,* a manifestation of *secondary syphilis.* They are contagious.

Carcinoma of the Vulva

An ulcerated or raised red vulvar lesion in an elderly woman may indicate vulvar carcinoma.

TABLE 14-2 Shapes of the Cervical Os

Normal Variations

Oval	Slitlike

Lacerations

Unilateral Transverse	Bilateral Transverse

Stellate

TABLE 14-3 Abnormalities of the Cervix

Endocervical polyp. A bright red, smooth mass that protrudes from the os suggests a polyp. It bleeds easily.

Mucopurulent cervicitis. A yellowish exudate emerging from the cervical os suggests this diagnosis. Causes include *Chlamydia* and gonococcal infections.

Carcinoma of the cervix. An irregular, hard mass suggests cancer. Early lesions cannot be detected by physical examination alone.

Columnar epithelium   Vaginal adenosis
Collar

Fetal exposure to diethylstilbestrol (DES). Several changes may be seen: a collar of tissue around the cervix, columnar epithelium that covers the cervix or extends to the vaginal wall (then termed *vaginal adenosis*), and, rarely, carcinoma of the vagina.

TABLE 14-4 Vaginal Discharge

Note: Accurate diagnosis depends on laboratory assessment and cultures.

Trichomonas vaginitis	**Discharge:** Yellowish green, often profuse, may be malodorous
	Other Symptoms: Itching, vaginal soreness, dyspareunia
	Vulva: May be red
	Vagina: May be normal or red, with red spots, petechiae
	Laboratory Assessment: Saline wet mount for trichomonads
Candida vaginitis	**Discharge:** White, curdy, often thick, not malodorous
	Other Symptoms: Itching, vaginal soreness, external dysuria, dyspareunia
	Vulva: Often red and swollen
	Vagina: Often red with white patches of discharge
	Laboratory Assessment: KOH preparation for branching hyphae
Bacterial vaginosis	**Discharge:** Gray or white, thin, homogeneous, scant, malodorous
	Other Symptoms: Fishy genital odor
	Vulva: Usually normal
	Vagina: Usually normal
	Laboratory Assessment: Saline wet mount for "clue cells," "whiff test" with KOH for fishy odor

TABLE 14-5 Relaxations of the Pelvic Floor

When the pelvic floor is weakened, various structures may become displaced. These displacements are seen best when the patient strains down.

A **cystocele** is a bulge of the anterior wall of the upper part of the vagina, together with the urinary bladder above it.

A **cystourethrocele** involves both the bladder and the urethra as they bulge into the anterior vaginal wall throughout most of its extent.

A **rectocele** is a bulge of the posterior vaginal wall, together with a portion of the rectum.

A **prolapsed uterus** has descended down the vaginal canal. There are three degrees of severity: first, still within the vagina (as illustrated); second, with the cervix at the introitus; and third, with the cervix outside the introitus.

TABLE 14-6	**Positions of the Uterus and Uterine Myomas**

 An anteverted uterus lies in a forward position at roughly a right angle to the vagina. This is the most common position. *Anteflexion*—a forward flexion of the uterine body in relation to the cervix—often coexists.

 A retroverted uterus is tilted posteriorly with its cervix facing anteriorly.

 A retroflexed uterus has a posterior tilt that involves the uterine body but not the cervix. A uterus that is retroflexed or retroverted may be felt only through the rectal wall; some cannot be felt at all.

 A myoma of the uterus is a very common, benign tumor that feels firm and often irregular. There may be more than one. A myoma on the posterior surface of the uterus may be mistaken for a retrodisplaced uterus; one on the anterior surface may be mistaken for an anteverted uterus.

15

The Anus, Rectum, and Prostate

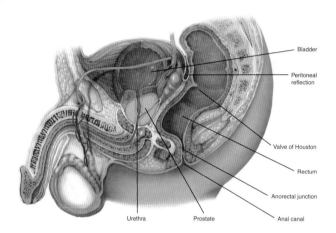

Bladder

Peritoneal reflection

Valve of Houston

Rectum

Anorectal junction

Anal canal

Urethra   Prostate

THE HEALTH HISTORY

Common or Concerning Symptoms

- Change in bowel habits
- Blood in the stool
- Pain with defecation; rectal bleeding or tenderness
- Anal warts or fissures
- Weak stream of urine
- Burning with urination

Ask about any change in bowel habits or problems with diarrhea or constipation. Is there any blood in the stool, or dark tarry stools?

Pencil-like stool or blood in stool in *colon cancer;* dark tarry stools in *gastrointestinal bleeding*

Any pain with defecation, or rectal bleeding or tenderness?

Hemorrhoids; proctitis from STDs

Any anal warts or fissures?

Human papillomavirus (HPV), condylomata lata in secondary syphilis; fissures in proctitis, Crohn's disease

In men, is there difficulty starting the urine stream or holding back urine? Is the flow weak? What about frequent urination, especially at night? Or pain or burning when passing urine? Any blood in the urine or semen or pain with ejaculation? Is there frequent pain or stiffness in the lower back, hips, or upper thighs?

These symptoms suggest urethral obstruction as in *benign prostatic hyperplasia (BPH)* or *prostate cancer,* especially in men older than 70 years. The American Urological Association (AUA) Symptom Index helps quantify BPH severity (see Table 15-1, p. 267).

HEALTH PROMOTION AND COUNSELING

Important Topics for Health Promotion and Counseling

- Screening for prostate cancer
- Screening for polyps and colorectal cancer
- Counseling for STDs

Prostate Cancer. Prostate cancer is the leading cancer diagnosed in men in the United States and the third leading cause of death in men. Risk factors are age, family history of prostate cancer, and African-American ethnicity.

Screening methods such as the digital rectal examination (DRE) and the prostate-specific antigen (PSA) test are not highly accurate, which complicates decisions about screening of patients *without symptoms*. The DRE reaches only the posterior and lateral surfaces of the prostate, missing 25% to 35% of tumors in other areas. Sensitivity of the DRE for prostate cancer is low, ranging from 20% to 68%, and the rate of false positives is high. Recommendations about an annual DRE vary.

The benefits of PSA testing are also unclear. The PSA can be elevated in benign conditions like hyperplasia and prostatitis, and its detection rate for prostate cancer is low, about 28% to 35% in asymptomatic men. Several groups recommend annual combined screening with PSA and DRE for men older than 50 years and for African-Americans and men older than 40 years with a positive family history. Some experts now recommend baseline PSA testing at age 40, reducing the threshold for biopsy from 4.0 ng/ml to 2.5 ng/ml, and tracking *PSA velocity*, or the rate of rise in 1 year.

For men *with symptoms* of prostate disorders, the clinician's role is more straightforward. Men with incomplete emptying of the bladder, urinary frequency or urgency, weak or inter-mittent stream or straining to initiate flow, hematuria, nocturia, or even bony pains in the pelvis should be encouraged to seek evaluation and treatment early.

Colorectal Cancer (CRC). Screening recommendations have recently been revised to promote more aggressive surveil-lance by clinicians:

- Clinicians should first identify whether patients are at average or increased risk for CRC, ideally by approximately age 20 years, but earlier if the patient has a family history of familial adenomatous polyposis.

- Average-risk patients 50 years or older should be offered a range of screening options to increase compliance: annual fecal occult blood testing (FOBT); flexible sigmoidoscopy

every 5 years, either alone or combined with annual
FOBT; double-contrast barium enema every 5 years; or
colonoscopy every 10 years.

- People at increased risk should undergo colonoscopy at
  intervals ranging from 3 to 5 years.

Clinicians should also use the 6-sample fecal occult blood
test (FOBT). Avoid single-sample FOBT and DRE, which
have inadequate detection rates.

Counseling for STDs.   Anal intercourse increases risk for HIV
and STDs. Promote abstinence, use of condoms, and good
hygiene.

TECHNIQUES OF EXAMINATION

EXAMINATION TECHNIQUES   POSSIBLE FINDINGS

○⌐   **Wear gloves.**

MALE

Position the patient on his
side, or standing leaning
forward over the examining
table and hips flexed.

EXAMINATION TECHNIQUES	POSSIBLE FINDINGS

Inspect the

- Sacrococcygeal area

    Pilonidal cyst or sinus

- Perianal area

    Hemorrhoids, warts, herpes, chancre, cancer, fissures from *proctitis* or *Crohn's disease*

Palpate the anal canal and rectum with a lubricated and gloved finger. Feel the:

Lax sphincter tone in some neurologic disorders; tightness in proctitis

- Walls of the rectum

    Cancer of the rectum, polyps

- Prostate gland, as shown below, including median sulcus

EXAMINATION TECHNIQUES	POSSIBLE FINDINGS

Try to **feel** above the prostate for irregularities or tenderness, if indicated.

Benign hyperplasia, cancer, tenderness in *acute prostatitis*

⚥ / ♀ **FEMALE**

The patient is usually in the lithotomy position or lying on her side.

Rectal shelf of peritoneal metastases; tenderness of inflammation

Inspect the anus.

Palpate the anal canal and rectum.

Hemorrhoids

Rectal cancer, normal uterine cervix or tampon (felt through the rectal wall)

RECORDING YOUR FINDINGS

Recording the Physical Examination—
The Anus, Rectum, and Prostate

"No perirectal lesions or fissures. External sphincter tone intact. Rectal vault without masses. Prostate smooth and nontender with palpable median sulcus. (Or in a female, uterine cervix nontender.) Stool brown and hemoccult negative."

OR

"Perirectal area inflamed; no ulcerations, warts, or discharge. Cannot examine external sphincter, rectal vault, or prostate because of spasm of external sphincter and marked inflammation and tenderness of anal canal." (*Raises concern of proctitis from infectious cause*)

OR

"No perirectal lesions or fissures. External sphincter tone intact. Rectal vault without masses. Left lateral prostate lobe with 1 × 1 cm firm hard nodule; right lateral lobe smooth; medial sulcus is obscured. Stool brown and hemoccult negative." (*Raises concern of prostate cancer*)

TABLE 15-1 BPH Symptom Score Index: American Urological Association (AUA)

Score or ask the patient to score each of the questions below. Higher scores (maximum 35) indicate more severe symptoms; scores ≤7 are considered mild and generally do not warrant treatment.

PART A	Not at All	Less Than 1 Time in 5
1. Over the past month, how often have you had a sensation of not emptying your bladder completely after you finished urinating?		
2. Over the past month, how often have you had to urinate again less than two hours after you finished urinating?		
3. Over the past month, how often have you stopped and started again several times when you urinated?		
4. Over the past month, how often have you found it difficult to postpone urination?		
5. Over the past month, how often have you had a weak urinary stream?		
6. Over the past month, how often have you had to push or strain to begin urination?		

PART B	None	1 Time
7. Over the past month, how many times did you most typically get up to urinate from the time you went to bed at night until the time you got up in the morning?		

(Adapted from: Madsen FA, Bruskewitz RC. Clinical manifestations of benign prostatic hyperplasia. Urol Clin North AM 1995:22:291–298.)

Less Than Half the Time	About Half the Time	More Than Half the Time	Almost Always	Total Points for Each Row

2 Times	3 Times	4 Times	5 Times	Points for Part B

TOTAL PARTS A and B (maximum 35) _____

TABLE 15-2 Abnormalities on Rectal Examination

External Hemorrhoids
  (*Thrombosed*). Dilated
  hemorrhoidal veins that
  originate below the
  pectinate line, covered
  with skin; a tender,
  swollen, bluish ovoid mass
  is visible at the anal
  margin.

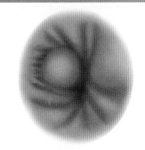

Polyps of the Rectum. A soft
  mass that may or may not
  be on a stalk; may not be
  palpable

Benign Prostatic Hyperplasia.
  An enlarged, nontender,
  smooth, firm but slightly
  elastic prostate gland; can
  cause symptoms without
  palpable enlargement

(table continues next page)

TABLE 15-2 **Abnormalities on Rectal Examination** (continued)

Acute Prostatitis. A prostate that is very tender, swollen, and firm because of acute infection

Cancer of the Prostate. A hard area in the prostate that may or may not feel nodular

Cancer of the Rectum. Firm, nodular, rolled edge of an ulcerated cancer

The Musculoskeletal System

16

FUNDAMENTALS FOR ASSESSING JOINTS

Assessing joints requires knowledge of their structure and function. Learn the surface landmarks and underlying anatomy of each major joint. Be familiar with the following terms:

- *Articular structures*—include the joint capsule and articular cartilage, synovium and synovial fluid, intra-articular ligaments, and juxta-articular bone

- *Extra-articular structures*—include periarticular ligaments, tendons, bursae, muscle, fascia, bone, nerve, and overlying skin

  - *Ligaments*—the ropelike bundles of collagen fibrils that connect bone to bone

  - *Tendons*—the collagen fibers that connect muscle to bone

  - *Bursae*—the pouches of synovial fluid that cushion the movement of tendons and muscles over bone or other joint structures

Review the three primary types of joint articulation—synovial, cartilaginous, and fibrous—and the varying degrees of movement each type allows.

● Joints

Synovial Joints

- Freely movable
- Separated by **articular cartilage** and a **synovial cavity**
- Lubricated by synovial fluid
- Surrounded by a joint capsule
- Example: knee, shoulder

SYNOVIAL

Cartilaginous Joints

- Slightly movable
- Contain fibrocartilaginous discs that separate the bony surfaces
- Have a central *nucleus pulposus* of discs that cushions bony contact
- Example: vertebral bodies

CARTILAGINOUS

Fibrous Joints

- No appreciable movement
- Consist of fibrous tissue or cartilage
- Lack a joint cavity
- Example: skull sutures

FIBROUS

Review the types of synovial joints and their associated features as well.

Note that joint structure determines joint function.

● Synovial Joints

Type of Joint	Articular Shape	Movement	Example
Spheroidal (ball and socket)	Convex surface in concave cavity	Wide-ranging flexion, extension, abduction, adduction, rotation, circumduction	Shoulder, hip
Hinge	Flat, planar	Motion in one plane; flexion, extension	Interphalangeal joints of hand and foot; elbow
Condylar	Convex or concave	Movement of two articulating surfaces, not dissociable	Knee; temporomandibular joint

THE HEALTH HISTORY

Common or Concerning Symptoms

- Low back pain
- Neck pain
- Monoarticular or polyarticular joint pain
- Inflammatory or infectious joint pain
- Joint pain with systemic features such as fever, chills, rash, anorexia, weight loss, and weakness
- Joint pain with symptoms from other organ systems

Assess the seven features of any joint pain.

TIPS FOR ASSESSING JOINT PAIN

- Ask the patient to *point to the pain*. This may save considerable time, because the patient's verbal description is often imprecise.

(continued)

TIPS FOR ASSESSING JOINT PAIN (CONTINUED)

- Clarify and record the *mechanism of injury,* particularly if there is a history of trauma.
- Determine whether the pain is *localized* or *diffuse, acute* or *chronic, inflammatory* or *noninflammatory.*

Low Back Pain. Ask "Any pains in your back?" *Back-ache* is the second most common reason for office visits. Ask if the pain is in the midline over the vertebrae, or off midline. If the pain radiates into the legs, ask about any associated numbness, tingling, or weakness.

See Table 16-1, Low Back Pain, pp. 301–302. Causes of *midline back pain* include vertebral collapse, disc herniation, epidural abscess, spinal cord compression, or spinal cord metastases. *Pain off the midline* in sacroiliitis, trochanteric bursitis, sciatica, or hip arthritis

Check for bladder or bowel dysfunction.

Present in *cauda equine syndrome* from S2–S4 tumor or disc herniation

Neck Pain. Ask about location, radiation into the arms, arm or leg weakness, bladder or bowel dysfunction.

Often from C7 or C6 spinal nerve compression from foraminal impingement

Joint Pain. Proceed with "Do you have any pain in your joints?"

Ask the patient to *point to the pain.* If *localized* and involving only one joint, it is *monoarticular.*

Consider trauma, monoarticular arthritis, tendonitis, or bursitis. Hip pain near the greater trochanter suggests trochanteric bursitis.

If *polyarticular*, does it migrate from joint to joint, or steadily spread from one joint to

Migratory pattern in *rheumatic fever* or *gonococcal arthritis*; progressive and symmetric in *rheumatoid arthritis*

multiple joint involve-
ment? Is the involvement
symmetric?

Ask if pain is extra-articular
(bones, muscles, and tissues
around the joint, such as
the tendons, bursae, or even
overlying skin). Are there
generalized "aches and
pains" (*myalgia* if in
muscles, *arthralgia* if in
joints with no evidence
of arthritis)?

Bursitis if inflammation of
bursae, *tendonitis* if in tendons,
and *tenosynovitis* if in tendon
sheaths; also *sprains* from
stretching or tearing of
ligaments

Assess the timing, quality,
and severity of joint symptoms. If from trauma, what
was the *mechanism of injury*
or the series of events that
caused the joint pain? Further, what aggravates or
relieves the pain? What are
the effects of exercise, rest,
and treatment?

Severe pain of rapid onset in a
red, swollen joint in *acute
septic arthritis* or *gout*

Is the problem *inflamma-
tory* or *noninflammatory*? Is
there *tenderness, warmth,* or
redness?

Fever, chills, warmth, redness
in *septic arthritis*; also consider
gout or *rheumatic fever*

Is the pain *articular* in origin, with *swelling, stiffness,*
or *decreased range of motion*?

Pain, swelling, loss of active
and passive motion, "locking,"
deformity in *articular joint pain*;
loss of active but not passive
motion, tenderness outside
the joint, no deformity in
nonarticular pain

Assess any *limitations of
motion*.

Transient stiffness after limited
activity in *degenerative arthritis*;
prolonged stiffness in *rheumatoid
arthritis, fibromyalgia,
polymyalgia rheumatica*

Ask about any *systemic* symptoms such as fever, chills, rash, anorexia, weight loss, and weakness.

Common in *rheumatoid arthritis, systemic lupus erythematosus, polymyalgia rheumatica,* and other inflammatory arthritides. High fever and chills suggest an infectious cause.

HEALTH PROMOTION AND COUNSELING

Important Topics for Health Promotion and Counseling

- Nutrition, exercise, and weight
- Low back: lifting and biomechanics
- Preventing falls
- Osteoporosis: screening and prevention

Nutrition and Exercise. Advise patients that a healthy lifestyle conveys direct benefits to the skeleton. Good nutrition supplies calcium for bone mineralization and bone density. Exercise appears to maintain and possibly supports bone mass, and improves outlook and stress management. Appropriate weight reduces excess mechanical wear on weight-bearing joints such as hips and knees.

Low Back. The low back is especially vulnerable, most notably at L5–S1, where the sacral vertebrae make a sharp posterior angle. Approximately 60% to 80% of the population experiences low back pain at least once. Exercises to strengthen the low back, especially in flexion and extension, and general fitness exercises appear equally effective. Education on lifting strategies, posture, and the biomechanics of injury is prudent for nurses, heavy-machinery operators, and construction workers.

Preventing Falls. Falls are the leading cause of nonfatal injuries and account for a dramatic rise in death rates after 65 years of age. Risk factors include unstable gait, imbalanced posture, reduced strength, cognitive loss and dementia, deficits in vision and proprioception, and osteoporosis. Urge patients to correct poor lighting, dark or steep stairs, chairs at awkward heights, slippery or irregular surfaces, and ill-fitting shoes. Scrutinize any medications affecting balance, especially benzodiazepines, vasodilators, and diuretics.

Osteoporosis. Osteoporosis is a major public health threat for postmenopausal women and some men. The World Health Organization defines osteoporosis as bone density equal to or greater than 2.5 standard deviations below the mean for young white adult women. A 10% drop in bone density, equivalent to one standard deviation, is associated with a 20% increase in risk of fracture.

The U.S. Preventive Services Task Force recommends routine bone density screening for women 65 years or older and for the risk factors below.

RISK FACTORS FOR OSTEOPOROSIS

- Postmenopausal status in white women
- Age older than 50 years
- Weight less than 70 kg
- Family history of fracture in a first-degree relative
- History of fracture
- Higher intakes of alcohol
- Women with delayed menarche or early menopause
- Current smokers
- Low levels of 25-hydroxyvitamin D
- Use of corticosteroids for more than 2 months
- Inflammatory disorders of the musculoskeletal, pulmonary, or gastrointestinal systems, including celiac sprue, chronic renal disease, organ transplantation, hypogonadism, anorexia nervosa

(Sources: NIH Consensus Development Panel on Osteoporosis Prevention, Diagnosis, and Therapy. Osteoporosis prevention, diagnosis, and therapy. JAMA 285(6):785–795, 2001; Raisz LG. Screening for osteoporosis. N Engl J Med 353(2):164–171, 2005.)

Several agents inhibit bone resorption: calcium, vitamin D, and antiresorptive agents such as bisphosphonates, selective estrogen-receptor modulators (SERMs), and calcitonin. Learn the therapeutic uses of the agents listed above and of exercise. The U.S. Preventive Services Task Force now recommends against the routine use of estrogen and progestin for the prevention of chronic conditions in postmenopausal women. Despite public interest, the natural estrogens, including the plant-derived phytoestrogens, have not been shown to reduce risk of fracture in humans.

TECHNIQUES OF EXAMINATION

GENERAL APPROACH

Inspect the joints and surrounding tissues as you examine the various body parts.

Identify joints with changes in structure and function, carefully assessing for:

- Symmetry of involvement—one or both sides of the body; one joint or several
- Deformity or malalignment of bones
- Changes in surrounding soft tissue—skin changes, subcutaneous nodules, muscle atrophy, crepitus
- Limitations in range of motion, ligamentous laxity
- Changes in muscle strength

Note signs of inflammation and arthritis: swelling, warmth, tenderness, redness.

EXAMINATION TECHNIQUES   POSSIBLE FINDINGS

TEMPOROMANDIBULAR JOINT (TMJ)

Inspect the TMJ for swelling or redness.

Palpate the TMJ as the patient opens and closes the mouth.

Palpate the muscles of mastication: the *masseters, temporal muscles,* and *pterygoid muscles.*

EXAMINATION TECHNIQUES

POSSIBLE FINDINGS

SHOULDERS

Inspect the contour of the shoulders and shoulder girdles from front and back.

Muscle atrophy; anterior or posterior dislocation of humeral head; scoliosis if shoulder heights asymmetric

PALPATE

• The clavicle from the sternoclavicular joint to the acromioclavicular joint

"Step-offs" if fracture from trauma

• The subacromial and subdeltoid bursae after lifting arm posteriorly

Subacromial or subdeltoid bursitis

Subacromial bursa

Rotator cuff

Assess range of motion.

• Flexion—"Raise your arm in front of you and overhead."

Intact glenohumeral motion if patient raises arms to shoulder level, palms facing *down*

• Extension—"Move your arms behind you."

Intact scapulothoracic motion if patient raises arms an additional 60 degrees, palms facing *up*

• Abduction—"Raise your arms out to the side and overhead."

EXAMINATION TECHNIQUES	POSSIBLE FINDINGS

- Adduction—"Cross your arm in front of your body, keeping the arm straight."

- External and internal rotation

Shoulder arthritis

TESTS ABDUCTION AND EXTERNAL ROTATION　　**TESTS ADDUCTION AND INTERNAL ROTATION**

Perform **maneuvers** to assess rotator cuff—supraspinatus, infraspinatus, teres minor, and subscapularis muscles and tendon insertions.

- "Empty can test" for supraspinatus strength

Weakness in *rotator cuff tear*

EXAMINATION TECHNIQUES	POSSIBLE FINDINGS

● Infraspinatus strength

Weakness in *rotator cuff tear* or *bicipital tendonitis*

● Forearm supination

Pain in *rotator cuff tear*

● "Drop arm" test

If patient cannot hold arm fully abducted at shoulder level, possible rotator cuff tear

EXAMINATION TECHNIQUES   POSSIBLE FINDINGS

ELBOWS

Inspect and palpate

- Olecranon process

  Olecranon bursitis; posterior dislocation from direct trauma or supracondylar fracture

- Medial and lateral epicondyles

  Tenderness distal to epicondyle in epicondylitis (medial → "tennis elbow"; lateral → "pitcher's elbow")

- Extensor surface of the ulna

  Rheumatoid nodules

- Grooves between the epicondyles and the olecranon

  Tender in arthritis

Ask patient to

- Flex and extend elbows

- Turn palms up and down (supination and pronation)

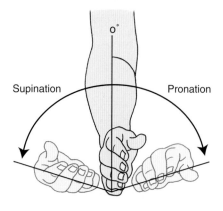

EXAMINATION TECHNIQUES   POSSIBLE FINDINGS

WRISTS AND HANDS
Inspect

- Movement of the wrist
(flexion, extension, ulnar
and medial deviation),
hands, and fingers

  Guarded movement in injury

- Contours of wrists, hands,
and fingers

  Deformities in *rheumatoid* and
degenerative arthritis; swelling
in arthritis, ganglia; impaired
alignment of fingers in flexor
tendon damage; flexion
contractures in Dupuytren's
contractures

- Contours of palms

  Thenar atrophy in median
nerve compression (*carpal
tunnel syndrome*); hypothenar
atrophy in ulnar nerve
compression

Palpate

- Wrist joints

  Swelling and tenderness
in *rheumatoid arthritis,
gonococcal infection* of joint
or extensor tendon sheaths

- Distal radius and ulna

  Tenderness over ulnar styloid
in *Colles' fracture*

EXAMINATION TECHNIQUES	POSSIBLE FINDINGS

- "Anatomic snuffbox," the hollow space distal to the radial styloid bone; thumb extensor and abductor tendons.

Tenderness suggests *scaphoid fracture.* Tenderness over extensor and abductor tendons in DeQuervain's tenosynovitis.

- Metacarpophalangeal joint

Swelling in *rheumatoid arthritis*

- Proximal and distal interphalangeal joint

Proximal nodules in rheumatoid arthritis (*Bouchard's nodes*), distal nodules in osteoarthritis (*Heberden's nodes*)

EXAMINATION TECHNIQUES	POSSIBLE FINDINGS

Assess range of motion.

- **Wrists:** Flexion, extension, adduction (radial deviation), abduction (lateral deviation)

  Arthritis, tenosynovitis

- **Fingers:** Flexions, extension, abduction/ adduction (spread fingers apart and back)

  Trigger finger, Dupuytren's contracture

- Thumbs

FLEXION

EXTENSION

ABDUCTION AND ADDUCTION

OPPOSITION

Perform selected maneuvers.

- Hand grip strength

Decreased grip strength if weakness of finger flexors or intrinsic hand muscles

EXAMINATION TECHNIQUES

POSSIBLE FINDINGS

- Thumb movement

Pain if DeQuervain's
tenosynovitis

- Carpal tunnel

  - Thumb adduction

Weakness of abductor pollicis
longus specific to median nerve

EXAMINATION TECHNIQUES	POSSIBLE FINDINGS

- Tinel's sign: Tap lightly over median nerve at volar wrist

Aching, tingling, and numbness in 2nd, 3rd, and 4th fingers

- Phalen's sign: Patient flexes wrists for 60 seconds

Aching, tingling, and numbness in 2nd, 3rd, and 4th volar fingers

SPINE

Inspect spine from the side and back, noting any abnormal curvatures.

Kyphosis, scoliosis, lordosis, gibbus, list curvatures

Look for asymmetric heights of shoulders, iliac crests, or buttocks.

Pelvic tilt

EXAMINATION TECHNIQUES   POSSIBLE FINDINGS

Spinous process of L5 vertebra

Intervertebral joint between L5 and sacrum

Posterior superior iliac spine

Sacroiliac joint

Ischial tuberosity and site of ischial bursa

Paravertebral muscles

Sacroiliac notch

Sciatic nerve

Identify and palpate

• Spinous processes of each vertebra	Tender if trauma, infection
	"Step-offs" in spondylolisthesis, fracture
• Sacroiliac joints	Sacroiliitis
• Paravertebral muscles, if painful	Paravertebral muscle spasm in abnormal posture, degenerative and inflammatory muscle disorders
• Sciatic nerve (midway between greater trochanter and ischial tuberosity)	Herniated disc or nerve root compression

Sciatic nerve

Greater trochanter

Ischial tuberosity

EXAMINATION TECHNIQUES	POSSIBLE FINDINGS

Test the range of motion in the neck and spine in: flexion, extension, rotation, and lateral bending.

Decreased mobility in arthritis

HIPS

Inspect gait for

- *Stance* (see below) and *swing* (foot moves forward, does not bear weight)

Most problems arise during the weight-bearing stance phase.

Heelstrike   Foot flat   Midstance   Push-off

PHASES OF GAIT: STANCE (Right Leg) AND SWING (Left Leg)

- *Width of base* (usually 2 to 4 inches from heel to heel), shift of pelvis, flexion of knee

Cerebellar disease or foot problems if wide base; impaired shift of pelvis in arthritis, hip dislocation, abductor weakness; disrupted gait if poor knee flexion

Palpate

- Along the inguinal ligament

Bulges in inguinal hernia, aneurysm

- The *iliopectineal bursa*, lateral to the femoral pulse

Tender in synovitis, bursitis, iliopsoas abscess

- The *trochanteric bursa*, on the greater trochanter of the femur

Focal tenderness in *trochanteric bursitis*, often described by patients as "low back pain"

EXAMINATION TECHNIQUES

POSSIBLE FINDINGS

- The *ischiogluteal bursa*, superficial to the ischial tuberosity

Tender in bursitis ("weaver's bottom")

Trochanteric bursa

Ischiogluteal bursa

TROCHANTERIC AND ISCHIOGLUTEAL BURSA

Check range of motion, including

- Flexion—"Bend your knee and pull it against your abdomen."

Flexion of opposite leg suggests deformity of that hip.

- Extension

Painful in iliopsoas abscess

- Abduction

Restricted in hip arthritis

EXAMINATION TECHNIQUES	POSSIBLE FINDINGS

- Adduction

- Internal and external rotation

Restricted in hip arthritis

KNEES

Review the structures of the knee.

Medial femoral condyle

Adductor tubercle

Medial femoral epicondyle

Patellar tendon

Medial collateral ligament

Medial tibial plateau

Pes anserine bursa

Tibial tuberosity

Inspect

- Gait for knee extension at heel strike, flexion during all other phases of swing and stance

Stumbling or pushing knee into extension in *quadriceps weakness*

EXAMINATION TECHNIQUES	POSSIBLE FINDINGS
• Alignment of knees	Bowlegs, knock-knees; flexion contractures in limb paralysis
• Contours of knees, including any atrophy of the quadriceps muscles	Quadriceps atrophy with *patellofemoral disorder*

Inspect and **palpate:**

The tibiofemoral joint—with knees flexed

• Joint line—place thumbs on either side of the patellar tendon.	Irregular, bony ridges in osteoarthritis.
• Medial and lateral meniscus	Tenderness if meniscus tear
• Medial and lateral collateral ligaments	Tenderness if MCL tear (LCL injuries less common)

The patellofemoral compartment

• Patella	Swelling over the patella in prepatellar bursitis ("housemaid's knee")
• Palpate the patellar tendon and ask patient to extend the leg.	Tenderness or inability to extend the leg in partial or complete tear of the patellar tendon
• Press the patella against the underlying femur.	Pain, crepitus, and a history of knee pain in *patellofemoral disorder*
• Push patella distally and ask patient to tighten knee against table.	Pain during contraction of quadriceps in *chondromalacia*

EXAMINATION TECHNIQUES	POSSIBLE FINDINGS

Also:

- Suprapatellar pouch

  Swelling in synovitis and arthritis

- Infrapatellar spaces (hollow areas adjacent to patella)

  Swelling in arthritis

- Medial tibial condyle

  Swelling in *pes anserine* bursitis

- Popliteal surface

  Popliteal or Baker's cyst

Assess any effusions.

- *Bulge Sign* (minor effusions): Compress the suprapatellar pouch, stroke downward on medial surface, apply pressure to force fluid to lateral surface, and then tap knee behind lateral margin of patella.

  A fluid wave returning to the medial surface after a lateral tap confirms an effusion—a positive "bulge sign."

Milk downward   Apply medial pressure   Tap and watch for fluid wave

EXAMINATION TECHNIQUES	POSSIBLE FINDINGS

- *Balloon Sign* (major effusions): Compress suprapatellar pouch with one hand; with thumb and finger of other hand, feel for fluid entering the spaces next to the patella.

A palpable fluid wave is a positive sign.

- *Lateral collateral ligament:* With knee slightly flexed, push laterally along medial surface of knee with one hand and pull medially at the ankle with the other hand (an *adduction* or *varus stress*).

Pain or a gap in the lateral joint line points to a partial or complete LCL tear.

- *Anterior cruciate ligament (ACL):* (1) With knee flexed, place thumbs on medial and lateral joint line and place fingers on hamstring insertions. Pull tibia forward, observe if tibia slides forward "like a drawer." Compare to opposite knee.

Forward slide of proximal tibia is a positive *anterior drawer sign* in ACL laxity or tear.

EXAMINATION TECHNIQUES	POSSIBLE FINDINGS

(2) *Lachman test:* Grasp the distal femur with one hand and the proximal tibia with the other (place the thumb on the joint line). Move the femur forward and the tibia back.

Significant forward excursion of tibia in ACL tear

• *Ballotte the patella* (major effusion): Push the patella sharply against the femur; watch for fluid returning to the suprapatellar space.

Visible wave is a positive sign.

EXAMINATION TECHNIQUES	POSSIBLE FINDINGS

If painful, use maneuvers to **assess** ligaments.

- *Medial meniscus and lateral meniscus—McMurray test:* With the patient supine, grasp the heel and flex the knee. Cup your other hand over the knee joint with fingers and thumb along the medial and lateral joint line. From the heel, rotate the lower leg internally and externally. Then push on the lateral side to apply a valgus stress on the medial side of the joint and rotate leg externally and slowly extend it.

Click or pop along the medial joint with valgus stress, external rotation, and leg extension in tear of posterior medial meniscus

Medial meniscus and lateral meniscus

- *Medial collateral ligament:* With knee slightly flexed, push medially against lateral surface of knee with one hand and pull laterally at the ankle with the other hand (*abduction* or *valgus stress*).

Pain or a gap in the medial joint line points to a partial or complete MCL tear.

- *Posterior cruciate ligament (PCL):* Position patient and hands as in the ACL test. Push the tibia posteriorly and observe for posterior movement, like a drawer sliding posteriorly.

Isolated PCL tears are rare.

Posterior cruciate ligament (PCL)

EXAMINATION TECHNIQUES   POSSIBLE FINDINGS

ANKLES AND FEET

Inspect ankles and feet.   Hallux valgus, corns, calluses

Palpate

- Ankle joint   Tender joint in arthritis

- Ankle ligaments: medial-deltoid; lateral-anterior and posterior talofibular, calcaneofibular   Tenderness in sprain: lateral ligaments weaker, inversion injuries (ankle bows outward) more common

- Achilles tendon   Rheumatoid nodules, tenderness in tendonitis

- **Compress** the metatarsophalangeal joints; then **palpate** each joint between the thumb and forefinger.   Tenderness in arthritis and other conditions

Assess range of motion.

- Dorsiflex and plantar flex the ankle (*tibiotalar joint*).   Arthritic joint often painful when moved in any direction; sprain, when injured ligament is stretched

EXAMINATION TECHNIQUES	POSSIBLE FINDINGS

- Stabilize the ankle and invert and evert the heel (*subtalar* or *talocalcaneal joint*).

Ankle sprain

INVERSION　　　　**EVERSION**

- Stabilize the heel and invert and evert the forefoot (*transverse tarsal joints*).

Trauma, arthritis

INVERSION　　　　**EVERSION**

- Flex toes at metatarsophalangeal joints.

EXAMINATION TECHNIQUES	POSSIBLE FINDINGS

SPECIAL TECHNIQUES

○— **Measuring Leg Length.** Patient's legs should be aligned symmetrically. With a tape, measure distance from anterior superior iliac spine to medial malleolus. Tape should cross knee medially.

Unequal leg length may be the cause of *scoliosis.*

/○— **Measuring Range of Motion.** To measure range of motion precisely, a simple pocket goniometer is needed. Estimates may be made visually. Movement in the elbow at the right is limited to range indicated by red lines.

A flexion deformity of 45° and further flexion to 90° (45° → 90°)

Recording the Physical Examination—
The Musculoskeletal System

"Good range of motion in all joints. No evidence of swelling or deformity."

OR

"Good range of motion in all joints. Hand with degenerative changes of Heberden's nodes at the distal interphalangeal joints, Bouchard's nodes at proximal interphalangeal joints. Mild pain with flexion, extension, and rotation of both hips. Good range of motion in the knees, with moderate crepitus; no effusion but boggy synovium and osteophytes along the tibiofemoral joint line bilaterally. Both feet with hallux valgus at the first metatarsophalangeal joints." (*Suggests osteoarthritis*)

AIDS TO INTERPRETATION

TABLE 16-1 Low Back Pain

Patterns	Physical Signs
Mechanical Low Back Pain Aching pain in the lumbo-sacral area; may radiate into lower leg, along L5 or S1 dermatomes. Usually acute, work-related, in age group 30 to 50 years; no underlying pathology	Paraspinal muscle or facet tenderness, muscle spasm or pain with back movement, loss of normal lumbar lordosis but no motor or sensory loss or reflex abnormalities. In osteoporosis, check for thoracic kyphosis, percussion tenderness over a spinous process, or fractures in the thoracic spine or hip.
Sciatica (Radicular Low Back Pain) Usually from disc herniation; more rarely from nerve root compression, primary or metastatic tumor	Disc herniation most likely if calf wasting, weak ankle dorsiflexion, absent ankle jerk, positive *crossed straight-leg raise* (pain in affected leg when healthy leg tested); negative straight-leg raise makes diagnosis highly unlikely.
Lumbar Spinal Stenosis Pseudoclaudication pain in the back or legs that improves with rest, forward lumbar flexion. Pain vague but usually bilateral, with paresthesias in one or both legs; usually from arthritic narrowing of spinal canal	Posture may be flexed forward with lower-extremity weakness and hyporeflexia; straight-leg raise usually negative

(table continues next page)

TABLE 16-1 Low Back Pain (continued)

Patterns	Physical Signs
Chronic Back Stiffness Consider ankylosing spondylitis in inflammatory polyarthritis, most common in men <40 years. Diffuse idiopathic skeletal hyperostosis (DISH) affects men more than women, usually aged >50 years.	Loss of the normal lumbar lordosis, muscle spasm, limited anterior and lateral flexion; improves with exercise. Lateral immobility of the spine, especially thoracic segment
Nocturnal Back Pain Unrelieved by Rest Consider metastatic malignancy to the spine from cancer of the prostate, breast, lung, thyroid, and kidney, and multiple myeloma.	Findings vary with the source. Local vertebral tenderness may be present.
Pain Referred from the Abdomen or Pelvis Usually a deep, aching pain, the level of which varies with the source (1% of low back pain)	Spinal movements are not painful and range of motion is not affected. Look for signs of the primary disorder, such as peptic ulcer, pancreatitis, dissecting aortic aneurysm.

TABLE 16-2 Pains in the Neck

Patterns	Physical Signs
Mechanical Neck Pain	
Aching pain in the cervical paraspinal muscles and ligaments with associated muscle spasm, with stiffness and tightness in the upper back and shoulder, lasting up to 6 weeks. No associated radiation, paresthesias, or weakness. Headache may be present.	Local muscle tenderness, pain on movement. No neurological deficits. Possible trigger points in *fibromyalgia*. *Torticollis* if prolonged abnormal neck posture and muscle spasm.
Mechanical Neck Pain—Whiplash	
Also mechanical neck pain with aching paracervical pain and stiffness, often beginning the day after injury. Occipital headache, dizziness, malaise, and fatigue may be present. Chronic whiplash syndrome if symptoms last more than 6 months, present in 20%–40% of injuries.	Localized paracervical tenderness, decreased neck range of motion, perceived weakness of the upper extremities. Causes of cervical cord compression such as fracture, herniation, head injury, or altered consciousness are excluded.
Cervical Radiculopathy— from nerve root compression	
Sharp burning or tingling pain in the neck and one arm, with associated paresthesias and weakness. Sensory symptoms often in myotomal pattern, deep in muscle, rather than dermatomal pattern.	C7 nerve root affected most often (~45%–60%), with weakness in triceps and finger flexors and extensors. C6 nerve root involvement also common, with weakness in biceps, brachioradialis, wrist extensors.

(table continues next page)

TABLE 16-2 **Pains in the Neck** (continued)

Patterns	Physical Signs
Cervical Myelopathy—from cervical cord compression	
Neck pain with bilateral weakness and paresthesias in both upper and lower extremities, often with urinary frequency. Hand clumsiness, palmar paresthesias, and gait changes may be subtle. Neck flexion often exacerbates symptoms.	Hyperreflexia; clonus at the wrist, knee, or ankle; extensor plantar reflexes (positive Babinski signs); and gait disturbances. May also see *Lhermitte's sign:* neck flexion with resulting sensation of electrical shock radiating down the spine. Confirmation of cervical myelopathy warrants neck immobilization and neurosurgical evaluation.

TABLE 16-3	**Patterns of Pain in and Around the Joints**	
	Rheumatoid Arthritis	Osteoarthritis (Degenerative Joint Disease, or DJD)
Process	Chronic inflammation of synovial membranes with secondary erosion of adjacent cartilage and bone, and damage to ligaments and tendons	Degeneration and progressive loss of cartilage within the joints, damage to underlying bone, and formation of new bone at the margins of the cartilage
Common Locations	Hands (proximal interphalangeal and metacarpophalangeal joints), feet (metatarsophalangeal joints), wrists, knees, elbows, ankles	Knees, hips, hands (distal, sometimes proximal interphalangeal joints), cervical and lumbar spine, and wrists (first carpometacarpal joint); also joints previously injured or diseased
Pattern of Spread	Symmetrically additive: progresses to other joints while persisting in the initial ones	Additive; however, sometimes only one joint is involved
Onset	Usually insidious	Usually insidious
Progression and Duration	Often chronic, with remissions and exacerbations	Slowly progressive, with temporary exacerbations after periods of overuse

(table continues next page)

TABLE 16-3	**Patterns of Pain in and Around the Joints** (continued)	

	Rheumatoid Arthritis	Osteoarthritis (Degenerative Joint Disease, or DJD)
Associated Symptoms	Frequent swelling of synovial tissue in joints or tendon sheaths; also sub-cutaneous nodules Tender, often warm, but seldom red Prominent stiffness, often for 1 hour or more in the mornings, also after inactivity Limitation of motion common Weakness, fatigue, weight loss, and low fever	Small effusions in the joints may be present, especially in the knees; also bony enlargement Possibly tender, seldom warm, and rarely red Frequent but brief stiffness (usually 5–10 min), in the morning and after inactivity Limitation of motion often develops

TABLE 16-4 Painful Tender Shoulders

Acromioclavicular Arthritis

Tenderness over the acromioclavicular joint, especially with adduction of the arm across the chest. Pain often increases with shrugging the shoulders, due to movement of scapula.

Subacromial and Subdeltoid Bursitis

Pain over anterior superior aspect of shoulder, particularly when raising the arm overhead. Tenderness common anterolateral to the acromion, in hollow recess formed by the acromiohumeral sulcus. Often seen in overuse syndromes.

Rotator Cuff Tendinitis

Tenderness over the rotator cuff, when elbow passively lifted posteriorly or with "drop-arm" maneuver.

Bicipital Tendinitis

Tenderness over the long head of the biceps when rolled in the bicipital groove or when flexed arm is supinated against resistance suggests *bicipital tendinitis*.

TABLE 16-5 Painful Tender Knees

Arthritis. *Degenerative arthritis* usually occurs after age 50; associated with obesity. Often with medial joint line tenderness, palpable osteophytes, bowleg appearance, suprapatellar bursae and joint effusion. Systemic involvement, swelling, and subcutaneous nodules in *rheumatoid arthritis.*

Prepatellar bursa

Pes anserine

Bursitis. Inflammation and thickening of bursa seen in repetitive motion and overuse syndromes. Can involve *prepatellar bursa* ("housemaid's knee"), *pes anserine* bursa medially (runners, osteoarthritis), *iliotibial band* laterally (over lateral femoral condyle), especially in runners.

Iliotibial band

(table continues next page)

TABLE 16-5 Painful Tender Knees (continued)

Patella moves up and lateral

Leg extends and foot raises

Patellofemoral instability. During flexion and extension of knee, due to subluxation and/or malalignment, patella tracks laterally instead of centrally in trochlear groove of femoral condyle. Inspect or palpate for lateral motion with leg extension. May lead to chondromalacia, osteoarthritis.

Lateral meniscus

Medial meniscus torn

Meniscal tear. Commonly arises from twisting injury of knee; in older patients may be degenerative, often with clicking, popping, or locking sensation. Check for tenderness along joint line over medial or lateral meniscus and for effusion. May have associated tears of medial collateral of anterior cruciate ligaments.

Anterior cruciate ligament torn

Anterior cruciate tear or sprain. In twisting injuries of the knee, often with popping sensation, immediate swelling, pain with flexion/extension, difficulty walking, and sensation of knee "giving way." Check for anterior drawer sign, swelling of hemarthrosis, injuries to medial meniscus or medial collateral ligament. Consider evaluation by an orthopedic surgeon.

(table continues next page)

TABLE 16-5 Painful Tender Knees (continued)

Medial collateral ligament torn

Collateral ligament sprain or tear. From force applied to medial or lateral surface of knee (valgus or varus stress), producing localized swelling, pain, stiffness. Patients able to walk but may develop an effusion. Check for tenderness over affected ligament and ligamentous laxity during valgus or varus stress.

Baker's cyst

Posterior knee

Baker's cyst. Cystic swelling palpable on the medial surface of the popliteal fossa, prompting complaints of aching or fullness behind the knee. Inspect, palpate for swelling adjacent to medial hamstring tendons. If present, suggests involvement of posterior horn of medial meniscus. In rheumatoid arthritis, cyst may expand into calf or ankle.

The Nervous System

The *central nervous system* (CNS) consists of the brain and
spinal cord. The *peripheral nervous system* consists of the
12 pairs of cranial nerves and the spinal and peripheral
nerves. Most peripheral nerves contain both motor and
sensory fibers.

 CENTRAL NERVOUS SYSTEM

The Brain

- *Gray matter,* or aggregations of neuronal cell bodies; rims
  the surfaces of the cerebral hemispheres, forming the
  cerebral cortex

- *White matter,* or neuronal axons coated with myelin,
  allowing nerve impulses to travel more rapidly

- *Basal ganglia,* which affect movement

- *Thalamus,* which processes and relays sensory impulses to
  the cerebral cortex

- *Hypothalamus,* which maintains homeostasis and regulates
  temperature, heart rate, and blood pressure; affects
  endocrine system, and governs emotional behaviors such
  as anger and sex drive; and contains hormones that act
  directly on the pituitary gland

- *Brainstem,* which connects the upper part of the brain
  with the spinal cord and has three sections: midbrain,
  pons, and medulla

- *Reticular activating (arousal) system,* in the diencephalon and upper brainstem; activation linked to consciousness

- *Cerebellum,* at the base of the brain, which coordinates all movement and helps maintain the body upright in space

The Spinal Cord

- A cylindrical mass of nerve tissue encased within the bony vertebral column, extending from medulla to first or second lumbar vertebra

- Contains important motor and sensory nerve pathways that exit and enter the cord via anterior and posterior nerve roots and spinal and peripheral nerves

- Mediates reflex activity of the deep tendon (or spinal nerve) reflexes

- Divided into five segments: cervical (C1–8), thoracic (T1–12), lumbar (L1–5), sacral (S1–5), and coccygeal

- Roots fan out like a horse's tail at L1–2, the *cauda equina*

 PERIPHERAL NERVOUS SYSTEM

The Cranial Nerves

- Cranial Nerves III through XII arise from the diencephalon and brainstem.

- Cranial Nerves I and II are actually fiber tracts emerging from the brain.

The Peripheral Nerves

- Thirty-one pairs of nerves carry impulses to and from the cord: 8 cervical, 12 thoracic, 5 lumbar, 5 sacral, and 1 coccygeal.

- Each nerve has an anterior (ventral) root containing motor fibers, and a posterior (dorsal) root containing sensory fibers.

- These merge to form a short (<5 mm) *spinal nerve.*

- Spinal nerve fibers commingle with similar fibers in plexuses outside the cord—from these emerge *peripheral nerves.*

THE HEALTH HISTORY

Common or Concerning Symptoms

- Headache
- Dizziness or vertigo
- Generalized, proximal, or distal weakness
- Numbness, abnormal or lost sensations
- Loss of consciousness, syncope, or near-syncope
- Seizures
- Tremors or involuntary movements

Headache: ask about location, severity, duration, and any associated symptoms, such as visual changes, weakness, or loss of sensation. Ask if coughing, sneezing, or sudden movements of the head affect the headache.

See Table 7-1, Primary Headaches, p. 125, and Table 7-2, Secondary Headaches, pp. 126–129. *Subarachnoid hemorrhage* may evoke "the worst headache of my life." Dull headache affected by maneuvers, especially on awakening and in the same location, in mass lesions such as brain tumors

Dizziness can have many meanings. Is the patient lightheaded or feeling faint? Or is there *vertigo*, a perception that the room is spinning or rotating?

Lightheadedness in palpitations; near-syncope from vasovagal stimulation, low blood pressure, febrile illness, and others; vertigo in inner ear conditions, brainstem tumor

Are any medications contributing to dizziness? Are associated symptoms present, such as double vision (*diplopia*), difficulty forming words (*dysarthria*), or difficulty with gait or balance (*ataxia*)? Is there any weakness?

Diplopia, dysarthria, ataxia in vertebrobasilar *transient ischemic attack (TIA)* or *stroke*

Weakness or paralysis in *TIA* or *stroke*

Distinguish *proximal* from *distal* **weakness.** For *proximal weakness,* ask about combing hair, reaching for things on a high shelf, difficulty getting out of a chair or taking a high step up. For *distal weakness* ask about hand movements such as opening a jar or can or using hand tools (e.g., scissors, pliers, screwdriver). Ask about frequent tripping.

Bilateral proximal weakness in *myopathy;* bilateral, predominantly distal weakness in *polyneuropathy;* weakness worsened by repeated effort and improved by rest in *myasthenia gravis*

Is there any **loss of sensation,** difficulty moving a limb, or altered sensation such as tingling or pins and needles? Peculiar sensations without an obvious stimulus (*paresthesias*)? *Dysesthesias,* or disordered sensations in response to a stimulus, may last longer than the stimulus itself.

Loss of sensation, paresthesias, and dysesthesias in brain and spinal cord lesions; also in disorders of peripheral sensory roots and nerves; paresthesias in hands and around mouth in hyperventilation

"Have you ever fainted or passed out?" leads the discussion to any *loss of consciousness.*

Syncope if sudden but temporary loss of consciousness from decreased cerebral blood flow commonly called *fainting.*

Get a complete description of the event. What brought on the episode? Were there any warning symptoms? Was the patient standing, sitting, or lying down when it began? How long did it last? Could voices be heard while passing out and coming to? How rapid was recovery? Were onset and offset slow or fast?

Young people with emotional stress and warning symptoms of flushing, warmth, or nausea may have *vasodepressor (or vasovagal) syncope* of slow onset, slow offset. *Cardiac syncope* from dysrhythmias, more common in older patients, often with sudden onset, sudden offset.

Also ask if anyone observed the episode. What did the patient look like before, during, and after the episode? Was there any seizure-like movement of the arms or legs? Any incontinence of the bladder or bowel?

A **seizure** is a paroxysmal disorder caused by sudden excessive electrical discharge in the cerebral cortex or its underlying structures. Depending on the type, there may be loss of consciousness or abnormal feelings, thought processes, and sensations, including smells, as well as abnormal movements.

Tonic–clonic motor activity, incontinence, and *postictal state* in generalized *seizures*. Unlike syncope, injury such as tongue biting or bruising of limbs may occur.

HEALTH PROMOTION AND COUNSELING

Important Topics for Health Promotion and Counseling

- Preventing stroke or transient ischemic attack (TIA)
- Preventing risk of peripheral neuropathy

Preventing Stroke or TIA.   Cerebrovascular disease is the third leading cause of death in the United States. Decreased vascular perfusion results in sudden focal but transient brain dysfunction in *TIA,* or in permanent neurological deficits in *stroke.*

Counsel patients about the warning signs of stroke attacks: sudden numbness or weakness of the face, arm, or leg; sudden confusion or trouble speaking or understanding; sudden difficulty walking, dizziness, or loss of balance or coordination; sudden trouble seeing in one or both eyes; or sudden severe headache. Detecting TIAs is important—in the first 3 months after a TIA, subsequent stroke occurs in approximately 15% of patients.

Stroke prevention requires aggressive management of risk factors and patient education. Risk factors include smoking, excess weight, hypertension, dyslipidemia, heavy alcohol use, physical inactivity, obesity, and diabetes. Blood pressure should be ≤ 140/90 mm Hg and ≤ 130/80 mm Hg for those with diabetes or nondiabetic renal disease with proteinuria. Lipid-lowering agents may reduce risk of stroke. Urge patients to replace saturated and transunsaturated fats, found in dairy products, meat, and stick margarine, with polyunsaturated and unhydrogenated monosaturated fats, found in soybeans, liquid margarine, and fish oils. Or recommend increased intake of fruits, vegetables, and fiber. Counsel patients to maintain regular exercise and body weight and to control their intake of alcohol. Aim for optimal control of blood glucose levels, at approximately 100 mg/dL for patients with diabetes.

Preventing Risk of Peripheral Neuropathy. Promote optimal glucose control in diabetes to reduce risk of sensorimotor polyneuropathy, autonomic dysfunction, mononeuritis multiplex, or diabetic neuropathy.

TECHNIQUES OF EXAMINATION

● Cranial Nerves and Function

No.	Cranial Nerve	Function
I	Olfactory	Sense of smell
II	Optic	Vision
III	Oculomotor	Pupillary constriction, opening the eye (lid elevation), and most extraocular movements

● Cranial Nerves and Function (continued)

No.	Cranial Nerve	Function
IV	Trochlear	Downward, inward movement of the eye
VI	Abducens	Lateral deviation of the eye
V	Trigeminal	*Motor*—temporal and masseter muscles (jaw clenching), also lateral pterygoid's (lateral jaw movement) *Sensory*—facial. The nerve has three divisions: (1) ophthalmic, (2) maxillary, and (3) mandibular.
VII	Facial	*Motor*—facial movements, including those of facial expression, closing the eye, and closing the mouth *Sensory*—taste for salty, sweet, sour, and bitter substances on the anterior two thirds of the tongue
VIII	Acoustic	Hearing (cochlear division) and balance (vestibular division)
IX	Glossopharyngeal	*Motor*—pharynx *Sensory*—posterior portions of the eardrum and ear canal, the pharynx, and the posterior tongue, including taste (salty, sweet, sour, bitter)
X	Vagus	*Motor*—palate, pharynx, and larynx *Sensory*—pharynx and larynx
XI	Spinal accessory	*Motor*—the sternomastoid and upper portion of the trapezius
XII	Hypoglossal	*Motor*—tongue

EXAMINATION TECHNIQUES	POSSIBLE FINDINGS

CRANIAL NERVES
CN I (OLFACTORY)

Test sense of smell on each side.

Loss in frontal lobe lesions

CN II (OPTIC)

Assess visual acuity.

Blindness

Check visual fields.

Hemianopsia

Inspect optic discs.

Papilledema, optic atrophy

CN II, III (OPTIC AND OCULOMOTOR)

Test pupillary reactions to light. If abnormal, test reactions to near effort.

Blindness, CN III paralysis, tonic pupils; Horner's syndrome may affect light reactions

CN III, IV, VI (OCULOMOTOR, TROCHLEAR, AND ABDUCENS)

Assess extraocular movements.

Strabismus from paralysis of CN III, IV, or VI; nystagmus

CN V (TRIGEMINAL)

Test pain and light touch sensations on face in ophthalmic, maxillary, and mandibular zones.

CN V—SENSORY

EXAMINATION TECHNIQUES	POSSIBLE FINDINGS

Feel the contractions of temporal and masseter muscles.

Motor or sensory loss from lesions of CN V or its higher motor pathways

TEMPORAL MUSCLES   **MASSETER MUSCLES**

Check corneal reflexes.

CN VII (FACIAL)

Ask patient to raise both eyebrows, frown, close eyes tightly, show teeth, smile, and puff out cheeks.

Weakness from lesion of peripheral nerve, as in Bell's palsy, or of CNS, as in a stroke. See Table 17-3, Facial Paralysis, p. 339.

CN VIII (ACOUSTIC)

Assess hearing. If decreased:

- Test for lateralization (**Weber test, p. 122**).

Sensorineural loss causes lateralization to affected ear where AC > BC. Conduction loss causes lateralization to affected ear and BC > AC.

EXAMINATION TECHNIQUES	POSSIBLE FINDINGS

- Compare air and bone conduction (**Rinne test**).

See p. 122.

CN IX, X (GLOSSOPHARYNGEAL AND VAGUS)

Observe any difficulty swallowing.

A weakened palate or pharynx impairs swallowing.

Listen to the voice.

Hoarseness or nasality

Watch soft palate rise with "ah."

Palatal paralysis in CVA

Test gag reflex on each side.

Absent reflex

CN XI (SPINAL ACCESSORY)

Trapezius Muscles. **Assess** muscles for bulk, involuntary movements, and strength of shoulder shrug.

Atrophy, fasciculations, weakness

Sternomastoid Muscles. **Assess** strength as head turns against your hand.

Weakness of sternomastoid muscle when head turns to *opposite* side

CN XII (HYPOGLOSSAL)

Listen to patient's articulation.

Dysarthria from damage to CN X or CN XII

Inspect the resting tongue.

Atrophy, fasciculations

Inspect the protruded tongue.

Deviation to weak side

EXAMINATION TECHNIQUES   POSSIBLE FINDINGS

⏚/○— *THE MOTOR SYSTEM*

BODY POSITION

Observe the patient's body   Hemiplegia in stroke
position during movement
and at rest.

INVOLUNTARY MOVEMENTS

If present, **observe** location,   Tremors, fasciculations, tics,
quality, rate, rhythm,   chorea, athetosis, oral–facial
amplitude, and setting.   dyskinesias

MUSCLE BULK

Inspect muscle contours.   Atrophy

MUSCLE TONE

Assess resistance to passive   Spasticity, rigidity, flaccidity
stretch of arms and legs.

MUSCLE STRENGTH

Test and grade the major
muscle groups:

● Grading Muscle Strength	
Grade	**Description**
0	No muscular contraction detected
1	A barely detectable trace of contraction
2	Active movement with gravity eliminated
3	Active movement against gravity
4	Active movement against gravity and some resistance
5	Active movement against full resistance (normal)

Look for a pattern in any detectable weakness. It may suggest
a lower motor neuron lesion affecting a peripheral nerve or
nerve root. Weakness of one side of body suggests an upper

EXAMINATION TECHNIQUES	POSSIBLE FINDINGS

motor neuron lesion. A *polyneuropathy* causes symmetric distal weakness, and a *myopathy* usually causes proximal weakness. Weakness that worsens with repeated effort and improves with rest suggests *myasthenia gravis*.

- Elbow flexion (C5, C6)— biceps

- Elbow extension (C6, C7, C8)—triceps

- Wrist extension (C6, C7, C8)—radial nerve

  Radial nerve damage: *stroke* or *multiple sclerosis* if hemiplesia

- Grip (C7, C8, T1)

  Weak grip in *cervical radiculopathy, DeQuervain's tenosynovitis, carpal tunnel syndrome*

- Finger abduction (C8, T1)—ulnar nerve

  Weak in ulnar nerve disorders

- Thumb opposition (C8, T1)—median nerve

  Carpal tunnel syndrome

EXAMINATION TECHNIQUES   POSSIBLE FINDINGS

- ⫯ Trunk—flexion, extension, lateral bending

- ⫯ /○— Hip flexion (L2, L3, L4)—iliopsoas

- Hip extension (S1)— gluteus maximus

- Hip adduction (L2, L3, L4)—adductors

- Hip abduction (L4, L5, S1)—sulcus medius and minimus

- Knee extension (L2, L3, L4)—quadriceps

- Knee flexion (L4, L5, S1, S2)— hamstrings

- Ankle dorsiflexion (L4, L5)

- Ankle plantar flexion (S1)

COORDINATION

Check:

Rapid alternating movements in arms and legs (tap foot)

Clumsy, slow movements in cerebellar disease

EXAMINATION TECHNIQUES	POSSIBLE FINDINGS
Point-to-point movements in arms and legs	Clumsy, unsteady movements in cerebellar disease

Gait. **Ask** patient to

- Walk away, turn, and come back

  CVA, cerebellar ataxia, parkinsonism, or loss of position sense may all affect performance.

- Walk heel to toe

  Corticospinal tract injury

- Walk on toes, then on heels

- Hop in place on each foot; do one-legged shallow knee bends. Substitute rising from a chair and climbing on a stool for hops and bends as indicated.

  Proximal hip girdle weakness increases risk of falls.

Stance

- **Do** a *Romberg test* (a sensory test of stance). **Ask** patient to stand with feet together and eyes open, then closed for 20 to 30 seconds. Mild swaying may occur. Stand close by to prevent falls.

  Loss of balance that appears when eyes are closed is a *positive* Romberg test, suggesting poor position sense.

- Look for a *pronator drift*. Watch as patient holds arms forward, with eyes closed, for 20 to 30 seconds.

  Flexion and pronation at elbow and downward drift of arm from *contralateral corticospinal tract lesion*

EXAMINATION TECHNIQUES	POSSIBLE FINDINGS
Ask patient to keep arms up and **tap** them downward. A smooth return to position is normal.	Weakness, incoordination, poor position sense

THE SENSORY SYSTEM

/○— Using an object such as a broken cotton swab to test sharp and dull sensation, compare **symmetric areas on the two sides of the body.** Do not reuse the object on another patient.	Hemisensory deficits
Also **compare** proximal and distal areas of arms and legs for *pain, temperature,* and *touch sensation.* Scatter stimuli to sample most dermatomes and major peripheral nerves.	"Glove-and-stocking" loss of peripheral neuropathy
Map any area of abnormal response, including dermatomes, if present.	Dermatomal sensory loss in *herpes zoster, nerve root compression.* See Table 17-7, pp. 344–345, for dermatomes.
Assess response to the following stimuli. Except when you are explaining the tests, patient's eyes should be closed.	
• *Pain.* Use the sharp end of a pin or other suitable tool. The dull end serves as a control.	Analgesia, hypalgesia, hyperalgesia

EXAMINATION TECHNIQUES	POSSIBLE FINDINGS

- *Temperature* (if indicated). Use test tubes with hot and ice-cold water, or other objects of suitable temperature.

Temperature and pain senses usually correlate.

- *Light touch.* Use a fine wisp of cotton.

Anesthesia, hyperesthesia

Check for *vibration and position senses.* If responses are abnormal, test more proximally.

Loss of vibration and position senses in peripheral neuropathy from diabetes or alcoholism and in posterior column disease from syphilis or B_{12} deficiency

- *Vibration and position.* Vibration: Use a 128-Hz or 256-Hz tuning fork, held on a *bony* prominence. Vibration and position senses, both carried in the posterior columns, often correlate.

- *Position.* Holding patient's finger or big toe by its sides, move it up or down.

Assess one or more of the *discriminative* sensations:

- *Stereognosis.* Ask for identification of a common

Lesions in the posterior columns or sensory cortex

object placed in patient's hand.

impair stereognosis, number identification, and two-point discrimination.

- *Number identification.* Ask for identification of a number drawn on patient's palm with blunt end of a pen.

- *Two-point discrimination.* Find minimal distance on pad of patient's finger at which the sides of two points can be distinguished from one (normally <5 mm).

- *Point localization.* Touch skin briefly, and ask patient to open both eyes and identify the place touched.

A lesion in the sensory cortex may impair point localization on the opposite side and cause extinction of the touch sensation on that side.

- *Extinction.* Simultaneously touch opposite, corresponding areas of the body, and ask patient where the touch is felt.

EXAMINATION TECHNIQUES   POSSIBLE FINDINGS

🖉/○— *REFLEXES*

● Grading Reflexes	
Grade	**Description**
4+	Hyperactive (with clonus)
3+	Brisker than average, not necessarily abnormal
2+	**Average, normal**
1+	Diminished, low normal
0	No response

Biceps (C5, C6)

Hyperactive deep tendon reflexes, absent abdominal reflexes, and a Babinski response in *upper motor neuron lesions*

Triceps (C6, C7)

EXAMINATION TECHNIQUES

POSSIBLE FINDINGS

Supinator (brachioradialis)
(C5, C6)

/○— Knee (L2, L3, L4)

Ankle (S1)

Ankle jerks symmetrically;
decreased or absent in
peripheral polyneuropathy

EXAMINATION TECHNIQUES   POSSIBLE FINDINGS

Check for clonus if reflexes
seem hyperactive.

CUTANEOUS STIMULATION REFLEXES

○— Abdominals (upper   May be absent with upper or
T8, T9, T10; lower T10,   lower neuron lesions
T11, T12)

Plantar (L5, S1), normally   Babinski response from
flexor   corticospinal tract lesion

EXAMINATION TECHNIQUES	POSSIBLE FINDINGS

∘�216 ***Anal Reflex.*** With a dull object, stroke outward from anus in four quadrants. Watch for anal contraction.

Loss of reflex suggests lesion at S2–3–4 level.

SPECIAL TECHNIQUES

∘── **Meningeal Signs.** With patient supine, flex head and neck toward chest. Note resistance or pain, and watch for flexion of hips and knees (*Brudzinski's sign*).

Meningeal irritation may cause resistance or pain on flexion during both maneuvers.

Flex one of patient's legs at hip and knee, then straighten knee. Note resistance or pain (*Kernig's sign*).

A compressed lumbosacral nerve root also causes pain on straightening the knee of the raised leg.

∘── **Lumbosacral Radiculopathy.** Straight leg raise.

With patient supine, raise relaxed and straightened leg, flexing the leg at the hip. Then dorsiflex the foot.

Pain and muscle weakness if herniated disc; may also see calf wasting and weak ankle dorsiflexion

EXAMINATION TECHNIQUES	POSSIBLE FINDINGS

Asterixis. Ask patient to hold both arms forward, with hands cocked up and fingers spread. Watch for 1 to 2 minutes.

Sudden brief flexions in liver disease, uremia hypercapnia.

Winging of the Scapula. Ask patient to push against the wall of your hand with a partially straightened arm. Inspect scapula. It should stay close to the chest wall.

Winging of scapula away from chest wall suggests weakness of the serratus anterior muscle.

The Stuporous or Comatose Patient. ○— **Assess** ABCs (airway, breathing, and circulation).

Take pulse, blood pressure, and rectal temperature.

Establish level of consciousness with escalating stimuli.

Lethargy, obtundation, stupor, coma

Don't dilate pupils, and **don't flex patient's neck** if cervical cord may have been injured.

EXAMINATION TECHNIQUES   POSSIBLE FINDINGS

⬤ Levels of Consciousness

Alertness	Patient is awake and aware of self and environment. When spoken to in a normal voice, patient looks at you and responds fully and appropriately to stimuli.
Lethargy	When spoken to in a loud voice, patient appears drowsy but opens eyes and looks at you, responds to questions, and then falls asleep.
Obtundation	When shaken gently, patient opens eyes and looks at you but responds slowly and is somewhat confused. Alertness and interest in environment are decreased.
Stupor	Patient arouses from sleep only after painful stimuli. Verbal responses are slow or absent. Patient lapses into unresponsiveness when stimulus stops. Patient has minimal awareness of self or environment.
Coma	Despite repeated painful stimuli, patient remains unarousable with eyes closed. No evident response to inner need or external stimuli is shown.

Observe

- Breathing pattern   Cheyne-Stokes, ataxic breathing

- Pupils   Asymmetric if structural lesions or possible brain herniation

- Ocular movements   Deviation to affected side in hemispheric stroke

Note posture of body.   Decorticate rigidity, decerebrate rigidity, flaccid hemiplegia

EXAMINATION TECHNIQUES

POSSIBLE FINDINGS

Check for the *oculocephalic reflex (doll's eye movements)*. Holding upper eyelids open, turn head quickly to each side, and then flex and extend patient's neck. This patient's head will be turned to her right.

In a comatose patient with an **intact** brainstem, the eyes move in the opposite direction, in this case to her left (doll's eye movements) as below.

Test for flaccid paralysis.

Very deep coma or a lesion in midbrain or pons abolishes this reflex, so eyes do not move.

- Hold forearms vertically; note wrist positions.

A flaccid hand droops to the horizontal.

- From 12 to 18 inches above bed, drop each arm.

A flaccid arm drops more rapidly.

- Support both knees in a somewhat flexed position, and then extend each knee and let lower leg drop to the bed.

The flaccid leg drops more rapidly.

- From a similar starting position, release both legs.

A flaccid leg falls into extension and external rotation.

Complete the neurologic and general physical examination.

RECORDING YOUR FINDINGS

Recording the Physical Examination—
The Nervous System

"*Mental Status:* Alert, relaxed, and cooperative. Thought process coherent. Oriented to person, place, and time. Detailed cognitive testing deferred. *Cranial Nerves:* I—not tested; II through XII intact. *Motor:* Good muscle bulk and tone. Strength 5/5 throughout. *Cerebellar:* Rapid alternating movements (RAMs), finger-to-nose (F→N), heel-to-shin (H→S) intact. Gait with normal base. Romberg—maintains balance with eyes closed. No pronator drift. *Sensory:* Pinprick, light touch, position, and vibration intact. *Reflexes:* 2+ and symmetric with plantar reflexes downgoing."

Alternatively, record reflexes using table or stick figure:

	Biceps	Triceps	Brach	Knee	Ankle	Pl
RT	2+	2+	2+	2+	2+	↓
LT	2+	2+	2+	2+	1+	↓

AIDS TO INTERPRETATION

TABLE 17-1 Types of Stroke

Assessing patients with stroke involves three fundamental questions based on a careful history and detailed physical examination: *What brain area and related vascular territory explain the patient's findings? Is the stroke ischemic or hemorrhagic? If ischemic, is the mechanism thrombus or embolus?* Stroke is a medical emergency, and timing is of the essence. Answers to these questions are critical to patient outcomes and use of antithrombotic therapies in acute ischemic stroke.

In *acute ischemic stroke*, ischemic brain injury begins with a central core of very low perfusion and often irreversible cell death. This core is surrounded by an *ischemic penumbra* of metabolically disturbed cells that are still potentially viable, depending on restoration of blood flow and duration of ischemia. Because most irreversible damage occurs in the first 3 to 6 hours after onset of symptoms, therapies targeted to the 3-hour window achieve the best outcomes, with recovery in up to 50% of patients in some studies.

Clinician performance in diagnosing stroke improves with training. Understanding the pathophysiology of stroke takes dedication, expert supervision to improve techniques of neurological examination, and perseverance. *This brief overview is intended to prompt further study and practice.* Accuracy in clinical examination is achievable, and more important than ever in determining patient therapy.

(table continues next page)

TABLE 17-1 Types of Stroke (continued)

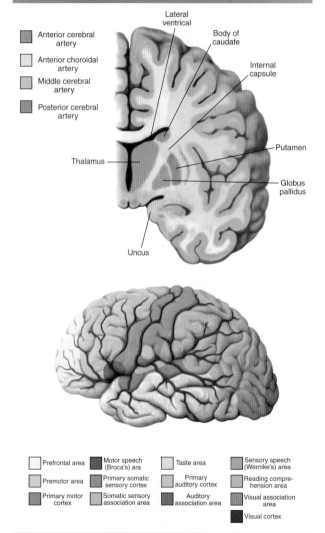

Anterior cerebral artery

Anterior choroidal artery

Middle cerebral artery

Posterior cerebral artery

Lateral ventrical

Body of caudate

Internal capsule

Putamen

Globus pallidus

Thalamus

Uncus

Prefrontal area

Premotor area

Primary motor cortex

Motor speech (Broca's) ara

Primary somatic sensory cortex

Somatic sensory association area

Taste area

Primary auditory cortex

Auditory association area

Sensory speech (Wernike's) area

Reading comprehension area

Visual association area

Visual cortex

TABLE 17-2 **Clinical Features and Vascular Territories of Stroke**

Major Clinical Features	Vascular Territory	Additional Comments
Contralateral leg weakness	*Anterior circulation*—anterior cerebral artery (ACA)	Includes stem of circle of Willis connecting internal carotid artery to ACA, and the segment distal to ACA and its anterior choroidal branch
Contralateral face, arm > leg weakness, sensory loss, field cut, aphasia (left MCA) or neglect, apraxia (right MCA)	*Anterior circulation*—middle cerebral artery (MCA)	Largest vascular bed for stroke
Contralateral motor or sensory deficit without cortical signs	*Subcortical circulation*—lenticulostriate deep penetrating branches of MCA	Small vessel subcortical *lacunar infarcts* in internal capsule, thalamus, or brainstem. Four common syndromes: pure motor hemiparesis; pure sensory hemianesthesia; ataxic hemiparesis; clumsy hand–dysarthria syndrome
Contralateral field cut	*Posterior circulation*—posterior cerebral artery (PCA)	Includes paired vertebral arteries, the basilar artery, paired posterior cerebral arteries. Bilateral PCA infarction causes cortical blindness but preserved pupillary light reaction.
Dysphagia, dysarthria, tongue/palate deviation and/or ataxia with crossed sensory/motor deficits (= ipsilateral face with contralateral body)	*Posterior circulation*—brainstem, vertebral, or basilar artery branches	
Oculomotor deficits and/or ataxia with crossed sensory/motor deficits	*Posterior circulation*—basilar artery	Complete basilar artery occlusion—"locked-in syndrome" with intact consciousness but inability to speak and quadriplegia

(Source: Adapted from American College of Physicians. Stroke, in Neurology. Medical Knowledge Self-Assessment Program (MKSAP) 14. Philadelphia: American College of Physicians, 2006. pp. 52–68.)

TABLE 17-3 Facial Paralysis

Distinguish peripheral from central lesions of CN VII by closely observing movements of the *upper face*. Because of innervation from both hemispheres, the movements are *preserved* in central lesions

	Lesion of Peripheral Nervous System	Lesion of Central Nervous System
Side of face affected	Same side as the lesion	Side opposite the lesion
Upper face	Unable to wrinkle forehead, raise eyebrow, close eye	Movements normal or slightly weak
Lower face	Unable to smile, show teeth	Same

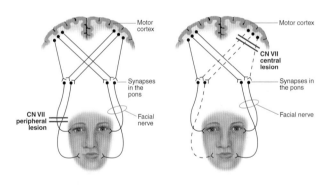

Common cause	Bell's palsy (injury to CN VII)	CVA

TABLE 17-4   **Motor Disorders**

	Peripheral Nervous System Disorder	Central Nervous System Disorder*	Parkinsonism (Basal Ganglia Disorder)	Cerebellar Disorder
Involuntary movements	Often fasciculations	No fasciculations	Resting tremors	Intention tremors
Muscle bulk	Atrophy	Normal or mild atrophy (disuse)	Normal	Normal
Muscle tone	Decreased or absent	Increased, spastic	Increased, rigid	Decreased
Muscle strength	Decreased or lost	Decreased or lost	Normal or slightly decreased	Normal or slightly decreased
Coordination	Unimpaired, though limited by weakness	Slowed and limited by weakness	Good, though slowed and often tremulous	Impaired, ataxic
Reflexes *Deep tendon*	Decreased or absent	Increased	Normal or decreased	Normal or decreased
Plantar	Flexor or absent	Extensor	Flexor	Flexor
Abdominals	Absent	Absent	Normal	Normal

*Upper motor neuron

TABLE 17-5 **Involuntary Movements**

Resting static tremors. Seen at rest, usually disappear with movement; seen in Parkinsonism

Postural tremor. Seen when maintaining active posture; in anxiety, hyperthyroidism; also familial

Intention tremor. Seen with intentional movement, absent at rest; in cerebellar disorders, including multiple sclerosis

Fasciculations. Fine, rapid flickering of muscle bundles

Chorea. Brief, rapid, irregular, jerky; face, head, arms, or hands

Athetosis. Slow, twisting, writhing; face, distal limbs

(table continues next page)

| TABLE 17-5 | **Involuntary Movements** (continued) |

Oral-facial dyskinesias. Rhythmic, repetitive, bizarre movements of face, mouth. Tardive dyskinesias with prolonged use of psychotropic drugs such as phenothiazines

Tics. Brief, irregular, repetitive, coordinated movements (e.g., winking, shrugging); in Tourette's syndrome, users of phenothiazines, amphetamines

Dystonia. Grotesque, twisted postures, often in trunk or, as shown, in neck (*spasmodic torticollis*)

TABLE 17-6 Disorders of Muscle Tone

Spasticity	Rigidity
Location. Upper motor neuron of the corticospinal tract at any point from the cortex to the spinal cord	**Location.** Basal ganglia system
Description. Increased muscle tone (*hypertonia*) that is rate-dependent. Tone is greater when passive movement is rapid, and less when passive movement is slow. Tone is also greater at the extremes of the movement arc. During rapid passive movement, initial hypertonia may give way suddenly as the limb relaxes. This spastic "catch" and relaxation is known as "clasp-knife" resistance.	**Description.** Increased resistance that persists throughout the movement arc, independent of rate of movement, is called *lead-pipe rigidity*. With flexion and extension of the wrist or forearm, a superimposed rachet-like jerkiness is called *cogwheel rigidity*.
Common Cause. Stroke, especially late or chronic stage	**Common Cause.** Parkinsonism

Flaccidity	Paratonia
Location. Lower motor neuron at any point from the anterior horn cell to the peripheral nerves	**Location.** Both hemispheres, usually in the frontal lobes
Description. Loss of muscle tone (*hypotonia*), causing the limb to be loose or floppy. The affected limbs may be hyper-extensible or even flaillike.	**Description.** Sudden changes in tone with passive range of motion. Sudden loss of tone that increases the ease of motion is called *mitgehen* (moving with). Sudden increase in tone making motion more difficult is called *gegenhalten* (holding against).
Common Cause. Guillain–Barré syndrome; also initial phase of spinal cord injury (spinal shock) or stroke	**Common Cause.** Dementia

TABLE **17-7** Dermatomes

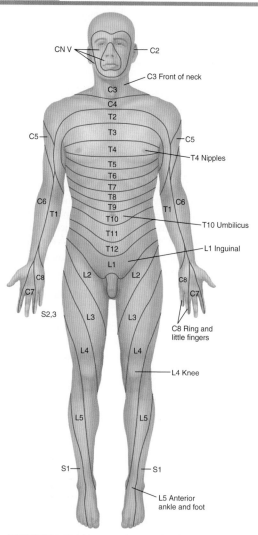

DERMATOMES INNERVATED BY POSTERIOR ROOTS

(table continues next page)

TABLE 17-7 **Dermatomes** (continued)

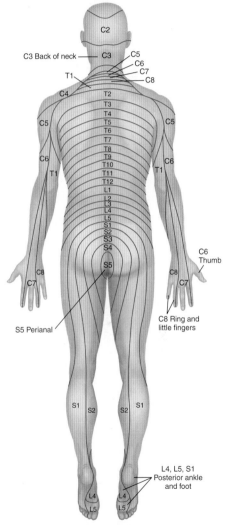

C2

C3 Back of neck — C3
C5
C6
C7
C8
T1
C4
T2
T3
T4
T5
T6
T7
T8
T9
T10
T11
T12
L1
L2
L3
L4
L5
S1
S2
S3
S4
S5
C5
C5
C6
C6
T1
T1

C6
Thumb

C8
C7
C8
C7

C8 Ring and
little fingers

S5 Perianal

S1
S2
S2
S1

L4, L5, S1
Posterior ankle
and foot

L4
L5
L4
L5

DERMATOMES INNERVATED BY POSTERIOR ROOTS

TABLE 17-8 Metabolic and Structural Coma

	Toxic–Metabolic	Structural
Pathophysiology	Arousal centers poisoned or critical substrates depleted	Lesion destroys or compresses brainstem arousal areas, either directly or secondary to more distant expanding mass lesions.
Clinical Features		
• Respiratory pattern	If regular, may be normal or hyperventilation. If irregular, usually Cheyne-Stokes	Irregular, especially Cheyne-Stokes or ataxic breathing. Also with selected stereotypical patterns like "apneustic" respiration (peak inspiratory arrest) or central hyperventilation.
• Pupillary size and reaction	Equal, reactive to light. If *pinpoint* from opiates or cholinergics, you may need a magnifying glass to see the reaction. May be unreactive if *fixed and dilated* from anticholinergics or hypothermia	Unequal or unreactive to light (fixed) *Midposition, fixed*—suggests midbrain compression *Dilated, fixed*—suggests compression of CN III from herniation
• Level of consciousness	Changes *after* pupils change	Changes *before* pupils change
Examples of Cause	Uremia, hyperglycemia	Epidural, subdural, or intracerebral hemorrhage
	Alcohol, drugs, liver failure	Cerebral infarct or embolus
	Hypothyroidism, hypoglycemia	Tumor, abscess
	Anoxia, ischemia	Brainstem infarct, tumor, or hemorrhage
	Meningitis, encephalitis	Cerebellar infarct, hemorrhage, tumor, or abscess
	Hyperthermia, hypothermia	

TABLE 17-9 **Pupils in Comatose Patients**

Small or Pinpoint Pupils

Bilaterally small pupils (1–2.5 mm) suggest (1) damage to the sympathetic pathways in the hypothalamus or (2) metabolic encephalopathy (a diffuse failure of cerebral function that has many causes, including drugs). Light reactions are usually normal.

Pinpoint pupils (<1 mm) suggest (1) a hemorrhage in the pons or (2) the effects of morphine, heroin, or other narcotics. The light reactions may be seen with a magnifying glass.

Midposition Fixed Pupils

Midposition or *slightly dilated pupils* (4–6 mm) and *fixed to light* suggest damage in the midbrain.

Large Pupils

Bilaterally fixed and dilated pupils in severe anoxia with sympathomimetic effects, may be seen with cardiac arrest. They also result from atropine-like agents, phenothiazines, or tricyclic antidepressants.

One Large Pupil

One fixed and dilated pupil warns of herniation of the temporal lobe, causing compression of the oculomotor nerve and midbrain.

Assessing Children: Infancy Through Adolescence

CHILD DEVELOPMENT

Children display tremendous variations in physical, cognitive, and social development compared with adults.

Key Principles of Child Development

- Child development proceeds along a predictable pathway marked by developmental milestones.
- The range of normal development is wide. Children mature at different rates.
- Various physical, psychological, social, and environmental factors, as well as diseases, can affect child development and health. For example, chronic diseases, child abuse, and poverty can contribute to detectable physical abnormalities and influence the rate and course of developmental advancement.
- The child's developmental level affects how you conduct the medical history and physical examination.

THE HEALTH HISTORY

The child's history follows the same outline as the adult's history, with certain *additions* presented here.

Identifying Data. Record date and place of birth, nickname, and first names of parents (and last name of each, if different).

Chief Complaints. Determine if they are the concerns of the child, the parent(s), a schoolteacher, or some other person.

Present Illness. Determine how each family member responds to the child's symptoms, why he or she is concerned, and whether the illness may provide for the child any secondary gain.

Past History
Birth History. This is especially important when neurologic or developmental problems are present. Get hospital records if necessary.

- Prenatal—maternal health: medications; tobacco, drug, and alcohol use; weight gain; duration of pregnancy
- Natal—nature of labor and delivery, birth weight, Apgar scores at 1 and 5 minutes
- Neonatal—resuscitation efforts, cyanosis, jaundice, infections, bonding

Feeding History. This is particularly important with either undernutrition or obesity.

- Breast-feeding—frequency and duration of feeds, difficulties, timing and method of weaning
- Bottle-feeding—type; amount; frequency; vomiting; colic; diarrhea
- Vitamins, iron, and fluoride supplements; introduction of solid foods
- Eating habits—types and amounts of food eaten, parental attitudes and responses to feeding problems

Growth and Developmental History. This is particularly important with delayed growth or development and behavioral disturbances.

- Physical growth—weight and height at all ages; head circumference at birth and less than 2 years; periods of slow or rapid growth
- Developmental milestones—ages child held head up, rolled over, sat, stood, walked, and talked
- Speech development, performance in preschool and school
- Social development—day and night sleeping patterns; toilet training; habitual behaviors; discipline problems; school behavior; relationships with family and peers

Current Health Status
Allergies. Pay particular attention to history of eczema, urticaria, perennial allergic rhinitis, asthma, food intolerance, insect hypersensitivity, and recurrent wheezing.

Immunizations. Include dates given and any untoward reactions.

Screening Tests.   These are likely to vary according to the child's medical and social conditions. Include newborn screening results, anemia screening, blood lead, sickle cell disease, vision, hearing, developmental screening, and others (e.g., tuberculosis).

HEALTH PROMOTION AND COUNSELING

1. Age-appropriate developmental achievement of the child
   - Physical (maturation, growth, puberty)
   - Motor (gross and fine motor skills)
   - Cognitive (achievement of milestones, language, school performance)
   - Emotional (self-efficacy, self-esteem, independence, morality)
   - Social (social competence, self-responsibility, integration with family and community)

2. Health supervision visits (per health supervision schedule)
   - Periodic assessment of medical and oral health
   - Adjustment of frequency for children or families with special needs

3. Integration of physical examination findings

4. Immunizations

5. Screening procedures

6. Anticipatory guidance
   - Healthy habits
   - Nutrition and healthy eating
   - Emotional and mental health
   - Oral health
   - Safety and prevention of injury
   - Sexual development and sexuality
   - Self-responsibility and efficacy
   - Family relationships (interactions, strengths, supports)
   - Prevention or recognition of illness
   - Prevention of risky behaviors and addictions
   - School and vocation
   - Peer relationships
   - Community interactions

7. Partnership between health care provider and child, adolescent, and family

TECHNIQUES OF EXAMINATION

Sequence of Examination

> The sequence of examination varies according to the child's age and comfort level.
>
> - For infants and young children, *perform nondisturbing maneuvers early and potentially distressing maneuvers toward the end.* For example, palpate the head and neck and auscultate the heart and lungs early; examine the ears and mouth and palpate the abdomen near the end. If the child reports pain in an area, examine that part last.
> - For older children and adolescents, use the same sequence as with adults, except examine the most painful areas last.

ASSESSING NEWBORNS

EXAMINATION TECHNIQUES   POSSIBLE FINDINGS

IMMEDIATE ASSESSMENT AT BIRTH

Listen to the anterior thorax with your stethoscope. **Palpate** the abdomen. **Inspect** the head, face, oral cavity, extremities, genitalia, and perineum.

Apgar Score. Score each newborn according to the following table, at 1 and 5 minutes after birth, according to the 3-point scale (0, 1, or 2) for each component.

If the 5-minute score is 8 or more, proceed to a more complete examination.

EXAMINATION TECHNIQUES   POSSIBLE FINDINGS

● The Apgar Scoring System

Assigned Score

Clinical Sign	0	1	2
Heart rate	Absent	<100	>100
Respiratory effort	Absent	Slow and irregular	Good; strong
Muscle tone	Flaccid	Some flexion of the arms and legs	Active movement
Reflex irritability*	No responses	Grimace	Crying vigorously, sneeze, or cough
Color	Blue, pale	Pink body, blue extremities	Pink all over

1-Minute Apgar Score		5-Minute Apgar Score	
8–10	Normal	8–10	Normal
5–7	Some nervous system depression	0–7	High risk for subsequent central nervous system and other organ system dysfunction
0–4	Severe depression, requiring immediate resuscitation		

*Reaction to suction of nares with bulb syringe.

Gestational Age and Birth Weight. Classify newborns according to their gestational age and birth weight.

CLASSIFICATION BY GESTATIONAL AGE AND BIRTH WEIGHT

Gestational Age

Classification	Gestational Age
● Preterm	<37 wks (<259th day)
● Term	37–42 wks
● Postterm	>42 wks (>294th day)

Birth Weight

Classification	Weight
● Extremely low birth weight	<1,000 grams
● Very low birth weight	<1,500 grams
● Low birth weight	<2,500 grams
● Normal birth weight	≥2,500 grams

● Newborn Classifications

Category	Abbreviation	Percentile
Small for gestational age	SGA	<10th
Appropriate for gestational age	AGA	10–90th
Large for gestational age	LGA	>90th

EXAMINATION SEVERAL HOURS AFTER BIRTH

During the first day of life, newborns should have a comprehensive examination following the technique outlined under "Infants." Wait until 1 or 2 hours after a feeding, when the newborn is more responsive. Ask parents to remain.

EXAMINATION TECHNIQUES | POSSIBLE FINDINGS

Observe the baby's color, size, body proportions, nutritional status, posture, respirations, and movements of the head and extremities.

Normally findings are spontaneous motor activity, flexion and extension of the extremities, and brief body tremors.

Most newborns are *bowlegged,* reflecting their curled up intrauterine position.

Inspect the newborn's *umbilical cord* to detect abnormalities. Normally, there are two thick-walled umbilical arteries and one larger but thin-walled umbilical vein, which is usually located at the 12 o'clock position.

A *single umbilical artery* may be associated with congenital anomalies. *Umbilical hernias* in infants are from a defect in the abdominal wall.

The neurologic screening examination of all newborns should include assessment of mental status, gross and fine motor function, tone, cry, deep tendon reflexes, and primitive reflexes.

Signs of severe neurologic disease include *extreme irritability; persistent asymmetry of posture* or *extension of extremities; constant turning of head to one side; marked extension of head, neck, and extremities (opisthotonus); severe flaccidity;* and *limited pain response.*

ASSESSING INFANTS

MENTAL AND PHYSICAL STATUS

Observe the parents' affect when talking about the baby; their manner of holding,

Common causes of *developmental delay* include abnormalities in embryonic

EXAMINATION TECHNIQUES

POSSIBLE FINDINGS

moving, and dressing the baby; and their response to situations that may produce discomfort for the baby. **Observe** a breast or bottle feeding. **Determine** attainment of developmental milestones using the Denver Developmental Screening Test before conducting the physical examination.

development, hereditary and genetic disorders, environmental and social problems, other pregnancy or perinatal problems, childhood diseases such as infection (e.g., meningitis), trauma, and severe chronic disease.

GENERAL SURVEY

Growth, reflected in increases in height and weight within expected limits, is an excellent indicator of health during infancy and childhood. Deviations from normal may be early indications of an underlying problem. To assess growth, compare a child's parameters with respect to

Causes of *failure to thrive* can be environmental or psychosocial, or various gastrointestinal, neurologic, cardiac, endocrine, renal, and other diseases.

• Normal values according to age and sex

• Prior readings to assess trends

Measures above the 97th or below the 3rd percentile, or recent rises or falls from prior levels, require investigation.

Height and Weight. **Plot** each child's height and weight on standard growth charts to determine progress.

Reduced growth in height may indicate *endocrine disease,* other *causes of short stature,* or, if weight is also low, other *chronic diseases.*

EXAMINATION TECHNIQUES	POSSIBLE FINDINGS

Head Circumference.
Determine head
circumference at every
physical examination during
the first 2 years.

Premature closure of the sutures
or *microcephaly* may cause
small head size. *Hydrocephalus,*
subdural hematoma, or, rarely,
brain tumor or *inherited*
syndromes may cause
abnormally large head size.

VITAL SIGNS

Blood Pressure. Measure
blood pressure at least once
during infancy. Although
the hand-held method is
shown here, the most easily
used measure of systolic
blood pressure in infants and
young children is obtained
with the *Doppler method.*

● Causes of Sustained Hypertension in Children

Newborn	Middle Childhood
Renal artery disease (stenosis, thrombosis)	Renal parenchymal or arterial disease
Congenital renal malformations	Primary hypertension
Coarctation of the aorta	Coarctation of the aorta

Infancy and Early Childhood	**Adolescence**
Renal parenchymal or artery disease	Primary hypertension
Coarctation of the aorta	Renal parenchymal disease
	Drug induced

EXAMINATION TECHNIQUES	POSSIBLE FINDINGS

Pulse. The heart rate is quite variable. | Tachycardia (>180–200/min) usually indicates *paroxysmal supraventricular tachycardia.* Bradycardia may result from serious underlying disease.

Respiratory Rate. The respiratory rate has a greater range and is more responsive to illness, exercise, and emotion than in adults. | Respiratory diseases such as *bronchiolitis* or *pneumonia* may cause rapid respirations (up to 80–90/min), but *also* increased work of breathing.

THE SKIN

Assess

- *Texture* and *appearance* | *Cutis marmorata*

- Vasomotor changes | *Acrocyanosis; cyanotic congenital heart disease*

- Pigmentation (e.g., Mongolian spots) | *Café-au-lait spots*

- Hair (e.g., lanugo) | *Midline hair tuft on back*

- Common skin conditions (e.g., milia, erythema toxicum) | *Herpes simplex*

- Jaundice | *Hemolytic disease*

- Turgor | *Dehydration*

THE HEAD

Examine *sutures* and *fontanelles* carefully. | Head small with *microcephaly,* enlarged with *hydrocephaly;* fontanelles full and tense with *meningitis,* closed with *microcephaly,* separated with *increased intracranial pressure*

EXAMINATION TECHNIQUES   POSSIBLE FINDINGS

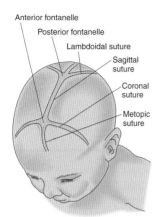

Anterior fontanelle
Posterior fontanelle
Lambdoidal suture
Sagittal suture
Coronal suture
Metopic suture

(hydrocephaly, subdural hematoma, and brain tumor)

Swelling from subperiosteal hemorrhage (cephalo-hematoma) does not cross suture lines; swelling from bleeding associated with a fracture does.

Check the *face* for symmetry. **Examine** for an overall impression of the *facies;* comparing with the faces of the parents is helpful.

PEARLS TO EVALUATE POTENTIALLY ABNORMAL FACIES

Carefully review the history, especially the *family history, pregnancy,* and *perinatal history.*

Note abnormalities, especially of *growth, development,* or *dysmorphic somatic features.*

Measure and plot percentiles, especially of *head circumference, height,* and *weight.*

Consider the three mechanisms of facial dysmorphogenesis:

● Deformations from intrauterine constraint
● Disruptions from amniotic bands or fetal tissue
● Malformations from an intrinsic abnormality (either face/head or brain)

Examine parents and siblings (similarity may be reassuring but might point to a familial disorder).

Determine whether facial features fit a recognizable syndrome. Compare against references, pictures, tables, and databases.

EXAMINATION TECHNIQUES   POSSIBLE FINDINGS

THE EYES

Newborns and young infants may look at your face and follow a bright light if you catch them while alert.
Normal visual milestones are as follows:

Nystagmus, strabismus

● Visual Milestones of Infancy	
Birth	Blinks, may regard face
1 month	Fixes on objects
1½–2 months	Coordinated eye movements
3 months	Eyes converge, baby reaches
12 months	Acuity around 20/50

THE EARS

Check *position*, *shape*, and *features*.

Small, deformed or low-set auricles may indicate associated *congenital defects,* especially renal disease.

● Signs That an Infant Can Hear	
Age	**Signs**
0–2 months	Startle response and blink to a sudden noise Calming down with soothing voice or music
2–3 months	Change in body movements in response to sound Change in facial expression to familiar sounds
3–4 months	Turning eyes and head to sound
6–7 months	Turning to listen to voices and conversation

EXAMINATION TECHNIQUES   POSSIBLE FINDINGS

THE NOSE

Test patency of the nasal passages by occluding alternately each nostril while holding the infant's mouth closed.

With *choanal atresia,* the baby cannot breathe if one nostril is occluded.

THE MOUTH AND PHARYNX

Inspect (with a tongue blade and flashlight) and **palpate.**

Supernumerary teeth, Epstein's pearls

You may see a whitish covering on the tongue. If this coating is from milk, you can easily remove it by scraping or wiping it away.

Oral candidiasis (thrush)

THE NECK

Palpate the *lymph nodes,* and **assess** for any additional masses (e.g., *congenital cysts*).

Lymphadenopathy is usually from viral or bacterial infections. Other neck masses include *malignancy, branchial cleft* or *thyroglossal duct cysts, periauricular cysts and sinuses.*

Preauricular
Posterior auricular
Tonsillar
Occipital
Anterior cervical
Posterior cervical
Submandibular
Deep cervical
Epidermoid cyst
Cystic hygroma
2nd branchial cleft cyst
Submental
Thyroglossal duct cyst
Supraclavicular

THE THORAX AND LUNGS

Carefully **assess** respirations and breathing pattern.

Apnea

Don't rush to the stethoscope, but observe the patient carefully first.

Upper respiratory infections may cause nasal flaring.

EXAMINATION TECHNIQUES   POSSIBLE FINDINGS

● Examination of the Lungs in Infants—Before You Touch the Child!

Assessment	Possible Findings	Explanation
General appearance	Inability to feed or smile Lack of consolability	*Lower respiratory infections* below the vocal cords (e.g., *bronchiolitis, pneumonia*) are common in infants.
Respiratory rate	Tachypnea	Cardiac or respiratory disease
Color	Pallor or cyanosis	Cardiac or pulmonary disease
Nasal component of breathing	Nasal flaring (enlargement of both nasal openings during inspiration)	Upper or lower respiratory infection
Audible breath sounds	Grunting (repetitive, short expiratory sound) Wheezing (musical expiratory sound) Stridor (high-pitched, inspiratory noise) Obstruction (lack of breath sounds)	*Acute stridor* is a potentially serious condition with causes such as *laryngotracheobronchitis (croup), epiglottitis, bacterial tracheitis, foreign body, vascular ring*
Work of breathing	Nasal flaring Grunting Retractions (or chest indrawing): Supraclavicular (motion of soft tissue above clavicles) Intercostal (indrawing of the skin between ribs) Subcostal (just below the costal margin)	In infants, abnormal work of breathing combined with abnormal findings on auscultation is the best finding for ruling in *pneumonia*.

EXAMINATION TECHNIQUES   POSSIBLE FINDINGS

● Distinguishing Upper Airway From Lower Airway Sounds

Technique	Upper Airway	Lower Airway
Compare sounds from nose/ stethoscope	Same sounds	Often different sounds
Listen to harshness of sounds	Harsh and loud	Variable
Note symmetry (left/right)	Symmetric	Often asymmetric
Compare sounds at different locations (higher or lower)	Sounds louder as stethoscope is moved up chest	Sounds louder lower in chest
Inspiratory vs. expiratory	Almost always inspiratory	Often has expiratory phase

---

THE HEART

Inspection. Observe carefully for any cyanosis.

At birth: *Transposition of the great arteries; pulmonary valve atresia or stenosis*

Within a few days of birth: The above; also *total anomalous pulmonary venous return, hypoplastic left heart*

Weeks, months, or years of life: The above; also *pulmonary vascular disease with atrial, ventricular, or great vessel shunting*

Palpation. Palpate the *peripheral pulses.* The *point of maximal impulse (PMI)* is not always palpable in

No or diminished femoral pulses suggest *coarctation of the aorta.* Weak or thready, difficult-to-feel pulses may

EXAMINATION TECHNIQUES	POSSIBLE FINDINGS
infants. *Thrills* are palpable when enough turbulence is within the heart or great vessels.	reflect *myocardial dysfunction* and *congestive heart failure.*
Auscultation. *Heart rhythm* is evaluated more easily in infants by listening to the heart than by feeling the peripheral pulses.	The most common dysrhythmia in children is *paroxysmal supraventricular tachycardia.*
Heart Sounds. **Evaluate** S_1 and S_2 carefully. They are normally crisp.	A louder-than-normal pulmonic component, particularly louder than the aortic sound, suggests *pulmonary hypertension.* Persistent splitting of S_2 may indicate a right ventricular volume load, such as *atrial septal defect.*

THE BREASTS

The breasts of males and females may be enlarged for months after birth as a result of maternal estrogen, and even engorged for 1 to 2 weeks with a white liquid.

THE ABDOMEN

You will find it easy to **palpate** an infant's abdomen, because infants like being touched.	Abnormal abdominal masses can be associated with kidney, bladder, or bowel tumors. In *pyloric stenosis,* deep palpation in the right upper quadrant or midline can reveal an "olive," or a 2-cm firm pyloric mass.

EXAMINATION TECHNIQUES   POSSIBLE FINDINGS

MALE GENITALIA

Inspect with the infant supine.

In 3% of infants, one or both testes cannot be felt in the scrotum or inguinal canal. Try to milk the testes into the scrotum.

Common scrotal masses are *hydroceles* and *inguinal hernias.*

FEMALE GENITALIA

In females, genitalia may be prominent for several months after birth from the effects of maternal estrogen.

Ambiguous genitalia involves masculinization of the female external genitalia.

THE MUSCULOSKELETAL SYSTEM

The focus is detecting congenital abnormalities, particularly in the hands, spine, hips, legs, and feet.

Skin tags, remnants of digits, polydactyly (extra fingers), or *syndactyly* (webbed fingers) are congenital defects. *Fracture of the clavicle* can occur during a difficult delivery.

Examine the *hips* carefully at each visit for signs of dislocation. There are two major techniques: one to test for a posteriorly dislocated hip (*Ortolani test*) and the other to test for the ability to sublux or dislocate an intact but unstable hip (*Barlow test*).

Congenital hip dysplasia may have a positive Ortolani or Barlow test, particularly during the first 3 months of age.

With a *hip dysplasia,* you feel a "clunk."

ORTOLANI TEST

BARLOW TEST

EXAMINATION TECHNIQUES | POSSIBLE FINDINGS

Some normal infants exhibit twisting or *torsion of the tibia* inwardly or outwardly on its longitudinal axis.

Pathologic tibial torsion occurs only in association with *deformities of the feet or hips*.

THE NERVOUS SYSTEM

Evaluate the developing central nervous system by assessing *infantile automatisms*, called *primitive reflexes*.

Suspect a *neurologic* or *developmental abnormality* if primitive reflexes are

- Absent at appropriate age

- Present longer than normal

- Asymmetric

- Associated with posturing or twitching

Some neurologic abnormalities produce deficits or slow cognitive and social development. Infants with developmental delay may have abnormal findings on neurologic examination because much of it is based on age-specific norms.

Children with *spastic diplegias* will often have hypotonia as infants.

ASSESSING CHILDREN (1 TO 10 YEARS)

Tips for Interviewing Children

- **Establish rapport.** Refer to children by name and meet them on their own level. Maintain eye contact at their level (e.g., sit on the floor if needed). Participate in play and talk about their interests.

EXAMINATION TECHNIQUES   POSSIBLE FINDINGS

- **Work with families.** Ask simple, open-ended questions such as "Are you sick? Tell me about it," followed by more specific questions. Once the parent has started the conversation, direct questions back to the child. Also observe how parents interact with the child.
- **Identify multiple agendas.** Your job is to discover as many perspectives and agendas as possible.
- **Use the family as the key resource.** View parents as experts in the care of their child and you as their consultant.
- **Note hidden agendas.** As with adults, the chief complaint may not relate to the real reason the parent has brought the child to see you.

The following discussion focuses on those areas of the comprehensive physical examination that are different for children than for infants and for adults.

MENTAL AND PHYSICAL STATUS

In *children 1 to 5 years,* **observe** the degree of sickness or wellness, mood, nutritional state, speech, cry, facial expression, and developmental skills. Note parent–child interaction, including separation tolerance, affection, and response to discipline.

This overall examination can uncover evidence of *chronic disease, developmental delay, social or environmental disorders, and family problems.*

In *children 6 to 10 years,* **determine** orientation to time and place, factual knowledge, and language and number skills. Observe motor skills used in writing, tying laces, buttoning, cutting, and drawing.

EXAMINATION TECHNIQUES	POSSIBLE FINDINGS

Body Mass Index for Age. Age- and sex-specific charts are now available to assess body mass index (BMI) in children.

Underweight is <5th percentile, at risk of over-weight is ≥85th percentile, and overweight is ≥95th percentile.

BLOOD PRESSURE

Hypertension during childhood is more common than previously thought. Recognizing, confirming, and appropriately managing it is important. Blood pressure readings should be part of the physical examination of every child older than 2 years. *Proper cuff size is essential for accurate determination of blood pressure in children.*

The most frequent "cause" of elevated blood pressure in children is probably an *improperly performed examination,* often from an incorrect cuff size.

Causes of *sustained hypertension* in childhood include renal disease, coarctation of the aorta, and primary hypertension.

THE EYES

The two most important aspects of the eye examination for young children are to test visual acuity in each eye and to determine whether the gaze is conjugate or symmetric.

Strabismus; amblyopia; myopia; or hyperopia

SPECIAL TECHNIQUES

The corneal light reflex test (*left*) and the cover-uncover test (*right*) are particularly useful in young children.

Any difference in visual acuity between eyes is abnormal.

EXAMINATION TECHNIQUES   POSSIBLE FINDINGS

● Visual Acuity

Age	Visual Acuity
3 months	Eyes converge, baby reaches
12 months	~20/200
Younger than 4 years	20/40
4 years and older	20/30

THE EARS

Examine the ear canal and drum. There are two positions for the child (lying down or sitting), and also two ways to hold the otoscope, as illustrated.

EXAMINATION TECHNIQUES   POSSIBLE FINDINGS

SPECIAL TECHNIQUE

Pneumatic Otoscope.
Learn to use a *pneumatic otoscope* to improve your accuracy of diagnosis of otitis media in children.

- Check for leaks by placing your finger over the tip of the speculum and squeezing the bulb.

- Insert the speculum, obtaining a proper seal.

Acute otitis media involves a red and bulging tympanic membrane.

- When air is introduced into the normal ear canal, the tympanic membrane and its light reflex move inward. When air is removed, the tympanic membrane moves outward toward you.

Diminished movement of tympanic membrane with *acute otitis media;* no movement with *otitis media with effusion.* Pain on movement of the pinna with *otitis externa.*

THE MOUTH AND PHARYNX

For anxious or young children, you may want to leave this examination until toward the end. If you need to use the tongue blade, the best technique is to push down and pull slightly forward toward you while the child says "ah." Be careful not to place the blade too far posteriorly, eliciting a gag reflex.

EXAMINATION TECHNIQUES

POSSIBLE FINDINGS

Examine the *teeth* for the timing and sequence of eruption, number, character, condition, and position.

Abnormalities of the enamel may reflect local or general disease.

Carefully **inspect** the inside of the upper teeth, as shown.

Nursing bottle caries; dental caries; staining of the teeth, which may be intrinsic or extrinsic

Dental caries are the most common health problem of children and are particularly prevalent in impoverished children.

Look for abnormalities of tooth position.

Malocclusion

Note the size, position, symmetry, and appearance of the *tonsils.*

Peritonsillar abscess

THE HEART

One of the most challenging aspects to cardiac examination of children is evaluation of *heart murmurs.* In addition to trying to listen to a squirming, perhaps uncooperative child, a major challenge is to

See Table 18-4, Characteristics of Pathologic Heart Murmurs, pp. 381–382.

EXAMINATION TECHNIQUES   POSSIBLE FINDINGS

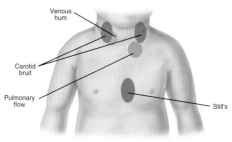

Location of Benign Heart Murmurs in Children

Venous hum

Carotid bruit

Pulmonary flow

Still's

distinguish common benign murmurs from unusual or pathologic ones. Most (indeed, some say nearly all) children will have one or more *functional*, or *benign*, *heart murmurs* before adulthood (see above).

THE ABDOMEN

Most children are ticklish when you first place your hand on their abdomens for **palpation.** This reaction tends to disappear, particularly if you distract the child.

A pathologically enlarged liver in children usually is palpable more than 2 cm below the costal margin, has a round, firm edge, and often is tender.

MALE GENITALIA

There is an art to **palpation** of the young boy's scrotum and testes, because many have an extremely active cremasteric reflex that may cause the testes to retract upward into the inguinal canal and thereby appear undescended. A useful

In *precocious puberty,* the penis and testes are enlarged, with signs of pubertal changes.

A painful testicle requires rapid treatment and may indicate *torsion.*

EXAMINATION TECHNIQUES | POSSIBLE FINDINGS

technique is to have the boy sit cross-legged on the examining table.

Inguinal hernias in older boys present as they do in adult men.

FEMALE GENITALIA

For the genital examination, use a calm, gentle approach, including a developmentally appropriate explanation.

Examine the genitalia in an efficient and systematic manner. The normal hymen can have various configurations.

Vaginal discharge in early childhood can result from *perineal irritation* (e.g., from bubble baths, soaps), *foreign body, vaginitis,* or *sexually transmitted diseases* from sexual abuse. *Vaginal bleeding* is always concerning. *Abrasions* or signs of trauma to the external genitalia can result from *sexual abuse.*

THE MUSCULOSKELETAL SYSTEM

In older children, abnormalities of the upper extremities are rare in the absence of injury. Observe the child standing and walking barefoot. You also can ask the child to touch the toes, rise from sitting, run a short distance, and pick up objects. You will detect most abnormalities by watching carefully.

A screening musculoskeletal examination for children participating in sports can detect injuries or abnormalities that may result in problems during athletics.

EXAMINATION TECHNIQUES	POSSIBLE FINDINGS

THE NERVOUS SYSTEM

Beyond infancy (when the primitive reflexes have disappeared), the neurologic examination includes the components evaluated in adults. Again, combine the neurologic and developmental assessments. You will need to turn this into a game with the child. The goal is to assess optimal development and neurologic performance, which requires the child's cooperation.

Delayed language or cognitive skills can be due to neurologic disease as well as developmental disorders.

ASSESSING ADOLESCENTS

The key to successfully examining teens is a comfortable, confidential environment that makes the examination relaxed and informative. Adolescents are more likely to open up when the interview focuses on them rather than on their problems.

Consider the patient's cognitive and social development when deciding issues of privacy, parental involvement, and confidentiality. Explain to both teen and parent that the purpose of confidentiality is to improve health care, not keep secrets. Your goal is to help adolescents bring their concerns or questions to their parents. Never make confidentiality unlimited, however. Always state to teens explicitly that you may need to act on information that makes you concerned about safety.

The physical examination of the adolescent is similar to that of the adult. Keep in mind issues particularly relevant to teens, such as puberty, growth, development, family and peer relationships, sexuality, decision making, and risk behaviors. For more details on specific techniques of examination, the reader should refer to the corresponding chapter for the regional examination of interest or concern. Following are special areas to highlight when examining adolescents.

EXAMINATION TECHNIQUES   POSSIBLE FINDINGS

THE BREASTS

Assess normal maturational development.

See Table 18-5, Sex Maturity Ratings in Girls: Breasts, p. 383

SPECIAL TECHNIQUE

Testing for Scoliosis.
Inspect any child who can stand for *scoliosis*. Make sure the child bends forward with the knees straight (*Adams bend test*). Evaluate any asymmetry in positioning or gait. If you detect scoliosis, use a *scoliometer* to test for the degree of scoliosis.

MALE AND FEMALE GENITALIA

An important goal when examining adolescent males and females is to assign a sexual maturity rating, regardless of chronologic age.

See Table 18-6, Sex Maturity Ratings in Boys, pp. 384–385, and Table 18-7, Sex Maturity Ratings in Girls: Pubic Hair, pp. 386–387.

RECORDING YOUR FINDINGS

The format of the pediatric medical record is the same as that of the adult. Thus, although the sequence of the physical examination may vary, convert your written findings back to the traditional format.

Recording the Physical Examination—
The Pediatric Patient

Brian is a chubby, active, and energetic toddler. He plays with the reflex hammer, pretending it is a truck. He appears closely bonded with his mother, looking at her occasionally for comfort. She seems concerned that Brian will break something. His clothes are clean.

Vital Signs. Ht 90 cm (90th percentile). Wt 16 kg (>95th percentile). BMI 19.8 (>95th percentile). Head circumference 50 cm (75th percentile). BP 108/58. Heart rate 90 and regular. Respiratory rate 30; varies with activity. Temperature (ear) 37.5°C. Obviously no pain. Skin: normal except for bruises on legs, and patchy, dry skin over external surface of elbows.

HEENT. *Head:* Normocephalic; no lesions. *Eyes:* Difficult to examine because he won't sit still. Symmetric with normal extraocular movements. Pupils 4 to 5 mm constricting. Discs difficult to visualize; no hemorrhages noted. *Ears:* Normal pinna; no external abnormalities. Normal external canals and tympanic membranes (TMs). *Nose:* Normal nares; septum midline. *Mouth:* Several darkened teeth on inside surface of upper incisors. One clear cavity on upper right incisor. Tongue normal. Cobblestoning of posterior pharynx; no exudates. Tonsils large but adequate gap (1.5 cm) between them.

Neck. Supple, midline trachea, no thyroid palpable.

Lymph Nodes. Easily palpable (1.5 to 2 cm) tonsillar lymph nodes bilaterally. Small (0.5 cm) nodes in inguinal canal bilaterally. All lymph nodes mobile and nontender.

Lungs. Good expansion. No tachypnea or dyspnea. Congestion audible, but seems to be upper airway (louder near mouth, symmetric). No rhonchi, rales, or wheezes. Clear to auscultation.

Cardiovascular. PMI in 4th or 5th interspace and midsternal line. Normal S1 and S2. No murmurs or abnormal heart sounds. Normal femoral pulses; dorsalis pedis pulses palpable bilaterally.

Breasts. Normal, with some fat under both.

Abdomen. Protuberant but soft; no masses or tenderness. Liver span 2 cm below right costal margin (RCM) and not tender. Spleen and kidneys not palpable.

Genitalia. Tanner I circumcised penis; no pubic hair, lesions, or discharge. Testes descended, difficult to palpate because of active cremasteric reflex. Normal scrotum both sides.

Musculoskeletal. Normal range of motion of upper and lower extremities and all joints. Spine straight. Gait normal.

Neurologic. *Mental Status:* Happy, cooperative child. *Developmental (DDST):* Gross motor—Jumps and throws objects. Fine motor—Imitates vertical line. Language—Does not combine words; single words only, three to four noted during examination. Personal–social—Washes face, brushes teeth, and puts on shirt. Overall—Normal, except for language, which appears delayed. *Cranial Nerves:* Intact, although several difficult to elicit. *Cerebellar:* Normal gait; good balance. *Deep tendon reflexes (DTRs):* Normal and symmetric throughout with downgoing toes. *Sensory:* Deferred.

AIDS TO INTERPRETATION

TABLE 18-1 **Classification of Newborn's Level of Maturity**

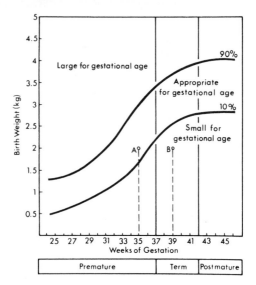

Weight Small for Gestational Age (SGA) = Birth weight <10th percentile on the intrauterine growth curve

Weight Appropriate for Gestational Age (AGA) = Birth weight within the 10th and 90th percentiles on the intrauterine growth curve

Weight Large for Gestational Age (LGA) = Birth weight >90th percentile on the intrauterine growth curve

Level of intrauterine growth based on birth weight and gestational age of liveborn, single, white infants. Point A represents a premature infant, while point B indicates an infant of similar birth weight who is mature but small for gestational age; the growth curves are representative of the 10th and 90th percentiles for all of the newborns in the sampling.

Classification of the low-birth-weight infant. In: Klaus MH, Fanaroff AA. Care of the High-Risk Neonate, 3rd ed. Philadelphia: WB Saunders, 1986.

TABLE 18-2 **Recommendations for Preventive Pediatric Health Care**

Each child and family is unique; therefore, these recommendations are designed for the care of children who are receiving competent parenting, have no manifestation of any important health problems, and are growing and developing in satisfactory fashion. Additional visits may become necessary if circumstances suggest variation from normal.

AGE	INFANCY										EARLY CHILDHOOD				MIDDLE CHILDHOOD		ADOLESCENCE									
	2-4 days¹	By 1 mo	2 mo	4 mo	6 mo	9 mo	12 mo	15 mo	18 mo	24 mo	3 y	4 y	5 y	6 y	8 y	10 y	11 y	12 y	13 y	14 y	15 y	16 y	17 y	18 y	19 y	20 y+
HISTORY Initial / Interval	•	•	•	•	•	•	•	•	•	•	•	•	•	•	•	•	•	•	•	•	•	•	•	•	•	•
MEASUREMENTS Height and Weight	•	•	•	•	•	•	•	•	•	•	•	•	•	•	•	•	•	•	•	•	•	•	•	•	•	•
Head Circumference	•	•	•	•	•	•	•	•	•	•																
Blood Pressure											•	•	•	•	•	•	•	•	•	•	•	•	•	•	•	•
SENSORY SCREENING Vision	S	S	S	S	S	S	S	S	S	S	O	S	S	S	O	O	S	S	S	S	O	S	S	O	S	S
Hearing	S	S	S	S	S	S	S	S	S	S	S	S	S	S	O	O	S	S	S	S	O	S	S	O	S	S
DEVELOPMENTAL / BEHAVIORAL ASSESSMENT²	•	•	•	•	•	•	•	•	•	•	•	•	•	•	•	•	•	•	•	•	•	•	•	•	•	•
PHYSICAL EXAMINATION³	•	•	•	•	•	•	•	•	•	•	•	•	•	•	•	•	•	•	•	•	•	•	•	•	•	•

1. For newborns discharged in less than 48 hours after delivery
2. By history and appropriate physical examination; if suspicious, by specific objective development testing
3. At each visit, a complete physical examination is essential, with infant totally unclothed, older child undressed and suitably draped

Key: • = to be performed   S = subjective, by history
O = objective, by a standard testing method

Adapted from *Recommendations For Preventive Pediatric Health Care* promulgated by the American Academy of Pediatrics Committee on Practice and Ambulatory Medicine, 1999.

TABLE 18-3 Hypertension in Childhood

Hypertension can start in childhood. While young children with elevated blood pressure are more likely to have a renal, cardiac, or endocrine cause, adolescents with hypertension are most likely to have primary or essential hypertension.

This child developed hypertension during adolescence, and it "tracked" into adulthood. Children tend to remain in the same percentile for blood pressure as they grow. This tracking of blood pressure continues into adulthood, supporting the concept that adult essential hypertension begins during childhood.

The consequences of untreated hypertension can be severe.

TABLE 18-4 Characteristics of Pathologic Heart Murmurs

Congenital Defect	Characteristics of Murmur
Pulmonary Valve Stenosis *Mild* *Moderate* *Severe* 	*Location.* Upper left sternal border *Radiation.* In mild degrees of stenosis, the murmur may be heard over the course of the pulmonary arteries in the lung fields. *Intensity.* Increases in intensity and duration as the degree of obstruction increases *Quality.* Ejection, peaking later in systole as the obstruction increases
Aortic Valve Stenosis 	*Location.* Midsternum, upper right sternal border *Radiation.* To the carotid arteries and suprasternal notch; may also be a thrill *Intensity.* Varies, louder with increasingly severe obstruction *Quality.* An ejection, often harsh, systolic murmur
Tetralogy of Fallot *With pulmonic stenosis* 	*General.* Variable cyanosis, increasing with activity *Location.* Mid to upper left sternal border. If pulmonary atresia, there is no systolic murmur but the continuous murmur of ductus arteriosus flow at upper left sternal border or in the back.

(table continues next page)

TABLE 18-4 **Characteristics of Pathologic Heart Murmurs** (continued)

Congenital Defect	Characteristics of Murmur
With pulmonic atresia	*Radiation.* Little, to upper left sternal border, occasionally to lung fields *Intensity.* Usually Grade III–IV *Quality.* Midpeaking, systolic ejection murmur
Transposition of the Great Arteries	*General.* Intense generalized cyanosis *Location.* No characteristic murmur. If a murmur is present, it may reflect an associated defect such as VSD or patent ductus arteriosus. *Radiation.* Depends on associated abnormalities *Quality.* Depends on associated abnormalities
Ventricular Septal Defect *Small to moderate*	*Location.* Lower left sternal border *Radiation.* Little *Intensity.* Variable, only partially determined by the size of the shunt. Small shunts with a high pressure gradient may have very loud murmurs. Large defects with elevated pulmonary vascular resistance may have no murmur. Grade II–IV/VI with a thrill if Grade IV/VI or higher.

TABLE 18-5 **Sex Maturity Ratings in Girls Breasts**

Stage 1

Preadolescent—elevation of nipple only

Stage 2

Breast bud stage. Elevation of breast and nipple as a small mound; enlargement of areolar diameter

Stage 3

Further enlargement and elevation of breast and areola, with no separation of the contours

Stage 4

Projection of areola and nipple to form a secondary mound above the level of the breast

Stage 5

Mature stage; projection of nipple only. Areola has receded to general contour of the breast (although in some normal individuals areola continues to form a secondary mound).

(Photos reprinted, with permission from the American Academy of Pediatrics.)

TABLE 18-6   Sex Maturity Ratings in Boys

In assigning SMRs in boys, observe each of the three characteristics separately. Record two separate ratings: pubic hair and genital. If the penis and testes differ in their stages, average the two into a single figure for the genital rating

| | Pubic Hair | Genitalia | |
		Penis	Testes and Scrotum
Stage 1	Preadolescent—no pubic hair except for the fine body hair (vellus hair) similar to that on the abdomen	Preadolescent—same size and proportions as in childhood	Preadolescent—same size and proportions as in childhood
Stage 2	Sparse growth of long, slightly pigmented, downy hair, straight or only slightly curled, chiefly at the base of the penis	Slight to no enlargement	Testes larger; scrotum larger, somewhat reddened, and altered in texture
Stage 3	Darker, coarser, curlier hair spreading sparsely over the pubic symphysis	Larger, especially in length	Further enlarged

| Stage 4 | | Coarse and curly hair, as in the adult; area covered greater than in stage 3 but not as great as in the adult and not yet including the thighs | Further enlarged in length and breadth, with development of the glans | Further enlarged; scrotal skin darkened |
| Stage 5 | | Hair adult quantity and quality, spread to the medial surfaces of the thighs but not up over the abdomen | Adult in size and shape | Adult in size and shape |

(Photos reprinted from *Pediatric Endocrinology and Growth*, 2nd ed., Wales & Wit, 2003, with permission from Elsevier.)

TABLE 18-7 Sex Maturity Ratings in Girls: Pubic Hair

Stage 1

Preadolescent—no pubic hair except for the fine body hair (vellus hair) similar to that on the abdomen

Stage 2

Sparse growth of long, slightly pigmented, downy hair, straight or only slightly curled, chiefly along the labia

Stage 3

Darker, coarser, curlier hair, spreading sparsely over the pubic symphysis

Stage 4

Coarse and curly hair as in adults; area covered greater than in stage 3 but not as great as in the adult and not yet including the thighs

(table continues next page)

TABLE 18-7 **Sex Maturity Ratings in Girls:
Pubic Hair** (continued)

Stage 5

Hair adult in quantity and quality, spread on the medial surfaces of the thighs but not up over the abdomen

Photos reprinted, with permission from the American Academy of Pediatrics.)

TABLE 18-8 **Physical Signs of Sexual Abuse**

Physical Signs that May Indicate Sexual Abuse in Children*

1. Marked and immediate dilatation of the anus in knee–chest position, with no constipation, stool in the vault, or neurologic disorders
2. Hymenal notch or cleft that extends greater than 50% of the inferior hymenal rim (confirmed in knee–chest position)
3. Condyloma acuminata in a child older than 3 years
4. Bruising, abrasions, lacerations, or bite marks of labia or perihymenal tissue
5. Herpes of the anogenital area beyond the neonatal period
6. Purulent or malodorous vaginal discharge in a young girl (all discharges should be cultured and viewed under a microscope for evidence of a sexually transmitted disease)

Physical Signs that Strongly Suggest Sexual Abuse in Children*

1. Lacerations, ecchymoses, and newly healed scars of the hymen or the posterior fourchette
2. No hymenal tissue from 3 to 9 o'clock (confirmed in various positions)
3. Healed hymenal transections, especially between 3 and 9 o'clock (complete cleft)
4. Perianal lacerations extending to external sphincter

A sexual-abuse expert must evaluate a child with concerning physical signs for a complete history and sexual abuse examination.

---

*Any physical sign must be evaluated in light of the entire history, other parts of the physical examination, and laboratory data.

The Pregnant Woman

THE HEALTH HISTORY

Common Concerns

- Symptoms of pregnancy
- Smoking, alcohol, use of illicit drugs, domestic violence
- Prior complications of pregnancy
- Chronic illnesses and family history
- Determining weeks of gestation by date and expected date of delivery

Focus the *initial prenatal visit* on confirming the pregnancy, assessing the health status of the mother and any risks for complications, and counseling to ensure a healthy pregnancy. Ask about the following topics:

- *Symptoms of pregnancy:* absence of menses, breast fullness or tenderness, nausea or vomiting, fatigue, and urinary frequency. Explain that serum or urine testing for beta human chorionic gonadotropin (HCG) offers the best confirmation of pregnancy.

- *Maternal concerns and attitudes:* Review the mother's feelings about the pregnancy and whether she plans to continue to term. Ask about any fears and about support from the father.

- *Current state of health:* risk factors that could adversely affect the mother or fetus. Ask about eating patterns and assess the quality of her nutrition. Does she smoke, drink alcohol, or use any illicit drugs? Does she take any medications? Or have any exposures to toxic substances? What about her income and her social support network? Are there any sources of unusual stress at home or in the work-place? Is there any history of physical abuse or domestic violence?

- *Past obstetric history:* Has she had any complications during past pregnancies, including labor and delivery? Has she had a premature or growth-retarded infant, or a baby large for gestational age? Has there been a prior fetal demise?

- *Past medical history:* Review any history of acute or chronic illnesses, especially hypertension, diabetes, cardiac conditions, asthma, systemic lupus erythematosus (SLE), and seizures, and any history of sexually transmitted diseases, exposure to diethylstilbestrol in utero, or HIV infection.

- *Family history* of chronic illnesses or genetically transmitted diseases: sickle cell anemia, cystic fibrosis, muscular dystrophy, and others.

Expected weeks of gestation by dates and the *expected date of delivery* (EDD):

- To establish *expected weeks of gestation,* count in weeks from either (1) the first day of the last menstrual period (LMP), known as *menstrual age,* or (2) the date of conception if this is known, termed *conception age.* The expected weeks of gestation can help with later assessment of uterine size, assuming that the LMP was normal, the dates were remembered accurately, and conception actually occurred. During the examination, compare your estimate of expected uterine size with the palpable size of the uterus if still within the pelvic cavity, or with the height of the fundus if above the symphysis pubis. If there are discrepancies, investigate possible causes.

- The first day of the LMP is also used to calculate the EDD, or the time projected to term labor and delivery assuming regular 28- to 30-day menstrual cycles. Using *Naegele's rule,* estimate the EDD by adding 7 days to the first day of the LMP, subtracting 3 months, and adding 1 year. This date may be one of the first questions the mother asks you.

- If the patient cannot remember her LMP or has irregular menstrual cycles, or if the dating is uncertain, vaginal probe ultrasound is used to confirm dating in the first trimester.

- Establish the desired frequency of *follow-up visits.* These visits will include measurement of blood pressure and weight, palpation of the uterine fundus to assess fetal growth, verification of fetal heart tones, and determination of fetal presentation and activity.

HEALTH PROMOTION AND COUNSELING

Important Topics for Health Promotion and Counseling

- Nutrition
- Weight gain
- Exercise
- Smoking cessation, alcohol, and illicit drugs
- Screening for domestic violence
- Immunizations

Nutrition and Weight Gain.   Evaluate nutritional status during the first prenatal visit, including: diet history; measurement of height, weight, and body mass index (BMI); and a hematocrit. Check use of needed vitamin and mineral supplements. Develop a nutrition plan appropriate to cultural preferences, typically three balanced meals each day, with increased intake as follows: 300 additional kcal; 5 to 6 g of protein; 15 mg of iron; 250 mg of calcium; and 400 to 800 mcg of folic acid, plus prenatal supplements. Caution against excess amounts of vitamin A, which can become toxic; fish with mercury exposure such as sharks, swordfish, or even canned tuna; unpasteurized dairy products; and undercooked meats.

Ideal *weight gain* in pregnancy follows a pattern: very little gain the first trimester, rapid increase in the second trimester, and mild slowing of the increase in the third trimester. Average weight gain is approximately 28 lbs, or ~10 kg. Weigh the woman at each visit, with the results plotted on a graph. Recommended weight gain ranges from the Institute of Medicine (1992), displayed next, are still current.

■ Recommended Total Weight Gain Ranges for Pregnant Women

Prepregnancy Weight-for-Height Category	Recommended Total Gain	
	lbs	kg
Low BMI <19.8	28–40	12.5–18
Normal BMI 19.8–26.0	25–35	11.5–16
High BMI 26.0–29.0	15–25	7.0–11.5
Obese BMI >29.0	~15	~7.0

Figures are for single pregnancies. The range for women carrying twins is 35–45 lb (16–20 kg). Young adolescents (<2 years after menarche) should strive for gains at the upper end of the range. Short women (<62 in. or <157 cm) should strive for gains at the lower end of the range.

Exercise.   The American College of Obstetricians and Gynecologists (2002) recommends that in conjunction with their physician and in the absence of contraindications, pregnant women should engage in moderate exercise for ~30 minutes most days of the week. Women initiating exercise during pregnancy should consider programs developed specifically for pregnant women. After the first trimester, women should avoid exercise in the supine position, which can compress the inferior vena cava and decrease blood flow to the placenta. The pregnant woman should stop exercise when she feels fatigued or uncomfortable and avoid overheating and dehydration.

Smoking Cessation.   Any smoking should be discontinued. Smoking has been linked to *complications of labor* such as placental abruption, placenta previa, preterm deliveries, low-birthweight babies, and even perinatal death.

Screening for Domestic Violence.   Prevalence during pregnancy ranges from 7% to 20% and may result in femicide, or murder of the mother and child. The American College of Obstetricians and Gynecologists recommends assessment of all women for any history of *domestic violence* that may escalate during the pregnancy. Clues include frequent changes in appointments at the last minute, behavior during the interview, chronic headache or abdominal pain, and bruises or other signs of injury.

Clinicians should ask direct questions in a nonjudgmental manner in a private setting **at each prenatal visit.** For example, ask "Since you've been pregnant, have you been slapped or otherwise physically hurt by anyone?" Women may need multiple opportunities to discuss abuse because of fears about safety and reprisal. Validate positive responses and mark the area of injury on a body diagram. Above all, in situations of admitted abuse, ask how you might help. Offer information on safe shelters, counseling centers, hotline telephone numbers, and other sources of assistance when she is ready to pursue these.* Assess the patient's safety and make any necessary referrals. Learn about requirements for mandatory reporting.

Immunizations.   Tetanus and influenza vaccines can be given in any trimester. Pneumococcal, meningococcal, and hepatitis B vaccines are also safe.

---

*National Domestic Violence Hotline: Web site: www.ncvh.org/index.html; 1-800-799-SAFE (7233); TTY for hearing impaired, 1-800-787-3224.

TECHNIQUES OF EXAMINATION

PREPARING FOR THE EXAMINATION

Show respect for the woman's comfort and privacy, as well as for her individual needs and sensitivities. Ask her to wear her gown with the opening in front to ease the examination of both breasts and the pregnant abdomen.

Positioning

- The semisitting position with the knees bent (see p. 396) affords the most comfort and protects abdominal organs and vessels from the weight of the gravid uterus.
- Avoid prolonged periods of lying on the back. Make your abdominal palpation efficient and accurate.
- The pelvic examination also should be relatively quick.

Equipment

- The examiner's hands should be warm and firm yet gentle in palpation. The fingers should be together and flat. Make palpation smooth and continuous rather than kneading, using the more sensitive palmar surfaces of the ends of the fingers.
- You may need a speculum larger than the usual size. Because of the increased vascularity of the vaginal and cervical structures, insert and open the speculum gently to avoid tissue trauma and bleeding.
- Avoid the cervical brush for Pap smears, because it often causes bleeding. Use the Ayre wooden spatula or "broom" sampling device.

VITAL SIGNS, HEIGHT, AND WEIGHT

Measure the blood pressure.
In midpregnancy, it may
be lower than in the
nonpregnant state.

EXAMINATION TECHNIQUES   POSSIBLE FINDINGS

> ## HYPERTENSION IN PREGNANCY
> ---
> - *Gestational hypertension* if systolic blood pressure (SBP) ≥140 mm Hg and diastolic blood pressure (DBP) ≥90 mm Hg, first occurring after week 20 and *without proteinuria*
> - *Chronic hypertension* if SBP ≥140 mm Hg and DBP ≥90 mm Hg prior to pregnancy, before week 20, and after 12 weeks postpartum
> - *Preeclampsia* if SBP ≥140 mm Hg and DBP ≥90 mm Hg after week 20 and *with proteinuria*

Measure the height and weight. Calculate BMI. First-trimester weight loss should not exceed 5% of prepartum weight.	Weight loss of more than 5% in excessive vomiting, or *hyperemesis*

HEAD AND NECK

- *Face.* Check for the mask of pregnancy, *chloasma,* or irregular brownish patches around the forehead and cheeks, across the bridge of the nose, or along the jaw.	Facial edema after 24 weeks in gestational hypertension
- *Hair*	Hair loss should not be attributed to pregnancy.
- *Eyes.* Note the conjunctival color.	Anemia of pregnancy may cause conjunctival pallor.
- *Nose,* including nasal congestion	Nosebleeds are more common.
- *Mouth*	Gingival enlargement common

EXAMINATION TECHNIQUES	POSSIBLE FINDINGS

- *Thyroid gland*. Inspect and palpate. Modest symmetric enlargement is common.

Significant enlargement is abnormal and should be investigated.

THORAX AND LUNGS

Inspect the thorax for contours. Observe the pattern of breathing.

Respiratory alkalosis in later trimesters

HEART

Palpate the apical impulse.

Impulse may be higher than normal in the 4th intercostal space because of transverse and leftward rotation of the heart from the higher diaphragm.

Auscultate the heart. A venous hum and systolic or continuous mammary souffle (see p. 180) are common.

New diastolic murmurs should be investigated.

BREASTS

Inspect the breasts and nipples for symmetry and color.

The venous pattern may be marked, the nipples and areolae are dark, and Montgomery's glands are prominent.

Palpate for masses.

During pregnancy, breasts are tender and nodular.

Compress each nipple between your index finger and thumb.

This may express colostrum from the nipples.

ABDOMEN

Place the pregnant woman in a semisitting position with her knees flexed.

EXAMINATION TECHNIQUES	POSSIBLE FINDINGS

- **Inspect** any scars or striae, the shape and contour of the abdomen, and the fundal height.

- **Assess** the shape and contour to estimate pregnancy size.

Purplish striae and linea nigra are normal.

36 wks
32 wks
28 wks
24 wks
20-22 wks
16 wks
12-14 wks

EXPECTED HEIGHT OF UTERINE FUNDUS BY WEEKS OF PREGNANCY

- **Palpate** for:

  Organs or masses

  Fetal movements, usually detected after 24 weeks

  Uterine contractility

Irregular contractions after 12 weeks or after palpation during the third trimester

Prior to 37 weeks, regular uterine contractions or bleeding are abnormal, suggesting *preterm labor.*

If woman is >20 weeks pregnant, **measure fundal height** with a tape measure from the top of the symphysis pubis to the top of the uterine fundus. After 20 weeks, measurement in centimeters should roughly equal the weeks of gestation.

If fundal height is more than 2 cm higher than expected, consider multiple gestation, a big baby, extra amniotic fluid, or uterine leiomyoma. If more than 4 cm lower, consider missed abortion, transverse lie, growth retardation, or false pregnancy.

Auscultate the fetal heart, noting its rate (FHR), location, and rhythm. A Doptone will detect the

Lack of an audible FHR may indicate pregnancy of fewer weeks than expected, fetal demise, or false pregnancy.

EXAMINATION TECHNIQUES	POSSIBLE FINDINGS

FHR after 10 weeks. The FHR is audible with a fetoscope after 18 weeks.

- From 12 to 18 weeks, listen in the midline of the lower abdomen.

- After 28 weeks, listen over the fetal back or chest. Use modified *Leopold's maneuvers* to palpate the fetal head and back and identify where to listen.

The *rate* usually is in the 160s during early pregnancy, and then slows to the 120s to 140s near term. After 32 to 34 weeks, the FHR should increase with fetal movement.

An FHR that drops noticeably near term with fetal movement could indicate poor placental circulation.

Rhythm. In the third trimester, expect a variance of 10 to 15 beats per minute (BPM) over 1 to 2 minutes.

Lack of beat-to-beat variability late in pregnancy warrants investigation with an FHR monitor.

GENITALIA, ANUS, AND RECTUM

Inspect the *external genitalia*.

Parous relaxation of the introitus, enlargement of the labia and clitoris, scars from an *episiotomy* or perineal lacerations

Inspect the *anus*.

Hemorrhoids may engorge later in pregnancy.

Palpate *Bartholin's* and *Skene's glands*.

Check for a *cystocele* or *rectocele*.

EXAMINATION TECHNIQUES	POSSIBLE FINDINGS
Speculum Examination. **Inspect** the *cervix* for color, shape, and healed lacerations.	Purplish color of pregnancy; lacerations from prior deliveries
Take *Pap smears*, if indicated.	Specimens may be needed for diagnosis of vaginal or cervical infection
Inspect the *vaginal walls*.	Bluish or violet color, deep rugae, leukorrhea in normal pregnancy; vaginal irritation, itching, and discharge in infection
Bimanual Examination. Insert two lubricated fingers into introitus, palmar side down, with slight pressure downward on the perineum. Slide fingers into the posterior vaginal vault. Maintaining downward pressure, gently turn fingers palmar side up.	
• **Assess** cervical os and degree of effacement. Place your finger gently in the os, and then sweep it around the *surface of the cervix*.	Closed os if nulliparous; os open to size of fingertip if multiparous
• **Estimate** the *length of the cervix*. **Palpate** the lateral surface from the cervical tip to the lateral fornix.	Prior to 34 to 36 weeks, cervix should retain normal length of ~1.5 to 2 cm.
• **Palpate** the *uterus* for size, shape, consistency, and position.	*Hegar's sign*, or early softening of the isthmus; pear-shaped uterus up to 8 weeks, then globular

EXAMINATION TECHNIQUES	POSSIBLE FINDINGS

- **Estimate** *uterine size*. With your internal fingers placed at either side of cervix, palmar surfaces upward, gently lift the uterus toward the abdominal hand. Capture the fundal portion of the uterus between your two hands and gently estimate size.

An irregularly shaped uterus suggests uterine myomata or a *bicornuate uterus,* two distinct uterine cavities separated by a septum.

- **Palpate** the *left and right adnexa*.

Early in pregnancy, it is important to rule out tubal (*ectopic*) pregnancy.

- Perform a *rectovaginal examination* to confirm uterine size or the integrity of the rectovaginal septum.

EXTREMITIES

Inspect the legs for *varicose veins*.

Inspect the hands and legs for *edema*.

Pathologic edema is often 3+ or more pretibially.

Check knee and ankle *reflexes*.

After 24 weeks, reflexes greater than 2+ may indicate pregnancy-induced hypertension.

SPECIAL TECHNIQUES

LEOPOLD'S MANEUVERS

Leopold's maneuvers help determine:

- *Fetal lie*, or where the fetus lies in relation to the woman's back (longitudinal or transverse)

Common deviations include *breech presentation* (fetal buttocks present at the outlet of the maternal pelvis) and absence of the presenting part well down into the maternal pelvis at term.

EXAMINATION TECHNIQUES	POSSIBLE FINDINGS

- *Presentation,* or the end of the fetus that is presenting at the pelvic inlet (head or buttocks)

- Location of the fetal back

- *Engagement,* or how far the presenting part of the fetus has descended into the maternal pelvis

- Estimated fetal weight

First Maneuver (Upper Pole)

Stand at the woman's side, facing her head. Keep the fingers of both examining hands together. Palpate gently with the fingertips to determine what part of the fetus is in the upper pole of the uterine fundus.

Second Maneuver (Sides of the Maternal Abdomen)

Place one hand on each side of the woman's abdomen, aiming to capture the body of the fetus between them. Use one hand to steady the uterus and the other to palpate the fetus.

EXAMINATION TECHNIQUES   POSSIBLE FINDINGS

Third Maneuver (Lower Pole)

Face the woman's feet. Palpate the area just above the symphysis pubis. Note whether the hands diverge with downward pressure or stay together to learn if the presenting part of the fetus, head or buttocks, is descending into the pelvic inlet.

Fourth Maneuver (Confirmation of the Presenting Part)

With your dominant hand, grasp the part of the fetus in the lower pole, and with your nondominant hand, the part of the fetus in the upper pole. Try to distinguish between the head and the buttocks.

RECORDING YOUR FINDINGS

Recording the Physical Examination— The Pregnant Woman

"*Abdomen:* No surgical scars. Active bowel sounds. Soft, nontender; no palpable hepatosplenomegaly or masses. Fundus palpable 2 fingerbreadths below the umbilicus; shape is ovoid and smooth. Fetal heart rate 144. No inguinal adenopathy. *External genitalia:* midline episiotomy scar present. No lesions, discharge, or signs of infection. *Bimanual examination:* cervix midline, soft, 4 cm in length; external os admits fingertip, internal os closed. No pain elicited on movement of cervix; no adnexal masses. Fundus enlarged to 20 weeks' size, midline, smooth; vaginal tone reduced." (*Describes examination of healthy pregnant woman at 20 weeks' gestation*)

The Older Adult

Older adults now number more than 27 million in the United States, growing to 86 million by 2050. Life span at birth is currently 79 years for women and 74 years for men. The "demographic imperative" is to maximize not only life span but also "health span" of our older population, so that seniors maintain full function for as long as possible, enjoying rich and active lives in their homes and communities.

- Assessing the older adult entails a focus on healthy or "successful" aging; the need to understand and mobilize family, social, and community supports; the importance of skills directed to functional assessment, "the sixth vital sign"; and promoting the older adult's long-term health and safety.

- The aging population displays marked heterogeneity. Investigators distinguish "usual" aging, with its complex of diseases and impairments, from optimal aging. Optimal aging occurs in those people who escape debilitating disease entirely and maintain healthy lives late into their 80s and 90s. Studies of centenarians show that genes account for approximately 20% of the probability of living to 100, with healthy lifestyles accounting for approximately 20% to 30%.

THE HEALTH HISTORY

APPROACH TO THE PATIENT

As you talk with older adults, convey respect, patience, and cultural awareness. Be sure to address patients by their last name.

Adjusting the Office Environment.   Make sure the office is neither too cool nor too warm. Face the patient directly, sitting at eye level. A well-lit room allows the older adult to see your facial expressions and gestures.

More than 50% of older adults have hearing deficits. Free the room of distractions or noise. Consider using a "pocket talker," a microphone that amplifies your voice and connects to an earpiece inserted by the patient. Chairs with higher seating and a wide stool with a handrail leading up to the examining table help patients with quadriceps weakness.

Shaping the Content and Pace of the Visit.   Older people often reminisce. Listen to this process of life review to gain important insights and help patients as they work through painful feelings or recapture joys and accomplishments.

Balance the need to assess complex problems with the patient's endurance and possible fatigue. Consider dividing the initial assessment into two visits.

Eliciting Symptoms in the Older Adult.   Older patients may overestimate healthiness even when increasing disease and disability are obvious. To reduce the risk of late recognition and delayed intervention, adopt more directed questions or *health screening tools.* Consult with family members and caretakers.

Acute illnesses present differently in older adults than in younger age groups. Be sensitive to changes in presentation of myocardial infarction and thyroid disease. Older patients with infections are less likely to have fever.

Recognize the symptom clusters typical of different *geriatric syndromes,* notable for the interaction and probable synergism among multiple risk factors, for example, falls, dizziness, depression, urinary incontinence, and functional impairment. Searching for the usual "unifying diagnosis" may pertain to fewer than 50% of older adults.

Cognitive impairment may affect the patient's history. Even elders with mild cognitive impairment, however, can provide sufficient history to reveal concurrent disorders. Use simple sentences with prompts to trigger necessary information. If impairments are more severe, confirm symptoms with family members or caretakers.

Addressing Cultural Dimensions of Aging.   By 2050, the older adult population will increase by 230%, and the minority older adult population by 510%. Cultural differences affect the epidemiology of illness and mental health, acculturation, the specific concerns of the elderly, the potential for misdiagnosis, and disparities in health outcomes. Review the components of self-awareness needed for cultural responsiveness, discussed in Chapter 3 (pp. 52–53). Ask about spiritual advisors and native healers. Cultural values particularly affect decisions about the end of life. Elders, family, and even an extended community group may make these decisions with or for the older patient.

 COMMON CONCERNS

- Activities of daily living
- Instrumental activities of daily living
- Medications
- Nutrition
- Acute and persistent pain
- Smoking and alcohol
- Advance directives and palliative care

Place symptoms in the context of your overall *functional assessment,* always focusing on helping the older adult to maintain optimal well-being and level of function.

Activities of Daily Living.   Daily activities provide an important baseline for the future. You might say "Tell me about your typical day" or "Tell me about your day yesterday." Then move to a greater level of detail: "You got up at 8 AM? How is it getting out of bed?"

ACTIVITIES OF DAILY LIVING AND INSTRUMENTAL ACTIVITIES OF DAILY LIVING

Physical Activities of Daily Living (ADLs)	Instrumental Activities of Daily Living (IADLs)
Bathing	Using the telephone
Dressing	Shopping
Toileting	Preparing food
Transferring	Housekeeping
Continence	Laundry
Feeding	Transportation
Managing money	Taking medicine

Medications.   Adults older than 65 take approximately 30% of all prescriptions. Roughly 30% take more than eight prescribed drugs each day! Take a thorough medication history, including name, dose, frequency, and indication for each drug. Explore all components of polypharmacy, or suboptimal prescribing, including concurrent use of multiple drugs, underuse, inappropriate use, and nonadherence. Ask about use of over-the-counter medications, vitamin and nutrition supplements, and mood-altering drugs. Medications are the most common modifiable risk factor associated with falls.

Nutrition.   Taking a diet history and using the Rapid Screen for Dietary Intake and the Nutrition Screening Checklist (pp. 71–72) are especially important in older adults.

Acute and Persistent Pain.   Pain and associated complaints account for 80% of clinician visits, usually for musculoskeletal complaints like back and joint pain. Older patients are less likely to report pain, leading to undue suffering, depression, social isolation, physical disability, and loss of function.

Inquire about pain each time you meet with the older patient. Ask specifically, "Are you having any pain right now? How about over the past week?" Unidimensional scales such as the Visual Analog Scale, graphic pictures, and the Verbal 0–10 Scale have all been validated and are easiest to use.

⬤ Characteristics of Acute and Persistent Pain

Acute Pain	Persistent Pain
Distinct onset	Lasts more than 3 months
Obvious pathology	Often associated with psychological or functional impairment
Short duration	Can fluctuate in character and intensity over time
Common causes: postsurgical, trauma, headache	Common causes: arthritis, cancer, claudication, leg cramps, neuropathy, radiculopathy

(Source: Reuben DB, Herr KA, Pacala JT, et al. Geriatrics at Your Fingertips: 2004, 6th ed. Malden, MA: Blackwell Publishing, for the American Geriatrics Society, 2004:149.)

Smoking and Alcohol. At each visit, advise elderly smokers to quit.

An estimated 5% to 10% of older adults have alcohol-related problems, and this percentage is expected to rise as the population ages in coming decades. Despite the prevalence of alcohol problems among the elderly, rates of detection and treatment are low. Use the CAGE questions to uncover problem drinking (see p. 50).

Advance Directives and Palliative Care. Providers should initiate these discussions before serious illness develops. Advance care planning involves providing information, invoking the patient's preferences, identifying proxy decision makers, and conveying empathy and support. Use clear, simple language. Ask about preferences relating to written "Do Not Resuscitate" orders specifying life support measures "if the heart or lungs were to stop or give out." Seek a written health care proxy or durable power of attorney for health care, "someone who can make decisions reflecting your wishes in case of confusion or emergency." Include these discussions in office settings rather than the uncertain and stressful environment of emergency or acute care.

The goal of *palliative care* is "to relieve suffering and improve the quality of life for patients with advanced illnesses and their families through specific knowledge and skills, including communication with patients and family members; management of pain and other symptoms; psychosocial, spiritual, and bereavement support; and coordination of an array of medical and social services."

HEALTH PROMOTION AND COUNSELING

Important Topics for Health Promotion and Counseling in the Older Adult

- When to screen
- Cancer screening
- Dementia and mild cognitive impairment
- Elder mistreatment

When to Screen. As the life span for older adults extends into the 80s, new issues for screening emerge. In general, base screening decisions on each older person's particular circumstances, rather than on age alone. Consider life expectancy, time interval until benefit from screening accrues, and patient preference. The American Geriatrics Society recommends that if life expectancy is short, give priority to treating conditions that will benefit the patient in the time that remains.

- Screen for age-related changes in *vision* and *hearing*. These are included in the 10-Minute Geriatric Screener (pp. 411–412).

- Recommend regular aerobic *exercise*. Resistance training and Tai Chi may help to improve balance.

- *Immunizations:* include the pneumococcal vaccine once after age 65, annual influenza vaccinations, and the herpes zoster vaccine.

- Promote *household safety*. Correct poor lighting, chairs at awkward heights, slippery or irregular surfaces, and environmental hazards.

Cancer Screening. *Cancer screening* can be controversial because of limited evidence about adults older than age 70 to 80:

- The American Geriatrics Society recommends annual or biennial *mammography* for breast cancer screening up to age 75, then every 2 to 3 years if life expectancy remains more than 4 years.

- 40% to 50% of deaths from cervical cancer are in women older than 65 years. Provide Pap smears every 1 to 3 years until age 65 to 70 when there is no history of cervical pathology.

- Colonoscopy is recommended for colon cancer screening every 10 years, beginning at age 50. This examination is difficult for many older patients, who may decline despite encouragement.

- Check for skin and oral cancers in high-risk patients.

Dementia and Mild Cognitive Impairment.   *Dementia* is "an acquired syndrome of decline in memory and at least one other cognitive domain such as language, visuospatial, or executive function sufficient to interfere with social or occupational functioning." It affects 16% of Americans over age 65. Prominent features include:

- Short- and long-term memory deficits and impaired judgment

- Impoverished thought processes

- Hesitant speech resulting from difficulty finding words

- Loss of orientation to place

Most dementias represent Alzheimer's disease (50% to 85%) or vascular multi-infarct dementia (10% to 20%). Dementia often has a slow, insidious onset. It may escape detection by both families and clinicians, especially in the early stages of *mild cognitive impairment,* which may be detected only on neurocognitive testing. Look for problems with memory, then later for changes in cognitive function or ADLs. Watch for family complaints of new or unusual behaviors. Investigate contributing factors such as medications, depression, metabolic abnormalities, or other medical and psychiatric conditions.

Elder Mistreatment.   Screen older patients for possible *elder mistreatment,* which includes abuse, neglect, exploitation, and abandonment. Prevalence is ~1% to 5% of the older population; however, many more cases may remain undetected.

TECHNIQUES OF EXAMINATION

Assessment of the older adult does not follow the traditional format of the history and physical examination. Enhanced techniques of interviewing, special emphasis on daily function and key topics related to elder health, and a focus on functional assessment are especially important.

Functional status is the ability to perform tasks and fulfill social roles associated with daily living across a wide range of complexity.

ASSESSING FUNCTIONAL STATUS: THE "SIXTH VITAL SIGN"

Assessing Functional Ability. Several performance-based assessment instruments are available. The screening tool below is brief, has high inter-rater agreement, and can be used easily by office staff. It covers the three important domains of geriatric assessment: physical, cognitive, and psychosocial function. It addresses key sensory modalities and urinary incontinence, an often unreported problem that greatly affects social interactions and self-esteem in the elderly. One mnemonic that helps students assess incontinence is DIAPERS: **D**elirium, **I**nfection, **A**trophic urethritis/vaginitis, **P**harmaceuticals, **E**xcess urine output (e.g., due to congestive heart failure, hyperglycemia), **R**estricted mobility, **S**tool impaction.

● 10-Minute Geriatric Screener	
Problem and Screening Measure	**Positive Screen**
Vision: 2 Parts: Ask: "Do you have difficulty driving, or watching television, or reading, or doing any of your daily activities because of your eyesight?	Yes to question and inability to read greater than 20/40 on Snellen chart

(continued)

● 10-Minute Geriatric Screener (continued)

Problem and Screening Measure	Positive Screen
If yes, then: Test each eye with Snellen chart while patient wears corrective lenses (if applicable).	
Hearing: Use audioscope set at 40 dB. Test hearing using 1,000 and 2,000 Hz.	Inability to hear 1,000 or 2,000 Hz in both ears or either of these frequencies in one ear
Leg mobility: Time the patient after instructing: "Rise from the chair. Walk 20 feet briskly, turn, walk back to the chair, and sit down."	Unable to complete task in 15 seconds

Urinary incontinence: 2 Parts:
  Ask: "In the last year, have you ever lost your urine and gotten wet?"
If yes, then ask:
  "Have you lost urine on at least 6 separate dates?"
	Yes to both questions

Nutrition/weight loss: 2 parts:
  Ask: "Have you lost 10 lbs over the past 6 months without trying to do so?"
  Weigh the patient.
	Yes to the question or weight <100 lbs

Memory: Three-item recall	Unable to remember all three items after 1 minute
Depression: Ask: "Do you often feel sad or depressed?"	Yes to the question

Physical disability: Six questions:
  "Are you able to . . . :
  "Do strenuous activities like fast walking or bicycling?"
	No to any of the questions

(continued)

Problem and Screening Measure	Positive Screen
"Do heavy work around the house like washing windows, walls, or floors?"	
"Go shopping for groceries or clothes?"	
"Get to places out of walking distance?"	
"Bathe, either a sponge bath, tub bath, or shower?"	
"Dress, like putting on a shirt, buttoning and zipping, or putting on shoes?"	

(Source: More AA, Siu AL. Screening for common problems in ambulatory elderly: clinical confirmation of a screening instrument. Am J Med 100:438–440, 1996.)

Further Assessment of Falls. Each year ~35% to 40% of healthy community-dwelling older adults experience falls. Incidence rates in nursing homes and hospitals are almost three times higher, with related injuries in approximately 25%.

The American Geriatrics Society recommends risk factor assessment for falls during routine primary care visits, with more intensive assessment in high-risk groups—those with first or recurrent falls, nursing home residents, and those prone to fall-related injuries. Assess how the fall occurred, seeking details from any witnesses, and identify risk factors, medical comorbidities, functional status, and environmental risks. Couple your assessment with interventions for prevention, including gait and balance training and exercise to strengthen muscles, reduction of home hazards, discontinuation of psychotropic medication, and multifactorial assessment with targeted interventions. Recommendations from the American Geriatrics Society are provided on the next page.

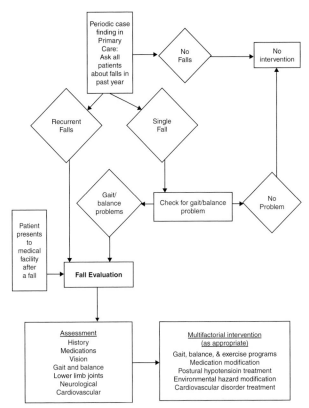

(Source: American Geriatrics Society, British Geriatrics Society, American Academy of Orthopaedic Surgeons. Guideline for the prevention of falls in older persons. Am Geriatr Soc 49(5):664–672, 2001.)

EXAMINATION TECHNIQUES   POSSIBLE FINDINGS

PHYSICAL EXAMINATION OF THE OLDER ADULT

Vital Signs. Measure blood pressure, checking for increased systolic blood pressure (SBP) and widened

Isolated systolic hypertension (SBP ≥140) after age 50 triples the risk of coronary heart disease in men. PP ≥60 is a risk

EXAMINATION TECHNIQUES	POSSIBLE FINDINGS
pulse pressure (PP), defined as SBP minus diastolic blood pressure (DBP).	factor for cardiovascular and renal disease and stroke.
Assess the patient for orthostatic hypotension, defined as a drop in SBP of ≥20 mm Hg or DBP of ≥10 mm Hg within 3 minutes of standing. Measure in two positions: supine after the patient rests for up to 10 minutes, then within 2 to 3 minutes after standing up.	*Orthostatic hypotension* in 10%–20% of older adults and in up to 30% of frail nursing home residents, especially when they first arise in the morning. Watch for light-headedness, weakness, unsteadiness, visual blurring, and, in 20% to 30% of patients, syncope.
Review the JNC VII categories of "pre-hypertension" to help with early detection and treatment.	Assess for medications, autonomic disorders, diabetes, prolonged bedrest, blood loss, and cardiovascular disorders.
Measure heart rate, respiratory rate, and temperature. The apical heart rate may yield more information about arrhythmias in older patients. Use thermometers accurate for lower temperatures.	Respiratory rate ≥25 breaths per minute indicates lower respiratory infection. Hypothermia is more common in elderly patients.
Weight and height are especially important and needed for calculation of the body mass index (p. 60). Weight should be measured at every visit.	Low weight is a key indicator of poor nutrition. Undernutrition in depression, alcoholism, cognitive impairment, malignancy, chronic organ failure (cardiac, renal, pulmonary), medication use, social isolation, and poverty

EXAMINATION TECHNIQUES	POSSIBLE FINDINGS
Skin. Note physiologic changes of aging, such as thinning, loss of elastic tissue and turgor, and wrinkling.	Dry, flaky, rough, and often itchy
Check the extensor surface of the hands and forearms.	White depigmented patches (*pseudoscars*); well-demarcated, vividly purple macules or patches that may fade after several weeks (*actinic purpura*)
Look for changes from sun exposure. There may be *actinic lentigines,* or "liver spots," and *actinic keratoses,* superficial flattened papules covered by a dry scale (p. 104).	Distinguish such lesions from a *basal cell carcinoma* and *squamous cell carcinoma* (p. 105). Dark, raised, asymmetric lesion with irregular borders in *melanoma*
Inspect for the benign *comedones,* or blackheads, on the cheeks or around the eyes; *cherry angiomas* (p. 103); and *seborrheic keratoses,* (p. 104).	
Inspect for painful vesicular lesions in a dermatomal distribution.	*Herpes zoster* from reactivation of latent varicella-zoster virus in the dorsal root ganglia
In older bedbound patients, especially when emaciated or neurologically impaired, inspect for damage or ulceration.	*Pressure sores* if obliteration of arteriolar and capillary blood flow to the skin or shear forces with movement across sheets or lifting upright incorrectly
HEENT. Inspect the eyelids, the bony orbit, and the eye.	*Senile ptosis* arising from weakening of the levator

EXAMINATION TECHNIQUES   POSSIBLE FINDINGS

palpebrae, relaxation of the skin, and increased weight of the upper eyelid

Ectropion or *entropion* of lower lids (p. 130)

Yellowing of the sclera and *arcus senilis,* a benign whitish ring around the limbus

Test visual acuity, using a pocket Snellen chart or wall-mounted chart.

More than 40 million Americans have refractive errors—*presbyopia.*

Examine the lenses and fundi.

Cataracts, glaucoma, and macular degeneration all increase with aging.

Inspect each lens for opacities.

Cataracts are the world's leading cause of blindness.

Assess the cup-to-disc ratio, usually ≤1:2.

Increased cup-to-disc ratio suggests open-angle *glaucoma* and possible loss of peripheral and central vision, and blindness. Prevalence is three to four times higher in African-Americans.

Inspect the fundi for colloid bodies causing alterations in pigmentation called *drusen.* These may be hard and sharply defined, or soft and confluent with altered pigmentation.

Macular degeneration causes poor central vision and blindness. Types include *dry atrophic* (more common but less severe) and *wet exudative,* or neovascular.

Test hearing by the whispered voice (see p. 121) or audioscope. Inspect ear canals for cerumen.

Removing cerumen often quickly improves hearing.

EXAMINATION TECHNIQUES	POSSIBLE FINDINGS

Examine the oral cavity for odor, appearance of the gingival mucosa, any caries, mobility of the teeth, and quantity of saliva.

Malodor in poor oral hygiene, periodontitis, or caries

Gingivitis if periodontal disease

Inspect for lesions on mucosal surfaces. Ask patient to remove dentures so you can check gums for denture sores.

Dental plaque and cavitation if caries. Increased tooth mobility; risk of tooth aspiration

Decreased salivation from medications, radiation, Sjögren's syndrome, or dehydration

Oral tumors, usually on lateral borders of tongue and floor of mouth

Thorax and Lungs. Note subtle signs of changes in pulmonary function.

Increased anteroposterior diameter, purse-lipped breathing, and dyspnea with talking or minimal exertion in *chronic obstructive pulmonary disease*

Cardiovascular System. Review blood pressure and heart rate.

Isolated systolic hypertension and a widened pulse pressure are cardiac risk factors. Search for *left ventricular hypertrophy (LVH)*.

Inspect the jugular venous pulsation (JVP), palpating the carotid upstrokes, and listen for any overlying carotid bruits.

A *tortuous atherosclerotic aorta* can raise pressure in the left jugular veins by impairing drainage into right atrium.

Carotid bruits in possible *carotid stenosis*.

Assess the point of maximal impulse (PMI), and then heart sounds.

Sustained PMI is found in LVH; diffuse PMI is found within congestive heart failure (see p. 170).

EXAMINATION TECHNIQUES	POSSIBLE FINDINGS
	In older adults, S_3 in dilatation of the left ventricle from congestive heart failure or cardiomyopathy; S_4 in hypertension
Listen for cardiac murmurs in all areas (see p. 172). Describe timing, shape, location of maximal intensity, radiation, intensity, pitch, and quality of each murmur.	A systolic crescendo–decrescendo murmur in the second right interspace in *aortic sclerosis* or *aortic stenosis*. Both carry increased risk of cardiovascular disease and death.
	A harsh holosystolic murmur at the apex suggests *mitral regurgitation*, also common in the elderly.
For systolic murmurs over the clavicle, check for delay between the brachial and radial pulses.	Delay during simultaneous palpation (but not compression) of brachial and radial pulses in *aortic stenosis*.
Breasts and Axillae. Palpate the breasts carefully for lumps or masses.	Possible breast cancer

Abdomen.

- Check for any bruits over the aorta, renal arteries, and femoral arteries.

  Bruits in atherosclerotic vascular disease

- Inspect the upper abdomen; palpate to the left of the midline for aortic pulsations.

  Widened aorta and pulsatile mass may be found in *abdominal aortic aneurysm*.

EXAMINATION TECHNIQUES   POSSIBLE FINDINGS

Female Genitalia and Pelvic Examination.

Take special care to explain the steps of the examination and allow time for careful positioning. For the woman with arthritis or spinal deformities who cannot flex her hips or knees, an assistant can gently raise and support the legs, or help the woman into the left lateral position.

Inspect the vulva for changes related to menopause; identify any labial masses. Bluish swellings may be varicosities.	Benign masses include condylomata, fibromas, leiomyomas, and sebaceous cysts.
	Bulging of the anterior vaginal wall below the urethra in urethrocele
Inspect the urethra for *caruncles*, or prolapse of fleshy erythematous mucosal tissue at the urethral meatus.	Clitoral enlargement in *androgen-producing tumors* or use of androgen creams
Speculum Examination. Inspect vaginal walls, which may be atrophic, and cervix.	Estrogen-stimulated cervical mucus with ferning in use of hormone replacement therapy, *endometrial hyperplasia,* and *estrogen-producing tumors*
Obtain endocervical cells for the Pap smear. Use a blind swab if the atrophic vagina is too small.	
Removing speculum, ask patient to bear down.	Uterine prolapse, cystocele, urethrocele, or rectocele.
Perform the bimanual examination.	See Table 14-6, Positions of the Uterus, and Uterine Myomas, p. 257.

EXAMINATION TECHNIQUES	POSSIBLE FINDINGS
	Mobility of cervix restricted if inflammation, malignancy, or surgical adhesion
	Palpable ovaries in *ovarian cancer.*
Perform the rectovaginal examination.	Enlarged, fixed, or irregular uterus if adhesions or malignancy. Rectal masses in *colon cancer.*
Male Genitalia and Prostate. Examine the penis; retract foreskin if present. Examine the scrotum, testes, and epididymis.	Smegma, penile cancer, and scrotal hydroceles
Do a rectal examination.	Rectal masses in *colon cancer. Prostate hyperplasia* if enlargement; *prostate cancer* if nodules or masses.
Peripheral Vascular System. Auscultate the abdomen for aortic, renal, femoral artery bruits.	Bruits over these vessels in *atherosclerotic disease.*
Palpate pulses.	Diminished or absent pulses in *arterial occlusion.* Confirm with an office ankle–brachial index.
Musculoskeletal System. Screen general range of motion and gait. If joint deformity, deficits in mobility, or pain with	Review the techniques for examining individual joints in Chapter 16.

Degenerative joint changes in *osteoarthritis;* joint |

EXAMINATION TECHNIQUES   POSSIBLE FINDINGS

movement, conduct a more thorough examination.

inflammation in *rheumatoid* or *gouty arthritis*. See Tables 16-1 to 16-4.

Nervous System. Begin evaluation with the 10-Minute Geriatric Screener, pp. 411–412.

Pursue further examination if any deficits. Focus especially on memory and affect.

Learn to distinguish delirium from depression and dementia. See Table 20-1.

Assess gait and balance, particularly standing balance; timed 8-foot walk; stride characteristics like width, pace, and length of stride; and careful turning.

Abnormalities of gait and balance, especially widening of base, slowing and lengthening of stride, and difficulty turning, are correlated with risk of falls.

Although neurologic abnormalities are common in older adults, their prevalence without identifiable disease increases with age, ranging from 30% to 50%.

Physiologic changes of aging: unequal pupil size, decreased arm swing and spontaneous movements, increased leg rigidity and abnormal gait, presence of the snout and grasp reflexes, and decreased toe vibratory sense.

Assess any tremor, rigidity, bradykinesia, micrographia, shuffling gait, and difficulty turning in bed, opening jars, and rising from a chair.

Tremor is slow frequency and at rest, with a "pill-rolling" quality, and aggravated by stress and inhibited during sleep or movement.

Essential tremor if bilateral, symmetric with positive family history, and diminished by alcohol

RECORDING YOUR FINDINGS

As you read through this physical examination, you will notice some atypical findings. Try to test yourself. See if you can interpret these findings in the context of all you have learned about the examination of the older adult.

Recording the Physical Examination—The Older Adult

2/1/08

Mr. J is an older adult who appears healthy but underweight, with good muscle bulk. He is alert and interactive, with good recall of his life history. He is accompanied by his son.

Vital Signs: Ht (without shoes) 160 cm (5′). Wt (dressed) 65 kg (143 lb). BMI 28. BP 145/88 right arm, supine; 154/94 left arm, supine. Heart rate (HR) 98 and regular. Respiratory rate (RR) 18. Temperature (oral) 98.6°F.

10-Minute Geriatric Screener: (see pp. 411–412)

Vision: Patient reports difficulty reading. Visual acuity 20/60 on Snellen chart.

Needs further evaluation for glasses and possibly hearing aid.

Hearing: Cannot hear whispered voice in either ear. Cannot hear 1,000 or 2,000 Hz with audioscope in either ear.

Leg Mobility: Can walk 20 feet briskly, turn, walk back to chair, and sit down in 14 seconds.

Urinary Incontinence: Has lost urine and gotten wet on 20 separate days.

Needs further evaluation for incontinence, including "DIAPER" assessment (see p. 410), prostate examination, and postvoid residual, which is normally ≤50 mL (requires bladder catheterization).

Nutrition: Has lost 15 lbs over the past 6 months without trying.

(continued)

Needs nutritional screen (see pp. 71–72).

Memory: Can remember three items after 1 minute.

Depression: Does not often feel sad or depressed.

Physical Disability: Can walk fast but cannot ride a bicycle. Can do moderate but not heavy work around the house. Can go shopping for groceries or clothes. Can get to places out of walking distance. Can bathe each day without difficulty. Can dress, including buttoning and zipping, and can put on shoes.

Consider exercise regimen with strength training.

Physical Examination: Record the vital signs and weight. Carefully describe your findings for each relevant segment of the peripheral examination, using terminology found in the "Recording Your Findings" section of the prior chapters.

AIDS TO INTERPRETATION

TABLE 20-1 Delirium and Dementia

	Delirium	Dementia
Clinical Features		
Onset	Acute	Insidious
Course	Fluctuating, with lucid intervals; worse at night	Slowly progressive
Duration	Hours to weeks	Months to years
Sleep/Wake Cycle	Always disrupted	Sleep fragmented
General Medical Illness or Drug Toxicity	Either or both present	Often absent, especially in Alzheimer's disease
Mental Status		
Level of Consciousness	Disturbed. Person less clearly aware of the environment and less able to focus, sustain, or shift attention	Usually normal until late in the course of the illness
Behavior	Activity often abnormally decreased (somnolence) or increased (agitation, hypervigilance)	Normal to slow; may become inappropriate
Speech	May be hesitant, slow or rapid, incoherent	Difficulty in finding words, aphasia
Mood	Fluctuating, labile, from fearful or irritable to normal or depressed	Often flat, depressed

(table continues next page)

TABLE 20-1 Delirium and Dementia (continued)

	Delirium	Dementia
Thought Processes	Disorganized, may be incoherent	Impoverished. Speech gives little information.
Thought Content	Delusions common, often transient	Delusions may occur.
Perceptions	Illusions, hallucinations, most often visual	Hallucinations may occur.
Judgment	Impaired, often to a varying degree	Increasingly impaired over the course of the illness
Orientation	Usually disoriented, especially for time. A known place may seem unfamiliar.	Fairly well maintained, but becomes impaired in the later stages of illness
Attention	Fluctuates. Person easily distracted, unable to concentrate on selected tasks	Usually unaffected until late in the illness
Memory	Immediate and recent memory impaired	Recent memory and new learning especially impaired
Examples of Cause	Delirium tremens (due to withdrawal from alcohol)	*Reversible:* Vitamin B_{12} deficiency, thyroid disorders
	Uremia	
	Acute hepatic failure	*Irreversible:* Alzheimer's disease, vascular dementia (from multiple infarcts), dementia due to head trauma
	Acute cerebral vasculitis	
	Atropine poisoning	

TABLE 20-2 **Screening for Dementia: The Mini-Cog**

Administration

The test is administered as follows:

1. Instruct the patient to listen carefully to and remember 3 unrelated words and then to repeat the words.
2. Instruct the patient to draw the face of a clock, either on a blank sheet of paper or on a sheet with the clock circle already drawn on the page. After the patient puts the numbers on the clock face, ask him or her to draw the hands of the clock to read a specific time.
3. Ask the patient to repeat the 3 previously stated words.

Scoring

Give 1 point for each recalled word after the clock drawing test (CDC) distractor.

Patients recalling none of the three words are classified as demented (Score = 0).

Patients recalling all three words are classified as nondemented (Score = 3).

Patients with intermediate word recall of 1–2 words are classified based on the CDT (Abnormal = demented; Normal = nondemented).

Note: The CDT is considered normal if all numbers are present in the correct sequence and position, and the hands readably display the requested time.

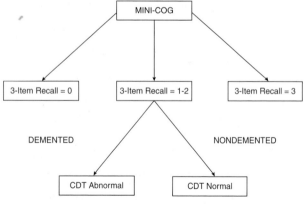

MINI-COG SCORING ALGORITHM

(From Borson S, Scanlan J, Brush M, et al. The Mini-Cog: a cognitive 'vital signs' measure for dementia screening in multi-lingual elderly. *Int J Geriatr Psychiatry* 15(11);1021–1027, 2000. Copyright John Wiley & Sons Limited. Reproduced with permission.)

INDEX

NOTE: Page numbers followed by *b* indicate boxed material; those followed by *t* indicate tables.

A

ABCD screen, 93, 106*t*
Abdomen, 193–213. *See also specific structures*
  back pain referred from, 302*t*
  in children, 364, 372
  common or concerning symptoms of, 193*b*
  disorders of, 209*t*–213*t*
  examination of, 14, 201–208
  fullness in, 195
  health history of, 193–199
  health promotion or counseling for, 199–200
  in older adults, 418
  painful or tender, 193–196, 198, 213*t*
  during pregnancy, 396–398
  recording exam findings of, 208*b*, 377*b*
Abdominal aortic aneurysm, 217–218, 418
Abdominal reflexes, 330, 340*t*
Abducens nerve, 317*b*, 318
Abduction stress test, 296
Abrasions, genital, 373
Abscess
  brain, 112
  lung, 157*t*
  peritonsillar, 371
Abstract thinking, 84
Abuse
  of alcohol, 2*b*, 4, 50–51, 199, 407
  of drugs, 4, 50–51, 80
  of older adults, 409
  physical, 51, 392–393
  sexual, 373, 388*b*
Achilles tendon, 297
Acoustic nerve, 317*b*, 319–320
Acquired immunodeficiency syndrome (AIDS), 105*t*. *See also* HIV
Acrocyanosis, 358

Acromioclavicular arthritis, 307*t*
Actinic keratoses, 104*t*, 415
Actinic lentigines, 415
Actinic purpura, 415
Activities of daily living, 405, 406*b*
Adams bend test, 375
Adduction stress test, 294
Adenomas, breast, 182*b*
Adnexa (ovaries), 15, 249, 400
Adolescents. *See also* Children
  examining, 352, 374–375
  hypertension in, 357*b*, 380*t*
  substance use in, 51
Advance directives, 407
Adventitious breath sounds, 146, 147*b*, 150, 161*t*
Affect, 79*b*, 81
Age
  gestational, 353, 354*b*
  of patient, 28
Agenda, for interview, 39–40
Agoraphobia, 90*t*
AIDS/HIV infection, 105*t*, 231–232
Air and bone conduction test, 122, 135*t*, 320
Airway sounds. *See* Breath sounds
Alcohol use and abuse
  health promotion and counseling for, 80, 199
  history of, 2*b*, 4, 50–51
  liver disease in, 193, 197*b*
  in older adults, 407
  screening for, 80
Alertness, patient, 77, 81, 333*b*
Alkalosis, respiratory, 396
Allen test, 222
Allergies, 2*b*, 4, 114, 350
Alopecia areata, 107*t*
Alternative health care, 5
Alzheimer's disease, 409
Amblyopia, 368
Amenorrhea, 242

Anal reflex, 331
Analgesic rebound headaches, 126*t*
"Anatomic snuffbox," 284
Androgen-producing tumors, 419
Anemia of pregnancy, 395
Aneurysm, aortic, 152*t*, 163, 418
Angina pectoris, 152*t*, 163
Angioedema, 136*t*
Angioma, 103*t*, 415
Angry patient, 47
Angular cheilitis, 136*t*
Anhedonia, 80
Ankle-brachial index, 217, 226*t*–227*t*
Ankles, 297–298
   muscles of, 323
   reflexes of, 329, 400
   ulcers on, 216, 225*t*
Ankylosing spondylitis, 302*t*
Anorexia, 60, 70*t*, 196, 242
Anteflexion, 257*t*
Anterior cruciate ligament (ACL),
   294–295, 309*t*
Anterior drawer sign, 294, 309*t*
Anus, 263, 264, 265*b*, 398
Anxiety, 57, 90*t*–91*t*, 153*t*
Aorta
   aneurysm of, 141, 152*t*, 163,
     217–218
   coarctation of, 363
   examination of, 14, 205
Aortic valve
   regurgitation of (insufficiency),
     169, 171, 173, 219
   sclerosis of, 418
   stenosis of, 169, 170, 174, 175,
     381*t*, 418
Apgar score, 352–353
Aphasia, 82
Aphthous ulcer, 138*t*
Apical pulse (impulse)
   in children, 363–364
   measuring, 64, 168, 170
   in older adults, 417
   in pregnancy, 396
Apnea, 361
Appearance
   of clinician, 38
   of patient, 58, 78, 81
Appendicitis, 194, 196, 207–208

Arcus senilis, 416
Argyll Robertson pupils, 117
Arms
   examination of, 218–219
   flaccid, 334
   pain in, 215
Arousal (reticular activating) system,
   312
Arrhythmias, 64, 176*t*–180*t*, 364.
   See also specific arrhythmias
Arterial insufficiency, 223, 224*t*, 225*t*
Arterial occlusion, 219
Arterial pulses, 218*b*
Arteries, retinal, 119, 120*b*
Arthralgia, 275
Arthritis
   acromioclavicular, 307*t*
   in ankles or feet, 297, 298
   degenerative, 275, 283, 305*t*–306*t*,
     308*t*, 421
   gonococcal, 274, 283
   gouty, 421
   in hips, 290, 291
   in knees, 293, 308*t*
   in older adults, 420–421
   patterns of pain in, 305*t*–306*t*
   rheumatoid, 274–275, 276, 283,
     284, 305*t*–306*t*, 308*t*, 421
   septic, 275
   in shoulders, 307*t*
   in spine, 289
   in wrists or hands, 283, 284
Articular structures, 271, 275
Asbestosis, 155*t*
Ascites, 206–207
Assessments, 17–36. *See also specific
   assessments*
   case study of, 19*b*–28*b*
   comprehensive *vs.* focused, 1*b*, 37
   organizing data for, 28–30
   and problem list, 36
   process of, 17–19
   recording, 33–36, 69
   test selection in, 30*b*–32*b*
   tips for, 29*b*
Asterixis, 332
Asthma, 154*t*, 158*t*, 161*t*
Astigmatism, 126*t*
Ataxia, 313

Ataxic (Biot's) breathing, 74t
Atelectasis, 161t
Atherosclerosis, 420
Athetosis, 341t
Atrial fibrillation, 64, 168
Atrial septal defect, 364
Attention, 77, 78, 83, 425t
Auditory acuity. *See* Hearing; Hearing loss
Auricles, 120–121, 360
Auscultation
    of abdomen, 201–202
    of chest, 146–148, 150
    of fetal heart, 397–398
    of heart, 171–173, 364, 396
Auscultatory gap, 62b, 168
Autonomy, 54
Axillae, 12, 186, 418
Axillary temperature, 65

B

Babinski response, 328, 330
Back
    examination of, 12, 287–289
    pain in, 274, 276, 301t–302t
Bacterial pneumonia, 156t
Bacterial vaginosis, 255t
"Baker's" (popliteal) cyst, 293, 310t
Balance, 313, 421
Balanitis, 232
Balloon sign, 294
Ballottement
    abdominal, 207
    patellar, 295
Barlow test, 365
Barrel chest, 159t
Bartholin's glands, 247, 398
Basal cell carcinoma, 105t, 415
Basal ganglia, 311, 340t
Behavior. *See also* Mental status
    of clinician, 38
    in delirium and dementia, 424t
    of patient, 46–47, 81
Bell's palsy, 339t
Beneficence, 54
Benign prostatic hyperplasia, 260, 264, 267t, 268t, 420
Biases, 52–53

Biceps reflexes, 328
Bicipital tendonitis, 281, 307t
Biliary obstruction, 198b
Bimanual examination, 15, 249
    in older adults, 419–420
    in pregnancy, 399–400
Biot's (ataxic) breathing, 74t
Birth control, 245
Birth history, 350
Birth weight, 353, 354b
Bladder disorders, 198–199, 211t–212t, 274
Bleeding
    gastrointestinal, 260
    nose, 114, 395
    postmenopausal, 243
    rectal, 260
    subarachnoid, 112, 127t, 313
    vaginal, 373
    vitreous, 112
Blindness, 129t
Bloating, abdominal, 195
Blood
    in stool, 260
    in urine, 198
Blood pressure. *See also* Hypertension; Hypotension, orthostatic
    adult classifications of, 63b, 164
    in children and adolescents, 357, 368, 380t
    cuffs for measuring, 61b, 368
    and diet, 73t
    health promotion for, 164
    measuring, 61–64, 168
    in older adults, 413–414
    in pregnancy, 394, 395b, 400
Body mass index (BMI)
    calculating, 59–61
    of children, 368
    excessively low, 70t
    of older adults, 414
    of pregnant women, 395
Body odors, 58
Body position
    observation of, 321
    for physical exam, 9b, 11, 394b, 396
Bone density, 277
Bottle-feeding, 350
Bouchard's nodes, 284

Bowel habits, 196, 260
Bowel sounds, 201*b*–202*b*
Bowlegs, 355
Brachial pulse, 219
Brachioradialis reflex, 329
Bradycardia, 358
Brain, 311–312
  abscess of, 112
  tumors of, 112, 127*t*–128*t*, 357
Brainstem, 311
Branchial cleft cyst, 361
Breast, 181–192
  cancer of, 182–183, 189*t*–192*t*,
    408–409
  in children and adolescents, 364,
    375, 383*t*
  common or concerning symptoms
    of, 181*b*
  discharge from, 186
  examination of, 12–13, 183–188
  health history of, 6, 181
  health promotion and counseling
    for, 181–183
  masses in, 181, 182*b*
  in older adults, 418
  in pregnancy, 396
  recording exam findings of, 189*b*,
    377*b*
  self-exam of, 183, 187*b*–188*b*
Breast-feeding, 350
Breath odor, 58
Breath sounds, 146, 147*b*
  in chest disorders, 161*t*
  in newborns, 362*b*, 363*b*
Breathing. *See also* Respiratory system
  abnormalities of, 74*t*
  in comatose patient, 332, 333
  in newborns, 358, 361, 362*b*
  in pregnancy, 396
  rate and rhythm of, 64–65, 143
  shortness of breath, 142,
    154*t*–155*t*, 163
Breech presentation, 400
Bronchi, 141
Bronchial breath sounds, 147*b*
Bronchiectasis, 157*t*
Bronchiolitis, 358, 362*b*
Bronchitis, 154*t*, 157*t*, 161*t*
Bronchophony, 148*b*

Bronchovesicular breath sounds, 147*b*
Brudzinski's sign, 331
Bruits
  abdominal, 201*b*–202*b*, 418, 420
  carotid, 169, 417
Bulge sign, 293
Bulimia, 60, 70*t*
Bullae, 99*t*
Burrows (scabies), 100*t*
Bursae, 271
Bursitis, 275
  in hips, 289–290
  in knees, 292, 293, 308*t*
  in shoulders, 307*t*

C

Café-au-lait spots, 358
CAGE questions, 50*b*, 199
Calcium, sources of, 72*t*
Calculating abilities, 84
Cancer
  breast, 182–183, 189*t*–192*t*
  cervical, 244, 254*t*, 409
  colorectal, 200, 209*t*, 261–262,
    420
  lung, 155*t*, 158*t*
  neck, 361
  oral, 136*t*, 138*t*, 417
  ovarian, 420
  penis, 232, 236*t*
  prostate, 260–261, 269*t*, 420
  rectal, 269*t*
  screening for, in older adults,
    408–409
  skin, 104*t*–105*t*, 106*t*, 415
  testicular, 238*t*
  vulvar, 252*t*
Candidiasis
  in infants, 361
  of tongue, 137*t*
  vaginitis, 255*t*
Canker sores, 138*t*
Capacity, altered, 46–47
Carcinoma. *See also* Cancer
  basal cell, 105*t*, 415
  of cervix, 254*t*
  of lip, 136*t*
  squamous cell, 104*t*, 105*t*, 415

of tongue or floor of mouth, 138*t*
of vulva, 252*t*
Cardiac syncope, 314
Cardiomyopathy, 170, 174, 175
Cardiovascular system, 163–180
    chest pain caused by disorders of,
        152*t*–153*t*
    common or concerning symptoms
        of, 57, 163*b*
    cough caused by disorders of,
        158*t*–159*t*
    disorders of, 176*t*–180*t*
    examination of, 13, 64, 168–175
    health history in, 6, 163–164
    health promotion and counseling
        for, 164–167
    in older adults, 417–418
    in pregnancy, 396
    recording exam findings, 175*b*,
        376*b*–377*b*
Carotid pulse, 169
Carotid stenosis, 417
Carpal tunnel syndrome, 283, 286,
        322
Cartilaginous joints, 272*b*
Caruncles, 247, 419
Cataracts, 113, 115, 416
Cauda equina, 274, 312
Caviar lesions, 138*t*
Cellulitis, 216
Central nervous system, 311–312,
        339*t*, 340*t*
Cephalohematoma, 359
Cerebellum, 14, 312, 340*t*
Cerebrovascular disease, 315
Cerumen, 416
Cervix
    abnormalities of, 254*t*
    cancer of, 244, 254*t*, 409
    examination of, 15, 247–249
    inflammation of (cervicitis), 254*t*
    in pregnancy, 399
    shapes of, 253*t*
Chalazion, 131*t*
Chancre
    lip, 136*t*
    penile, 232, 237*t*
    vulvar, 252*t*
Chart, medical. *See* Records, patient

Cheilitis, angular, 136*t*
Chemicals, irritating, 159*t*
Cherry angioma, 103*t*, 415
Chest pain, 141–142, 152*t*–153*t*,
        163–164. *See also* Thorax
Cheyne-Stokes breathing, 74*t*
Chief complaints, 2*b*, 3, 349
Children, 349–388
    development of, 349
    examining, 352–375 (*See also* spe-
        cific system or structure)
    head circumference in, 357
    health history of, 2*b*, 4, 349–351
    health promotion and counseling
        for, 351
    heart murmurs in, 371–372,
        381*t*–382*t*
    hypertension in, 357*b*, 368, 380*t*
    interviewing, 366*b*–367*b*
    newborn maturity level classifica-
        tion, 378*t*
    preventive care recommendations
        for, 379*t*
    recording exam findings for,
        375–377
    sex maturity ratings for, 383*t*–387*t*
    sexual abuse in, 388*t*
Chills, 198
Chloasma, 395
Choanal atresia, 361
Cholecystitis, 208
Cholesterol, 166
Chondromalacia, 292
Chorea, 341*t*
Chronic obstructive pulmonary dis-
        ease, 154*t*, 161*t*, 163, 417
Cirrhosis, 197*b*
"Clasp-knife" resistance, 343*t*
Claudication, 215, 224*t*
Clavicle fracture, 365
Clinical breast examination, 182
Clinical reasoning, 17–19. *See also*
        Assessments
Clinician
    behavior and appearance of, 38
    relationship with patient, sexuality
        in, 53
    self-awareness of, 52–53
Clitoris, 247

Clonus, 330
Clubbing, nail, 108t
Cluster headaches, 125t
Coarctation of the aorta, 363
Cognitive function
   assessment of, 83–84
   higher, 79b, 84
   in older adults, 404–405, 409
Cogwheel rigidity, 343t
Cold sore, 136t
Colitis, 210t
Colles' fracture, 283
Colonoscopy, 262, 409
Colorectal cancer
   and diarrhea, 209t
   in older adults, 420
   screening for, 200, 260, 261–262,
      409, 420
Coma, 332–334, 346t, 347t
Comedones, 415
Communication, with patient, 44,
   53
Complaints, chief, 2b, 3, 349
Comprehensive health history. See
   Health history
Comprehensive physical examination.
   See Physical examination
Concentration, difficulty with, 80
Conception age, 390
Conductive hearing loss, 113, 135t,
   319
Condylar joints, 273b
Confidentiality, patient, 39, 46–47, 54
Confusing patient, 46
Congestion, nasal, 114
Congestive heart failure, 170, 364
Conjunctiva, 117
Consciousness, level of
   assessing, 57, 78, 81
   defined, 78b, 333b
   in delirium or dementia, 424t
   loss of, 314
Consolidation (lung), 161t
Constipation, 196, 197, 260
Constructional ability, 84
Continuers, 40, 44
Contraception, 245
Convergence, eye, 117
Coordination, 323–325, 340t

Cornea, 117
Corneal light reflex test, 368
Corneal reflexes, 319
Coronary heart disease, 165–167
Costovertebral angle tenderness, 205
Cough, 142, 156t–159t
Counseling. See Health promotion
   and counseling
Cover-uncover eye test, 368
Crackles, 147b
Cranial nerves, 312
   assessment of, 14, 318–320
   function of, 316b–317b
Cranial neuralgias, 128t
Crohn's disease, 210t
Croup, 362b
Crust (skin), 101t
Crying patient, 47
Cryptorchidism, 233, 238t
Cultural differences, 52–53, 405
Cup-to-disc ratio, 416
Cutis marmorata, 358
Cyanosis, 363
Cyanotic congenital heart disease,
   358
Cyclothymic episode, 89t
Cystocele, 247, 256t, 398
Cystourethrocele, 247, 256t
Cysts
   "Baker's," 293, 310t
   branchial cleft, 361
   breast, 182b
   congenital, 361
   epidermoid, 251t
   epididymal, 239t
   periauricular, 361
   pilar, 116
   pilonidal, 263
   popliteal, 293
   skin, 98t
   thyroglossal, 361

D

Data
   identifying, 2b, 349
   organizing, 28–30
   subjective and objective, 2b
Deaf patient, 48

Death and dying, 51–52
Decision-making
  evidence-based, 18*b*
  patient's capacity for, 46–47, 80
Deep tendon reflexes, 328, 340t
Defecation, pain with, 260
Degenerative joint disease, 305t–306t, 308t
Dehydration, 358
Delirium, 46, 424t–425t
Delusional disorder, 92t
Dementia, 46, 409, 424t–426t
Dental caries, 115, 371, 417
Depression
  in older adults, 411*b*, 423*b*
  screening for, 57, 79–80, 411*b*
  symptoms of, 88*t*–89*t*
DeQuervain's tenosynovitis, 322
Dermatomes, 325, 344t–345t
Development of children, 350, 356
Diabetes, 199
Diabetic retinopathy, 133t
Diagnoses, establishing, 17*b*–19*b*
DIAPERS assessment, 410
Diaphragm, 146
Diarrhea, 196, 209t–210t, 260
Diastolic blood pressure, 63*b*, 414
Diet
  changes in, for hypertension, 73t
  in health history, 5, 350
  health promotion and counseling for, 56–57
  in older adults, 406
Diethylstilbestrol (DES), fetal exposure to, 254t
Diffuse esophageal spasm, 153t
Diffuse idiopathic skeletal hyperostosis, 302t
Diffuse interstitial lung diseases, 155t
Digit span, 83
Digital rectal examination, 261. *See also* Rectum
Diphtheria, 139t
Diplegias, spastic, 366
Diplopia, 113, 313
Disability, physical, 411*b*–412*b*, 423*b*

Disc, herniated, 301t
Discharge
  breast, 186
  penile, 231
  vaginal, 243, 255t, 373
Disease, defined, 42
Disease/illness model, 42
Disruptive patient, 47
Dissecting aortic aneurysm, 152t, 163
Distress, signs of, 57
Diverticulitis, 196
Dizziness, 313
Do Not Resuscitate (DNR) orders, 52, 407
Doll's eye movement, 334
Domestic violence, 51, 392–393
Dorsalis pedis pulse, 220
Double vision, 113, 313
Draping patient, 10
Drawer sign, anterior, 294, 309t
Dress, patient's, 58, 81
"Drop-arm" test, 281, 307t
Drugs
  abuse of, 4, 50–51, 80
  diarrhea due to, 209t
  incontinence due to, 212t
  medication history, 2*b*, 4
  use in older adults, 406
Drusen, 120*b*, 416
Dullness to percussion, 145*b*
Durable power of attorney for health care, 47, 407
Dying patient, 51–52
Dysarthria, 82, 313
Dysesthesias, 314
Dyskinesias, oral-facial, 342t
Dyslipidemias, 166
Dysmenorrhea, 242
Dyspareunia, 243
Dyspepsia, 195
Dysphagia, 196
Dysphonia, 82
Dyspnea, 142, 154t–155t, 163
Dysrhythmias, 64, 176t–180t, 364. *See also specific dysrhythmias*
Dysthymic disorder, 89t
Dystonia, 342t
Dysuria, 198

E

Ear canal, 121, 369
Eardrum, 121, 134*t*, 369–370
Ears. *See also* Hearing; Hearing loss
  in children, 360, 369–370
  disorders of, 135*t*
  examination of, 12, 120–122
  health history of, 6, 113–114
  in older adults, 416
  pain in (earache), 113
  recording exam findings, 124*b*, 376*b*
Eating disorders, 60, 70*t*
Ecchymosis, 104*t*
Echoing, 44
Ectopic pregnancy, 196, 400
Ectropion, 130*t*, 416
Edema, 164
  of breast skin, 192*t*
  dependent, 164
  pitting, 220
  in pregnancy, 395, 400
  scrotal, 236*t*
Effusion
  around knee, 293–294, 295
  behind eardrum, 134*t*
  pleural, 146, 161*t*
Egophony, 148*b*
Ejaculation, 230
Elbows, 282, 322
Elderly patients. *See* Older adults
Embolism, pulmonary, 155*t*, 158*t*
Emotional cues, of patient, 40
Empathy, for patient, 44
"Empty can test," 280
Endocervical polyp, 254*t*
Endocrine disorders, 7, 356
Endometrial hyperplasia, 419
Endometriosis, 242
Engagement (fetal), 401
Entropion, 130*t*, 416
Environment for examination, 10, 38,
      39, 404
Epidermoid cysts, 251*t*
Epididymis, 233, 239*t*, 420
Epiglottitis, 362*b*
Episcleritis, 130*t*
Episiotomy, 398
Epistaxis, 114

Epitrochlear nodes, 12, 219
Epstein's pearls, 361
Erectile dysfunction, 230
Erosion, skin, 102*t*
Esophagus, 142, 153*t*
Estrogen-producing tumors, 419
Ethics, 53–54
Ethnicity, 52
Evidence-based decision making, 18*b*
Excoriation, skin, 102*t*
Exercise
  health promotion and counseling
      for, 57, 276
  history of, 5
  in older adults, 408
  during pregnancy, 392
Expected date of delivery (EDD),
      390–391
Expiratory time, forced, 150
Expressions, facial, 58, 81
Extinction sensation, 327
Extra-articular structures, 271, 275
Extraocular muscles, 117, 318
Extremities, 14, 400. *See also specific
      structures*
Eyebrows, 116
Eyelids
  disorders of, 130*t*
  inspection of, 116
  in older adults, 415–416
Eyes. *See also* Vision
  in children, 360, 368–369
  disorders of, 115, 126*t*, 129*t*–133*t*
  examination of, 12, 116–120
  and headaches, 112, 126*t*
  health history of, 6, 112–113
  health promotion and counseling
      for, 115
  in older adults, 415–416
  during pregnancy, 395
  recording exam findings, 124*b*, 376*b*

F

Face
  edema of, 395
  examination of, 116
  expressions of, 58, 81

of infants, 359
  paralysis of, 116, 339*t*
  during pregnancy, 395
Facial nerve, 317*b*, 319
Failure to thrive, 356
Fainting, 314
Fallot, tetralogy of, 381*t*–382*t*
Falls, in older adults, 276, 412, 413*f*
False positive or negative results,
  30*b*, 31*b*
Family history, 3*b*, 5, 51, 390
Family planning, 245
Farsightedness (hyperopia), 112, 126*t*
Fasciculations, 341*t*
Fatigue, 55
Fecal occult blood test, 261–262
Feeding history, 350
Feet
  coldness, numbness or pallor in,
    216
  deformities of, 366
  examination of, 297–298
  swelling of, 216
  ulcers on, 225*t*
Females
  axillae in, 12, 186
  breast examination in, 12–13,
    183–185, 187*b*–188*b*
  epitrochlear nodes in, 12
  genital exams in, 7, 15, 241–257
    in children, 365, 373, 375
    in older adults, 419–420
    in pregnancy, 398–400
    recording results of, 250*b*, 377*b*
  Pap smears in, 244, 247–248,
    394, 399, 409, 419
  rectal exams in, 15, 250, 264
  sexual maturity of, 246, 383*t*,
    386*t*–387*t*
Femoral hernia, 234, 240*t*, 250
Femoral pulse, 220
Fetus
  engagement of, 401
  exposure to DES, 254*t*
  heart of, 397–398
  lie of, 400
  movement of, 397
  presentation of, 400–401
Fever, 56, 65–66, 198

Fever blister, 136*t*
Fibroadenoma of breast, 182*b*
Fibrocystic breast disease, 182*b*
Fibromyalgia, 275
Fibrous joints, 272*b*
Fingernails, 95, 108*t*–109*t*
Fingers, 216, 284–286, 322, 365
Fissures
  skin, 102*t*
  tongue, 137*t*
Flaccidity, 334, 343*t*
Flail chest, 160*t*
Flank pain, 198
Flatness to percussion, 145*b*
Folate, sources of, 72*t*
Fontanelles, 358–359
Forced expiratory time, 150
Foreign bodies
  in airway, 362*b*
  in vagina, 373
Fovea, 120*b*
Fractures
  of clavicle, 365
  Colles', 283
  scaphoid, 284
Fremitus, tactile, 145
Friction rubs, 171, 201
Fullness, abdominal, 195
Functional ability, 410
Fundal height, 397
Fundi, eye, 118–119, 416
Funnel chest (pectus excavatum),
  160*t*

G

Gag reflex, 320
Gait
  inspection of, 58, 289, 291, 313,
    324
  in older adults, 420–421
Gallbladder, 142
Gases, irritating, 159*t*
Gastroesophageal reflux disease, 158*t*,
  195
Gastrointestinal system
  bleeding in, 260
  chest pain caused by disorders of,
    153*t*

Gastrointestinal system (*continued*)
  common or concerning symptoms of, 193*b*
  examination of, 201–203
  health history of, 6, 193–197
Gaze, six cardinal directions of, 117
Gegenhalten, 343*t*
General survey, 55–61
  examination techniques for, 11, 57–66
  health history in, 5, 55–56
  health promotion and counseling in, 56–57
  in infants, 356–357
  interpreting findings of, 70*t*–74*t*
  recording findings of, 69
Genital examinations
  in females, 7, 15, 241–257
    in children, 365, 373, 375, 386*t*–387*t*, 388*b*
    common concerns of, 241*b*
    health promotion and counseling for, 244–245
    interpreting results of, 251*t*–257*t*
    in older adults, 419–420
    in pregnancy, 398–400
    recording results of, 250*b*, 377*b*
    techniques for, 246–250
  in males, 6–7, 15, 229–240
    in children, 365, 372–373, 375, 384*t*–385*t*, 388*b*
    common or concerning symptoms, 229*b*
    health promotion and counseling for, 231–232
    interpreting results of, 236*t*–240*t*
    in older adults, 420
    recording results of, 235*b*, 377*b*
    techniques for, 232–235
Genital herpes, 232, 237*t*, 251*t*
Genital warts, 232, 237*t*, 251*t*
Genitalia, ambiguous, 365
Geographic tongue, 137*t*
Geriatric syndromes, 404. *See also* Older adults
Gestation, expected weeks of, 390–391
Gestational age, 353, 354*b*, 378*t*
Gestational hypertension, 395*b*, 400

Giant cell (temporal) arteritis, 128*t*
Gingivitis, 417
Glaucoma, 113, 115, 126*t*, 416
Glaucomatous cupping, 132*t*
Glossopharyngeal nerve, 317*b*, 320
Goals for interview, 38
Goiter, 115, 124, 140*t*
Gonococcal infections, 231, 283
Gout, 275, 421
Granulomatous colitis, 210*t*
Graves' disease, 140*t*
Gray matter, 311
Great arteries, transposition of, 363, 382*t*
Grip, 322
Grooming, patient, 58, 81
Growth of children, 350, 356
Guarding, 202
Gums, 122
Gynecologic history, 4

H

Hair
  in infants, 358
  inspection of, 95, 116
  loss of, 93*b*, 107*t*–108*t*, 216
  during pregnancy, 395
  pubic, 384*t*–385*t*, 386*t*–387*t*
Hairy leukoplakia, 137*t*
Hairy tongue, 137*t*
Hand-washing, 16
Hands, 283–287
  arterial supply to, 222
  flaccid, 334
  in pregnancy, 400
Hashimoto's thyroiditis, 140*t*
Head
  circumference of, 357
  common or concerning symptoms of, 111*b*
  examination of, 12, 116
  health history of, 6, 111–112
  of infants, 357, 358–359
  in pregnancy, 395–396
  recording exam findings, 124*b*, 376*b*
Headaches, 111–112, 125*t*–129*t*, 313
Health care proxy, 48, 52, 407

Health history. *See also* Interview
  of children, 349–351
  components of, 1, 2*b*–3*b*
  comprehensive, 1, 3–7, 37
  focused, 1, 10, 37
  format of, 37
  interviewing process, 38–54
  of older adults, 403–405
  in pregnancy, 389–391
  recording findings of, 33–36
Health Insurance Portability and
      Accountability Act (HIPAA),
      46–47
Health maintenance, 4, 18*b*
Health promotion and counseling
  for abdominal aortic aneurysm,
      217–218
  for alcohol and substance abuse,
      80, 199
  for back pain, 276
  for breast health, 181–183
  for cardiovascular disease,
      164–167
  for children, 351
  for colon cancer screening, 200,
      261–262
  for depression, 79–80
  for diet, 56*b*
  for domestic violence, 392–393
  for dyslipidemias, 166
  for exercise, 56*b*, 276, 392
  for fall prevention, 276
  for family planning, 245
  for hearing loss, 115*b*
  for hepatitis, 199–200
  for hypertension, 164
  for immunizations, 393
  for menopause, 245
  for nutrition, 56*b*, 276, 391
  for older adults, 408–409
  for oral health, 115*b*
  for osteoporosis, 277
  for Pap smear screening, 244–245
  for peripheral arterial disease, 217
  for pregnancy, 391–393
  for prostate cancer, 260–261
  for renal artery disease, 217
  for skin care, 93*b*
  for smoking, 142, 392
  for STDs or HIV, 231–232, 245
  for stroke prevention, 165,
      315–316
  for suicidality, 80
  for testicular self-examination, 232
  for transient ischemic attacks,
      315–316
  for vision, 115*b*
  for weight, 56*b*
Hearing
  health history of, 113–114
  in infants, 360
  in older adults, 408, 411*b*, 416,
      422*b*
  testing, 12, 121–122, 319–320
Hearing loss and deafness
  history of, 113
  interviewing patient with, 48
  in older adults, 115
  patterns of, 135*t*
Heart. *See also* Cardiovascular system
  in children, 363–364, 371–372
  coronary heart disease, 165–167,
      358
  examination of, 13, 169–175
  health history of, 6
  in older adults, 417–418
  in pregnancy, 396
Heart failure
  congestive, 170
  left ventricular, 154*t*, 158*t*, 161*t*,
      163
Heart murmurs
  causes of, 180*t*
  in children, 371–372, 381*t*–382*t*
  gradations of, 173*b*
  identifying, 171–173
  in older adults, 418
  in pregnancy, 396
Heart rate
  fetal, 397–398
  in infants, 358
  measuring, 64, 168
  in older adults, 414
Heart rhythm, 64, 364, 398
Heart sounds
  in infants, 364

Heart sounds (*continued*)
  interpreting, 171, 176*t*–180*t*
  in older adults, 417–418
Heartburn, 195
Heberden's nodes, 284
HEENT (Head, eyes, ears, nose
    throat)
  examining, 12, 116–124
  health history of, 6, 111–115
  health promotion and counseling
    for, 115
  interpreting findings for, 125*t*–140*t*
  in older adults, 415–417
  recording findings for, 124*b*, 376*b*
Hegar's sign, 399
Height, 58
  of children and adolescents, 356
  of older adults, 414
  of pregnant women, 395
Hematologic system, 7
Hematoma, subdural, 357
Hemianopsia, 113
Hemolytic disease, 358
Hemoptysis, 142, 156*t*–159*t*
Hemorrhage
  subarachnoid, 112, 127*t*, 313
  vitreous, 112
Hemorrhoids, 268*t*, 398
Hepatitis
  alcoholic, 193, 197*b*
  health promotion and counseling
    for, 199–200
  and liver disease, 197*b*
  symptoms of, 195
  types of, 197*b*, 199–200
Hereditary hemorrhagic telangiecta-
    sia, 136*t*
Hernias
  in children, 355, 365, 372
  in females, 250
  femoral, 234, 240*t*, 250
  inguinal, 234, 236*t*, 240*t*, 250,
    365, 372
  in males, 15, 233, 234, 236*t*, 240*t*,
    365
  scrotal, 236*t*
  umbilical, 355
Herniated disc, 301*t*
Herpes simplex infection

  genital, 232, 237*t*, 251*t*
  in infants, 358
  oral (cold sore), 136*t*
Herpes zoster, 325, 415
Hinge joints, 273*b*
Hips, 289–291
  dysplasia of, 365
  muscles of, 323
  in newborns, 365–366
History. *See* Health history
HIV (human immunodeficiency
    virus), 231–232, 243, 245
Hoarseness, 114
"Housemaid's knee," 292, 308*t*
HPV (human papillomavirus), 244
Humility, cultural, 52
Hydrocele, 233, 236*t*, 365
Hydrocephalus, 116, 357, 358
Hygiene, personal, 58, 81
Hymen, 247, 373
Hyperemesis, 395
Hyperopia (farsightedness), 112,
    126*t*, 368
Hyperpnea, 74*t*
Hyperpyrexia, 65
Hyperresonance, 145*b*
Hypertension
  in children and adolescents, 357*b*,
    368, 380*t*
  chronic, 395*b*
  classification of, 63*b*, 164
  dietary changes for, 74*t*
  gestational, 395*b*, 400
  in older adults, 413–414
  pulmonary, 364
  screening for, 164
Hyperthyroidism, 115, 116
Hypertonia, 343*t*
Hypertrophic cardiomyopathy, 174,
    175
Hyperventilation, 74*t*
Hypoglossal nerve, 317*b*, 320
Hypomanic episode, 89*t*
Hypoplastic left heart syndrome, 363
Hypospadias, 232, 236*t*
Hypotension, orthostatic, 63*b*, 168,
    414
Hypothalamus, 311
Hypothermia, 65, 66

Hypotheses, generating and testing, 18*b*, 41–42
Hypothyroidism, 115
Hypotonia, 343*t*, 366
Hysterectomy, 244

I

Icterus (jaundice), 197, 358
Identifying data, 2*b*, 349
Iliopectineal bursa, 289
Iliotibial band bursitis, 308*t*
Illnesses. *See also specific illnesses*
  defined, 42
  history of, 2*b*, 4
  patient perspective on, 40*b*, 42*b*
  present, 2*b*, 3–4, 350
Immunizations, 4, 350, 393, 408
Impotence, 230
Incontinence, urinary
  in older adults, 410, 411*b*, 422*b*
  types of, 199, 211*t*–212*t*
Infants. *See also* Children
  examining, 352–366
  head circumference of, 357
  hypertension in, 357*b*, 368, 380*t*
  maturity classification of, 378*t*
Infections. *See also specific infections*
  and diarrhea, 209*t*, 210*t*
  sexually transmitted, 231–232, 243, 245, 373
Inflammation, 202, 275. *See also* Arthritis
Inflammatory bowel disease, 210*t*
Information assessment, 84
Inguinal hernia
  in children, 365, 372
  direct, 234, 240*t*
  indirect, 234, 236*t*, 240*t*, 250
Inguinal ligament, 289
Insight, patient, 77, 78*b*, 83
Intelligence, limited, 49
Intercourse, pain during, 243
Intermittent claudication, 215, 224*t*
Interpreters, 47, 48*b*
Interstitial lung diseases, diffuse, 155*t*
Interview, 37–54. *See also* Health history
  approach to, 38, 403–405

for children, 366*b*–367*b*
  comprehensive *vs.* focused, 1*b*, 37
  dealing with sensitive topics, 49–54
  sequence of, 39–43
  for specific situations, 46–49
  techniques for, 43–45
Intracranial pressure, 358
Introitus, 247
Involuntary movements, 321, 340*t*, 341*t*–342*t*
Iris, 117
Iron, sources of, 72*t*
Irritable bowel syndrome, 209*t*
Ischiogluteal bursa, 290
Isolated systolic hypertension, 64
Itching
  in eyes, nose, throat, 114
  vaginal, 243

J

Jaundice, 197, 358
Joints. *See also specific joints*
  assessing, 271–273
  common or concerning symptoms of, 273*b*
  examination of, 278–310
  health promotion and counseling for, 276–277
  pain in and around, 273–276, 305*t*–306*t*
Judgment, patient, 77, 78*b*, 83, 425*t*
Jugular veins, 168
Jugular venous pressure, 168, 417

K

Kaposi's sarcoma, 105*t*
Keloids, 101*t*
Keratoses, 104*t*–105*t*, 415
Kernig's sign, 331
Kidneys, 14, 198, 205
Klinefelter's syndrome, 238*t*
Knees
  examination of, 291–296
  extension and flexion of, 323
  painful, tender, 308*t*–310*t*
  reflexes, 329, 400
Koplik's spots, 139*t*

Korotkoff sounds, 62b, 174
Kubler-Ross stages of dying, 51
Kussmaul breathing, 74t
Kyphoscoliosis, thoracic, 160t

L

Labia, 246
Lachman test, 295
Lacrimal apparatus, 116
Lactating adenomas, 182b
Lactose intolerance, 210t
Language, 41, 79b, 82
Language barriers, 47, 48b
Laryngitis, 156t
Laryngotracheobronchitis (croup), 362b
Lateral collateral ligament (LCL), 292, 294
Lateralization test, 122, 319
Laxatives, abuse of, 210t
LDL (low-density lipoproteins), 166
Lead-pipe rigidity, 343t
Learning ability, 83
Left ventricular heart failure, 154t, 158t, 161t, 163
Left ventricular hypertrophy, 417
Legs
    coldness, numbness or pallor in, 216
    examination of, 14, 219–221
    flaccid, 334
    hair loss on, 216
    measuring length of, 299
    mobility in older adults, 411b, 422b
    pain in, 215
    in pregnancy, 400
    ulcers on, 216
    and vascular disease, 215–216, 224t–225t
Lens, eye, 117, 416
Leopold's maneuvers, 398, 400–402
Lesions
    oral, 136t–139t
    skin, 57, 94, 97t–104t
Lethargy, 333b
Leukonychia, 109t
Leukoplakia, hairy, 137t

Libido, 230
Lichenification, 101t
Lifestyle habits, 5, 167
Ligaments, 271
    knee, 294–295, 296, 309t–310t
Light reflex, 120b
Lighting for examination, 10
Lipid therapy, 166
Lips, 122, 136t
Listening, active, 43
Literacy, low, 48
Liver
    in children, 372
    disease of, 197–198
    examination of, 14, 203–204
    toxic damage to, 198b
"Liver spots," 415
LMP (last menstrual period), 390–391
Low-density lipoproteins (LDL), 166
Lumbar spinal stenosis, 301t
Lung sounds. *See* Breath sounds
Lungs
    abscess of, 157t
    assessing function of, 150
    cancer of, 155t, 158t
    common or concerning symptoms of, 141b
    disorders of, 154t–159t, 161t
    and dyspnea, 154t–155t
    examination of, 12, 13, 143–150
    health history of, 141–142
    health promotion and counseling for, 142
    of newborns, 361–363
    in older adults, 417
    in pregnant women, 396
    recording exam findings of, 151b, 376b
Lymph nodes
    axillary, 12, 186
    cervical, 12
    in children, 361, 376b
    epitrochlear, 12, 219
    examination of, 123, 124b
    inguinal, 221
Lymphadenopathy, 361

M

Macula, 119, 120*b*
Macular degeneration, 113, 115, 120*b*, 416
Macules, 97*t*
Malabsorption syndromes, 210*t*
Males
  axillae in, 12, 186
  breast exam in, 13, 186
  epitrochlear nodes in, 12
  genital exams in, 6–7, 15, 229–240
    in children, 365, 372–373, 375, 384*t*–385*t*, 388*b*
    common or concerning symptoms of, 229*b*
    health promotion and counseling for, 231–232
    interpreting results of, 236*t*–240*t*
    in older adults, 420
    recording results of, 235*b*, 377*b*
    techniques for, 232–235
  rectal exam in, 15, 262–264
  sexual maturity in, 384*t*–385*t*
Malocclusion, 371
Malodor, 417
Mammography, 182–183, 408–409
Manic episodes, 88*t*–89*t*
Manner, patient, 81
Masseter muscles, 278, 319
Mastitis, 182*b*
Mastoiditis, 121
McMurray test, 296
Medial collateral ligament (MCL), 292, 296, 310*t*
Median nerve compression (carpal tunnel syndrome), 283, 286, 322
Medical chart. *See* Records, patient
Medications. *See* Drugs
Melanoma, 93, 106*t*, 415
Melena, 197
Memory, 78*b*
  assessing, 77, 78, 83
  in delirium and dementia, 425*t*
  in older adults, 409, 411*b*, 423*b*
Ménière's disease, 114

Meningeal signs, 331
Meningitis, 112, 127*t*, 358
Menisci of knee, 292, 296, 309*t*
Menopause, 243, 245
Menstrual cycle, 242, 390
Mental status, 75–92
  of children, 355–356, 367, 377*b*
  common or concerning symptoms of, 77*b*
  in delirium and dementia, 424*t*–425*t*
  disorders of, 46–47, 75*b*–76*b*, 87*t*–92*t*
  examination of, 14, 77*b*, 78*b*–79*b*, 81–85
  health history of, 4, 7, 50, 77–79
  health promotion and counseling for, 79–80
  recording findings of, 86*b*, 377*b*
Microcephaly, 357, 358
Migraine headaches, 111, 112, 125*t*
Mini-Cog test, 426*t*
Mini-Mental State Examination, 85
Mitgehen, 343*t*
Mitral valve
  prolapse of, 174, 175
  regurgitation of, 171, 418
  stenosis of, 154*t*, 158*t*, 163, 171
Mixed mood disorder, 89*t*
Moles, 93, 106*t*
Mongolian spots, 358
Monoarticular joint pain, 274
Mood. *See also* Depression
  assessing, 77, 78, 82
  defined, 79*b*
  in delirium and dementia, 424*t*
  disorders of, 88*t*–89*t*
Motor system (motor activity)
  disorders of, 340*t*
  examination of, 14, 58, 321–325
  and mental status, 81
Mouth
  abnormalities of, 136*t*–139*t*
  cancers of, 138*t*, 409, 417
  candidiasis in, 137*t*, 361
  in children, 361, 370–371
  examination of, 12, 122–123
  health history of, 6, 114–115

Mouth (*continued*)
  health promotion and counseling
    for, 115
  in older adults, 417
  in pregnant women, 395
  recording exam findings of, 124*b*,
    376*b*
Movements
  coordinating, 323–324
  involuntary, 321, 340*t*, 341*t*–342*t*
MRSA precautions, 15–16
Multiple sclerosis, 322
Murmurs. *See* Heart murmurs
Murphy's sign, 208
Muscles
  bulk of, 321, 340*t*
  disorders of, 343*t*
  strength or weakness of, 55,
    321–323, 340*t*
  tone of, 321, 340*t*, 343*t*
Musculoskeletal system, 271–310.
    See also specific structures
  abnormalities of, 301*t*–310*t*
  assessing joints, 271–273
  in children, 365–366, 373
  common or concerning symptoms
    of, 273*b*
  examination of, 278–310
  health history of, 7, 273–276
  health promotion counseling for,
    276–277
  in older adults, 420–421
  range of motion in, 13, 275, 299
  recording exam findings, 300*b*, 377*b*
Myalgia, 275
Myasthenia gravis, 314, 322
Mycoplasma infections, 156*t*
Myelopathy, cervical, 304*t*
Myocardial infarction, 152*t*, 163, 194
Myocardium, 141, 364
Myoma, uterine, 257*t*
Myopathy, 314, 322
Myopia, 113, 368
Myxedema, 116

N

Naegele's rule, 390
Nails, 95, 108*t*–109*t*

Nasal congestion, 114
Nausea, 112, 195
Near reaction, 117
Near-sightedness, 113
Neck
  and chest pain, 142
  common or concerning symptoms
    of, 111*b*
  examination of, 12, 123–124
  health history of, 6, 114–115
  of infants, 361
  pain in, 274, 303*t*–304*t*
  range of motion in, 289
  recording exam findings of, 124*b*,
    376*b*
Negative predictive value, 31*b*–32*b*
Negatives, true and false, 30*b*, 31*b*
Neoplasms. *See* Cancer; Tumors
Nerves
  cranial, 14, 312, 316*b*–317*b*,
    318–320
  peripheral, 312
  root compression of, 325
  spinal, 312
Nervous system, 311–347
  in children, 355, 366, 374
  common or concerning symptoms
    of, 313–315
  components of, 311–312
  disorders of, 336*t*–347*t*
  examination of, 14, 316–334
  health history of, 7
  health promotion and counseling
    for, 315–316
  in older adults, 421
  recording exam findings, 335*b*, 377*b*
Neuralgias, cranial, 128*t*
Neuropathic ulcer, 225*t*
Neuropathy, peripheral, 316
Nevi, 93, 106*t*
Newborns. *See also* Children; Infants
  Apgar score of, 352–353
  assessing, 352–355
  birth weight of, 353, 354*b*, 378*t*
  gestational age of, 353, 354*b*, 378*t*
  head circumference of, 357
  height and weight of, 356
  hypertension in, 357*b*, 380*t*
  maturity classification of, 354*b*, 378*t*

vital signs in, 357–358
Night sweats, 56
Nipples
  discharge from, 186
  inspection of, 184, 185
  Paget's disease of, 192*t*
  in pregnancy, 396
  retraction and deviation of, 191*t*
Nocturia, 199
Nodules
  breast, 185
  in rheumatoid arthritis, 284
  skin, 98*t*
  thyroid, 140*t*
Nonarticular joint pain, 275
Nonmaleficence, 53
Nonverbal communication, 44
Nose
  bleeding from, 114, 395
  congestion in, 114
  examination of, 12, 122
  health history of, 6, 114
  in newborns, 361
  in pregnant women, 395
  recording exam results of, 124*b*,
    376*b*
Note-taking, 38
Nuchal rigidity, 361
Number identification, 327
Numbness, in legs or feet, 216
Nutrition
  health promotion and counseling
    for, 56–57, 72*t*–73*t*, 276
  and hypertension, 73*t*
  in older adults, 406, 411*b*,
    422*b*–423*b*
  during pregnancy, 391
  screening checklist for, 71*t*
  sources of nutrients, 72*t*
Nystagmus, 360

O

Obesity, 56–57
Objective data, 2*b*
Obsessive-compulsive disorder,
  90*t*–91*t*
Obstetric history, 4, 390
Obtundation, 333*b*

Obturator sign, 208
Occlusion, arterial, 420
Occult blood test, 261–262
Ocular fundus, 118–119
Ocular movements, 333
Oculocephalic reflex, 334
Oculomotor nerve, 316*b*, 318
Odors, body and breath, 58, 417
Odynophagia, 196
Older adults, 403–426
  adjusting environment for, 404
  common concerns of, 405–408
  content and pace of visit with, 404
  cultural differences in, 405
  delirium and dementia in, 409,
    424*t*–426*t*
  eliciting symptoms in, 404–405
  examining, 410–421
  falls in, 276, 412, 413*f*
  health history in, 403–405
  health promotion and counseling
    for, 408–409
  mistreatment of, 409
  osteoporosis in, 277
  recording exam findings of,
    422–423
Olfactory nerve, 316*b*, 318
Onycholysis, 109*t*
Open-angle glaucoma, 113, 416
Opening snap, 176*t*
Ophthalmoscope, 118*b*
Optic atrophy, 132*t*
Optic disc, 118, 119*b*–120*b*, 132*t*, 318
Optic nerve, 316*b*, 318
Oral cavity. *See* Mouth
Oral-facial dyskinesias, 342*t*
Oral temperature, 65–66
Orchitis, 238*t*
Orgasm, 230
Orientation to identity, place, and
    time, 78*b*
  assessing, 77, 83
  in delirium and dementia, 425*t*
  in older adults, 409
Orthopnea, 163
Orthostatic hypotension, 63*b*, 168,
    414
Ortolani test, 365
Osteoarthritis, 305*t*–306*t*, 420

Osteoporosis, 277
Otitis externa, 113, 120, 121, 370
Otitis media, 113, 121, 134*t*, 370
Otoscope, pneumatic, 370
Ovaries
  cancer of, 420
  examination of, 15, 249, 400
Overweight patients, 56–57
Ovulation, 245

P

Paget's disease of the nipple, 192*t*
Pain, 56, 57. *See also specific types of pain*
  acute and persistent, 67–69, 406, 407*b*
  response to, 325
Palliative care, 407–408
Palpitations, 163
Panic attack, 90*t*, 153*t*
Panic disorder, 90*t*
Pap smears
  in older adults, 244, 409, 419
  in pregnancy, 394, 399
  schedule of testing for, 244
  technique for, 247–248
Papilledema, 120*b*, 132*t*
Papillomavirus, human (HPV), 244
Papules, 97*t*
Paradoxical pulse, 174
Paralanguage, 44
Paralysis, 116, 313, 334
Paratonia, 343*t*
Paravertebral muscles, 288
Paresthesias, 314
Parietal pain, 194
Parkinsonism, 340*t*
Paronychia, 108*t*
Paroxysmal nocturnal dyspnea, 163
Paroxysmal supraventricular tachy-cardia, 358, 364
Partnering, with patient, 45, 53
Patches, skin, 97*t*
Patella, 292, 295
Patellofemoral disorder, 292, 309*t*
Pathologic processes, 17*b*
Pathophysiologic processes, 18*b*
Patient records. *See* Records, patient

Patients
  with altered capacity, 46–47
  angry or disruptive, 47
  approaching, 10, 403–405
  comfort of, 10, 39, 394*b*
  confidentiality of, 39, 46–47, 54
  confusing, 46
  crying, 47
  culture and ethnicity of, 52–53
  dying, 51–52
  emotional cues of, 40
  empowering, 45
  establishing rapport with, 39, 366*b*
  facilitating story of, 40, 41
  with impaired hearing, 48
  with impaired vision, 49
  interviewing, 37–54
  with language barriers, 47, 48*b*
  with limited intelligence, 49
  with low literacy, 48
  partnerships with, 45, 53
  with personal problems, 49
  perspective on illness, 40*b*, 42*b*
  position of, 9*b*, 11, 394*b*, 396
  sexual relationship with clinician, 53
  silent, 46
  talkative, 47
Peau d'orange sign, 192*t*
Pectoriloquy, whispered, 148*b*
Pectus carinatum (pigeon chest), 160*t*
Pectus excavatum (funnel chest), 160*t*
Pediatric patients. *See* Children
Pelvic examination, 246–250
  in older adults, 419–420
  in pregnancy, 399–400
Pelvic floor relaxations, 256*t*
Pelvic inflammatory disease, 196, 242, 249
Pelvis, back pain referred from, 302*t*
Penis
  abnormalities of, 231, 236*t*
  cancer of, 232, 236*t*
  in children and adolescents, 384*t*–385*t*
  discharge from, 231
  examination of, 15, 232
  in older adults, 420
Perceptions, patient's, 77, 78*b*, 83, 425*t*

Percussion, chest, 145–146, 149–150, 161*t*

Periauricular cysts and sinuses, 361

Pericardial friction rubs, 171

Pericarditis, 141, 152*t*

Perineal irritation, 373

Peripheral arterial disease, 215–216, 217

Peripheral nervous system, 311, 312. *See also* Nervous system
  disorders of, 340*t*
  lesion of, 339*t*

Peripheral neuropathy, 316

Peripheral vascular system, 215–227
  abnormalities of, 224*t*–225*t*
  common or concerning symptoms of, 215*b*
  examination of, 13, 218–223, 226*t*–227*t*
  health history of, 7, 215–216
  health promotion or counseling for, 216–218
  in older adults, 420
  recording exam results of, 223*b*

Peritoneal inflammation or tenderness, 202, 213*t*

Peritonsillar abscess, 371

Personal history, 3*b*, 5

Personal problems, patient with, 49

Pes anserine bursitis, 293, 308*t*

Petechia, 103*t*

Peutz-Jeghers syndrome, 136*t*

Peyronie's disease, 236*t*

Phalen's sign, 287

Pharynx
  abnormalities of, 139*t*
  in children, 361, 370–371
  examination of, 12, 123
  health history of, 6
  sore (pharyngitis), 114, 139*t*

Phimosis, 232

Phobias, 90*t*

Physical abuse, 51, 392–393

Physical examination, 8–16. *See also specific system or structure*
  approach to, 10, 403–405
  in children, 352–375
  comprehensive *vs.* focused, 1, 10
  health history in, 1*b*, 2*b*–3*b*, 3–7

interpreting findings of, 70*t*–74*t*

lighting and environment for, 10, 38, 39, 404

in older adults, 413–421, 423*b*

patient comfort in, 10, 394*b*

positions for, 9*b*, 11, 394*b*, 396

preparing for, 8

recording findings of, 33–36, 69

sequence for, 9*b*, 11, 352

Pigeon chest (pectus carinatum), 160*t*

Pigmentation, skin, 358

Pilar cysts, 116

Pilonidal cyst, 263

Pinguecula, 130*t*

Plan, developing, 19*b*, 42

Plantar reflexes, 330, 340*t*

Plaques, skin, 97*t*–98*t*

Pleura
  inflammation of (pleurisy), 194, 213*t*
  pain in, 141, 153*t*

Pleural effusion, 146, 161*t*

Pneumonia, 155*t*, 156*t*, 358, 362*b*

Pneumothorax, 155*t*, 161*t*

Point localization, 327

Point of maximal impulse (PMI)
  in children, 363–364
  measuring, 64, 168, 170
  in older adults, 417
  in pregnancy, 396

Polyarticular joint pain, 274–275

Polydactyly, 365

Polymyalgia rheumatica, 275, 276

Polyneuropathy, 314, 322

Polyps
  endocervical, 254*t*
  rectal, 268*t*

Polyuria, 199

Popliteal ("Baker's") cyst, 293, 310*t*

Popliteal pulse, 220

Position, patient's, 9*b*, 11, 394*b*, 396

Position sense, 326

Positive predictive value, 31*b*

Positives, true and false, 30*b*, 31*b*

Posterior cruciate ligament (PCL), 296

Posterior tibial pulse, 221

Postictal state, 315

Postnasal drip, 157*t*

Posttraumatic stress disorder, 91*t*

Postural hypotension, 63*b,* 168
Posture, 58, 81, 333
Precautions, standard and universal,
15–16
Precision, 30*b*
Precocious puberty, 372
Predictive value, 31*b*–32*b*
Preeclampsia, 395*b*
Pregnancy, 389–402
common concerns of, 389–391
ectopic, 196, 400
examination in, 394–402
health promotion and counseling
in, 391–393
planning or preventing, 245
recording exam findings in, 402*b*
symptoms of, 242, 389
Prehypertension, 63*b,* 164, 414
Premature ejaculation, 230
Prenatal care. *See* Pregnancy
Prepatellar bursitis, 292, 308*t*
Presbyopia, 112–113, 416
Present illness, 2*b,* 3–4, 350
Presentation, fetal, 401
Pressure sores, 415
Preventive care, pediatric, 379*t*
Primum non nocere (first, do no
harm), 53
Privacy, 10, 38
Problem identification, 17*b*–19*b,* 36
Pronator drift, 324
Prostate gland
benign hyperplasia of, 260, 264,
267*t,* 268*t,* 420
cancer of, 260–261, 269*t,* 420
examination of, 263–264
inflammation of (prostatitis), 198,
264, 269*t*
Prostate-specific antigen (PSA) test,
261
Prostatitis, 198, 269*t*
Proteinuria, 395*b*
Pseudoclaudication, 301*t*
Pseudoscars, 415
Psoas sign, 207–208
Psoriasis, 116
Psychiatric disorders. *See* Mental
status
Psychopathologic processes, 18*b*

Psychotic disorders, 92*t*
Pterygoid muscles, 278
Ptosis, 130*t,* 415–416
Puberty, 246, 372
Pubic hair, 246, 384*t*–385*t,*
386*t*–387*t*
Pulmonary embolism, 155*t,* 158*t*
Pulmonary fibrosis, idiopathic,
155*t*
Pulmonary function, 150
Pulmonary hypertension, 364
Pulmonary tuberculosis, 157*t*
Pulmonary valve
atresia of, 363, 382*t*
stenosis of, 170, 363, 381*t*
Pulse pressure, 414
Pulses
apical, 64, 168, 170
brachial, 219
carotid, 169
dorsalis pedis, 220
femoral, 220
in infants, 358, 363–364
in older adults, 420
palpation and grading of,
218–219, 220–221
paradoxical, 174
popliteal, 220
posterior tibial, 221
pulsus alternans, 174
radial, 64, 168, 219
Pulsus alternans, 174
Pupils, 117, 318, 333, 347*t*
Purging, 70*t*
Purpura, 103*t*
Pustules, 99*t*–100*t*
Pyelonephritis, 198
Pyloric stenosis, 364
Pyrexia (fever), 56, 65–66, 198

Q

Quadriceps, 291, 292
Questions, interview
adaptive questioning, 43–44
directed, 41, 43
open-ended, 40, 41
for sensitive topics, 49–53

R

Radial nerve, 322
Radial pulse, 64, 168, 219
Radiculopathy, 301t, 303t, 322, 331
Rales, 147b
Range of motion (ROM), 13
    at ankle, 297–298
    at hip, 290–291
    limitations to, 275
    measuring, 299
    at neck and spine, 289
    in older adults, 420–421
    at shoulder, 279–280
    at wrists and hands, 285–287
Rapport with patient, 39, 367b
Raynaud's phenomenon, 216
Reading ability, 48
Reasoning, clinical, 17–19. *See also*
        Assessments
Reassurance, of patient, 45
Rebound tenderness, 202–203
Records, patient. *See also specific*
        examinations
    checklist for, 33b–36b
    for children, 375b–377b
    of history and physical examina-
        tions, 33–36, 69
    for older adults, 422b–423b
    organizing, 33–36
    reviewing before exam, 38
Rectal temperature, 65, 66
Rectocele, 247, 256t, 398
Rectovaginal exam, 250, 400, 420
Rectum, 259–269
    bleeding in, 260
    cancer of, 269t
    examination of
        abnormalities in, 268t–269t
        in men, 15, 262–264
        in older adults, 420
        in women, 15, 250, 264
    polyps of, 268t
Red reflex, 118
Referral, source of, 2b
Referred pain, 194
Reflex esophagitis, 153t
Reflexes. *See also specific reflexes*
    assessing, 14, 328–331

grading, 328b
in infants, 366
and motor disorders, 340t
in pregnancy, 400
Regional enteritis, 210t
Reliability (test), 30b
Renal artery disease, 217
Renal system, 193b
Resonance, 145b
Respiratory alkalosis, 396
Respiratory infections, 361, 362
Respiratory rate and rhythm
    abnormalities of, 74t
    assessment of, 64–65, 143
    in children, 358, 361, 362b
    in older adults, 414
Respiratory system
    assessing function of, 150
    common or concerning symptoms
        of, 57, 141b
    disorders of, 153t, 154t–159t,
        161t, 163
    and dyspnea, 154t–155t, 163
    examination of, 12, 143–150
    health history of, 6, 142
    health promotion and counseling
        for, 142
    in pregnancy, 396
    recording findings of, 151b
Reticular activating system, 312
Retina, 112, 119b–120b
Retinal arteries and veins, 112, 119,
        120b
Retinopathy, diabetic, 133t
Review of systems, 3b, 5–7. *See also*
        specific systems
Rheumatic fever, 275
Rheumatoid arthritis
    in knees, 308t
    in older adults, 421
    pain in, 305t–306t
    symptoms of, 274–276
    in wrists or hands, 283, 284
Rhinitis, 114
Rhinorrhea, 114
Rhonchi, 147b
Rigidity, 343t
Ringworm (tinea capitis), 108t
Rinne test, 122, 135t, 320

Romberg test, 324
Rotator cuff, 280–281, 307*t*
Rovsing's sign, 207

S

Sacroiliac joints, 288
Safety, 5, 408
Salpingitis, 213*t*
Sarcoidosis, 155*t*
Sarcoma, Kaposi's, 105*t*
Satiety, early, 195
Scabies, 100*t*
Scales, skin, 100*t*
Scalp, 116
Scaphoid fracture, 284
Scapula, winging of, 332
Scars, 101*t*
Schizoaffective disorder, 92*t*
Schizophrenia, 92*t*
Schizophreniform disorder, 92*t*
Sciatic nerve, 288
Sciatica, 301*t*
Sclera, 117
Scoliosis, 299, 375
Screening tests
    for breast cancer, 182–183
    for cervical cancer, 244
    for children, 351
    for colorectal cancer, 200,
        261–262, 409, 420
    for depression, 57, 79–80, 411*b*
    history of, 4
    in older adults, 408–409,
        410*b*–412*b*, 422*b*
    for prostate cancer, 261–262
Scrotum
    abnormalities of, 236*t*
    in children, 365, 372
    edema in, 236*t*
    examination of, 15, 233
    hernia in, 236*t*
    in older adults, 420
Seborrheic keratoses, 104*t*–105*t*,
    415
Seizures, 315
Self-awareness, 52–53
Self-esteem, low, 80

Self-examinations
    breast, 182, 183, 187*t*–188*t*
    testicular, 232, 234*b*–235*b*
Self-reflection, 38
Senile ptosis, 415–416
Sensations
    discriminative, 326–327
    loss of, 314
    testing, 318, 325–326
Sensitivity (test), 30*b*–31*b*, 32*b*
Sensorineural hearing loss, 113, 135*t*,
    319
Sensory system, 14, 325–327
Serial 7s, 83
Sexual abuse, 373, 388*b*
Sexual history and function, 49
    in females, 243
    in males, 230–231
Sexual maturity
    in boys, 384*t*–385*t*
    in girls, 246, 383*t*, 386*t*–387*t*
Sexuality, in clinician-patient rela-
    tionship, 53
Sexually transmitted diseases
    in children, 373
    counseling for, 231–232, 245,
        263
    in females, 243, 245
    in males, 231–232, 237*t*
Shaking chills, 56
Shortness of breath, 142, 154*t*–155*t*,
    163
Shoulders, 279–281, 307*t*
Sighing breathing, 74*t*
Sigmoidoscopy, 261–262
Signs, 17*b*. *See also* Symptoms
Silent patient, 46
Sinuses, 6, 12, 114, 122
Sinusitis, 126*t*–127*t*
Skene's glands, 398
Skin
    cancer of, 93, 104*t*–105*t*, 106*t*,
        409, 415
    color of, 57, 94, 96*t*, 362*b*
    common or concerning symptoms
        of, 93*b*
    dimpling of, 191*t*
    examination of, 12, 94, 116
    health history of, 5

health promotion and counseling for, 93*b*
in infants, 358
lesions of, 57, 94, 97*t*–104*t*
nevi (moles), 93, 106*t*
in older adults, 415
recording exam results of, 95*b*
tags, 365
tumors of, 104*t*–105*t*
Skull, 116
Sleep disorders, 80
Smell, sense of, 318
Smoking
counseling for, 142
history of, 2*b*, 4
in older adults, 407
during pregnancy, 392
Smooth tongue, 137*t*
Sneezing, 114
Social development, 350
Social history, 3*b*, 5
Social phobia, 90*t*
Somatoform disorders, 46, 87*t*
Spasmodic torticollis, 342*t*
Spastic diplegias, 366
Spasticity, 343*t*
Specificity (test), 31*b*, 32*b*
Speculum examination, 247–248, 399, 419
Speech
aphasia, 82
in delirium and dementia, 424*t*
development of, in children, 350
and mental status, 78, 82
in older adults, 409
Spelling backwards, 83
Spermatic cord, 233, 239*t*, 372
Spermatocele, 239*t*
Spheroidal (ball and socket) joints, 273*b*
Spider angioma, 103*t*
Spider veins, 103*t*
Spinal accessory nerve, 317*b*, 320
Spinal cord, 312
Spinal nerve, 312
Spinal stenosis, 215, 301*t*
Spine, 12, 287–289
Spinous processes, 288
Spleen, 14, 204

Spontaneous pneumothorax, 155*t*
Sprains, 275, 297–298, 309*t*
Squamous cell carcinoma, 104*t*, 105*t*, 415
Stance, 289, 324
Standard precautions, 15–16
Staphylococcus aureus, methicillin-resistant, 15–16
Stereognosis, 326–327
Sternomastoid muscles, 143, 320
Stiffness, joint, 275, 302*t*
Stomach, 142
Stools, 197, 260
Strabismus, 360, 368
Strep throat, 114
Stress disorders, 91*t*
Stridor, 144, 362*b*
Stroke
facial paralysis in, 339*t*
health promotion and counseling for, 165, 315–316
symptoms of, 313, 322, 338*t*
types of, 336*t*–337*t*
vascular territories of, 338*t*
Stupor, 332–334
Sty, 131*t*
Subacromial bursa, 307*t*
Subarachnoid hemorrhage, 112, 127*t*, 313
Subdeltoid bursitis, 307*t*
Subdural hematoma, 357
Subjective data, 2*b*
Substance abuse, 2*b*, 4, 50–51, 80, 199
Subtalar joint, 298
Suicide, 80
Summarization, 45
Sun exposure, 93
Supinator reflex, 329
Surgical history, 4
Surrogate informant, 47
Sutures, cranial, 357, 358–359
Swallowing, 196, 320
Sweating, 56, 115
Swelling
of feet or legs, 216
in infant head, 359
in joints, 275

Symptoms. *See also specific structures or systems*
  characterization of, 4
  eliciting, 41, 404–405
  identifying, 17*b*
  multiple, 46
  sequence and time course of, 28–29, 41, 56
  seven attributes of, 41*b*
  unexplained, 75*b*–76*b*, 87*t*
Syncope, 314
Syndactyly, 365
Synovial joints, 272*b*, 273*b*
Syphilis
  lip chancre in, 136*t*
  mucous patch of, on tongue, 138*t*
  penile chancre in, 232, 237*t*
  secondary, 252*t*
  vulvar chancre in, 252*t*
Systemic lupus erythematosus, 276
Systems review, 3*b*, 5–7. *See also specific systems*
Systolic blood pressure, 63*b*, 168, 413–414
Systolic clicks, 171, 176*t*

T

Tachycardia, 358, 364
Tachypnea, 74*t*
Tactile fremitus, 145
Talkative patient, 47
Talocalcaneal joint, 298
Tavistock Principles, 54*b*
Teeth
  in children, 361, 371
  examination of, 122
  health promotion for, 115
Telangiectasia, hereditary hemorrhagic, 136*t*
Temperature
  intolerance to, 115
  measuring, 65–66
  in older adults, 414
  sensitivity to, 325, 326
Temporal muscles, 278, 319
Temporomandibular joint (TMJ), 278
Tenderness, 202–203, 213*t*
Tendonitis, 275, 307*t*

Tendons, 271
Tenosynovitis, 275
Tension headaches, 111, 125*t*
Terry's nails, 109*t*
Test selection, 30–32
Testes
  abnormalities of, 238*t*
  in children and adolescents, 372, 384*t*–385*t*
  examination of, 233
  in older adults, 420
  self-examination of, 232, 234*b*–235*b*
  tumor of, 238*t*
Tetralogy of Fallot, 381*t*–382*t*
Thalamus, 311
Thermometers, 65–66
Thoracic kyphoscoliosis, 160*t*
Thorax (chest), 141–161
  anterior, 13, 149–150
  common or concerning symptoms of, 141*b*
  disorders of, 152*t*–161*t*
  examination of, 12, 13, 143–150
  health history of, 141–142
  in newborns, 361–363
  in older adults, 417
  pain or discomfort in, 141–142, 152*t*–153*t*, 163–164
  posterior, 12, 144–148
  in pregnancy, 396
  recording findings of, 151*b*
  shape of, 143, 159*t*–160*t*
Thought content, 78*b*
  abstract, 84
  assessment of, 79, 82
  in delirium and dementia, 425*t*
Thought processes, 78*b*
  assessment or, 82
  in delirium and dementia, 409, 425*t*
Thoughts, recurring or unusual, 77, 79, 82
Thrills, 170, 364
Throat
  abnormalities of, 139*t*
  in children, 361, 370–371
  examination of, 12, 123, 124*b*
  health history of, 6, 114–115
  sore, 114, 139*t*

Thromboangiitis obliterans, 219

Thrush, 361

Thumbs, 285–286, 322

Thyroglossal duct cysts, 361

Thyroid gland, 115, 123–124, 140*t*, 396

TIA (transient ischemic attack), 313, 315–316

Tibeofemoral joint, 292

Tibial pulse, posterior, 221

Tibial torsion, 366

Tibiotalar joint, 297

Tics, 342*t*

Tinea capitis (ringworm), 108*t*

Tinel's sign, 287

Tinnitus, 114

Toenails, 95

Tongue, 123, 137*t*–138*t*, 320, 361

Tonsils, 123, 371

Torsion, spermatic cord, 239*t*, 372

Torticollis, spasmodic, 342*t*

Total anomalous pulmonary venous return, 363

Touch sensation, 325, 326

Trachea, 123, 141, 161*t*

Tracheal breath sounds, 147*b*

Tracheitis, bacterial, 362*b*

Tracheobronchitis, 153*t*, 156*t*

Transient ischemic attack, 313, 315–316

Transmitted voice sounds, 148, 150, 161*t*

Transposition of great arteries, 363, 382*t*

Transverse tarsal joints, 298

Trapezius muscles, 320

Tremors, 341*t*, 421

Triceps reflex, 328

Trichomonas vaginitis, 255*t*

Trichotillomania, 107*t*

Tricuspid regurgitation, 168

Trigeminal nerve, 317*b*, 318–319

Trigeminal neuralgia, 128*t*

Trochanteric bursa, 289, 290*f*

Trochlear nerve, 317*b*, 318

True negatives or positives, 30*b*, 31*b*

Trunk, 323

Tuberculosis, pulmonary, 157*t*

Tumors. *See also* Cancer

androgen-producing, 419

brain, 112, 127*t*–128*t*

estrogen-producing, 419

myoma of uterus, 257*t*

skin, 104*t*–105*t*

of testis, 238*t*

Turgor, skin, 358

Two-point discrimination, 327

Tympanic membrane, 66, 121, 134*t*, 369–370

Tympanosclerosis, 134*t*

Tympany, 145*b*

U

Ulcerative colitis, 210*t*

Ulcers

aphthous, 138*t*

of feet and ankles, 225*t*

on lower legs, 216

neuropathic, 225*t*

skin, 102*t*

venous stasis, 216

Ulnar nerve, 322

Umbilical artery, 355

Umbilical cord, 355

Umbilical hernias, 355

Universal precautions, 16

Urethra, 247

caruncle of, 247, 419

infection of (urethritis), 198, 231, 232, 247

Urgency, urinary, 198

Urinary incontinence

in older adults, 410, 411*b*, 422*b*

types of, 199, 211*t*–212*t*

Urinary system, 198–199

common or concerning symptoms of, 193*b*

health history of, 6, 198–199

Urination, 198–199, 260

Urine

blood in, 198

color of, 197

protein in, 395*b*

Uterus

bicornuate, 400

contractility of, 397

Uterus (*continued*)
  examination of, 15, 249
  myoma of, 257*t*
  positions of, 257*t*
  in pregnancy, 390, 397, 399–400
  prolapsed, 256*t*

V

Vagina
  adenosis of, 254*t*
  bleeding from, 373
  discharge from, 243, 255*t*, 373
  examination of, 15, 249
  infection of (vaginosis), 255*t*
  inflammation (vaginitis), 255*t*, 373
  walls of, during pregnancy, 399
Vagus nerve, 317*b*, 320
Valgus stress test, 296
Validation, of patient's feeling, 45
Validity (test), 30*b*
Valsalva maneuver, 174
Values, defined, 52
Varicocele, 239*t*
Varicose veins, 138*t*, 221, 400
Varus stress test, 294
Vascular disease, 363
Vascular ring, 362*b*
Vascular system, peripheral, 215–227
  abnormalities of, 224*t*–225*t*
  common or concerning symptoms
    of, 215*b*
  examination of, 13, 218–223,
    226*t*–227*t*
  health history of, 7, 215–216
  health promotion and counseling
    for, 216–218
  in older adults, 420
  recording exam results of, 223*b*
Vasodepressor syncope, 314
Vasomotor rhinitis, 114
Vasovagal syncope, 314
Veins
  jugular, 168
  retinal, 112, 119, 120*b*
  spider, 103*t*
  varicose, 138*t*, 221, 400
Venereal warts, 232, 237*t*, 251*t*, 260
Venous insufficiency, 224*t*, 225*t*

Venous pulsations, 120*b*
Venous stasis ulcers, 216
Ventricular failure, left, 154*t*, 158*t*,
    161*t*, 163
Ventricular hypertrophy, left, 417
Ventricular septal defect, 382*t*
Vertigo, 114, 313
Vesicles, 99*t*
Vesicular breath sounds, 147*b*
Vibration sense, 326
Violence, domestic, 51, 392–393
Viral infections, 156*t*, 209*t*
Visceral pain or tenderness,
    193–194, 213*t*
Vision
  acuity of, 116, 318, 368–369, 416
  changes in, 112–113
  in children, 360, 368–369
  disorders of, 115
  double vision, 113, 313
  examination of, 12, 116, 360,
    368–369, 416
  field defects, 129*t*
  and headaches, 112, 126*t*
  health history of, 112–113
  health promotion and counseling
    for, 115
  interviewing patient with impair-
    ment of, 49
  in older adults, 115, 408,
    410*b*–411*b*, 416, 422*b*
Vital signs
  blood pressure, 61–64
  heart rate and rhythm, 64
  measuring, 11, 61–66
  in newborns, 357
  in older adults, 413–414, 422*b*
  in pregnancy, 394–395
  recording findings of, 69, 376*b*
  respiratory rate and rhythm,
    64–65
  "sixth" (functional status), 410–413
  temperature, 65–66
Vitamin D, sources of, 72*t*
Vitreous floaters, 113
Vitreous hemorrhage, 112
Vocabulary assessment, 84
Voice sounds, 148, 150, 161*t*, 320
Vomiting, 112, 195, 395

Vulva, 251*t*–252*t*
Vulvovaginitis, 198

W

Waist circumference, 61
Warts, venereal, 232, 237*t*, 251*t*, 260
Weakness, muscle, 55, 313–314,
    321–322
"Weaver's bottom," 290
Weber test, 122, 135*t*, 319
Weight
    at birth, 353, 354*b*
    and body mass index, 59–61

changes in, 55
of children and adolescents, 356,
    368, 378*t*
general survey of, 59
health counseling for, 56–57
in older adults, 411*b*, 414
during pregnancy, 391, 392*b*, 395
Wheals, 98*t*
Wheezing, 142, 144, 147*b*
Whiplash, 303*t*
Whispered pectoriloquy, 148*b*
White lines in nails, 109*t*
White matter, 311
Wrists, 283–287, 322